W9-ARF-052

Healthy Heart Sourcebook for Women

Heart Diseases & Disorders Sourcebook, 2nd Edition

Household Safety Sourcebook

Immune System Disorders Sourcebook

Infant & Toddler Health Sourcebook

Infectious Diseases Sourcebook

Injury & Trauma Sourcebook

Kidney & Urinary Tract Diseases & Disorders Sourcebook

Learning Disabilities Sourcebook, 2nd Edition

Leukemia Sourcebook

Liver Disorders Sourcebook

Lung Disorders Sourcebook

Medical Tests Sourcebook, 2nd Edition

Men's Health Concerns Sourcebook, 2nd Edition

Mental Health Disorders Sourcebook, 2nd Edition

Mental Retardation Sourcebook

Movement Disorders Sourcebook

Obesity Sourcebook

Osteoporosis Sourcebook

Pain Sourcebook, 2nd Edition

Pediatric Cancer Sourcebook

Physical & Mental Issues in Aging Sourcebook

Podiatry Sourcebook

Pregnancy & Birth Sourcebook, 2nd Edition

Prostate Cancer

Public Health Sourcebook

Reconstructive & Cosmetic Surgery Sourcebook

Rehabilitation Sourcebook

Respiratory Diseases & Disorders Sourcebook

Sexually Transmitted Diseases Sourcebook, 2nd Edition

Skin Disorders Sourcebook

Sleep Disorders Sourcebook

Sports Injuries Sourcebook, 2nd Edition

Stress-Related Disorders Sourcebook

Stroke Sourcebook

Substance Abuse Sourcebook

Surgery Sourcebook

Transplantation Sourcebook

Traveler's Health Sourcebook

Vegetarian Sourcebook

Women's Health Concerns Sourcebook, 2nd Edition

Workplace Health & Safety Sourcebook

Worldwide Health Sourcebook

Teen Health Series

Cancer Information for Teens

Diet Information for Teens

Drug Information for Teens

Fitness Information for Teens

Mental Health Information for Teens

Sexual Health Information for Teens

Skin Health Information for Teens

Sports Injuries Information for Teens

Drug Abuse
SOURCEBOOK

Second Edition

Health Reference Series

Second Edition

Drug Abuse
SOURCEBOOK

Basic Consumer Health Information about Illicit Substances of Abuse and the Misuse of Prescription and Over-the-Counter Medications, Including Depressants, Hallucinogens, Inhalants, Marijuana, Stimulants, and Anabolic Steroids

Along with Facts about Related Health Risks, Treatment Programs, Prevention Programs, a Glossary of Abuse and Addiction Terms, a Glossary of Drug-Related Street Terms, and a Directory of Resources for More Information

Edited by
Catherine Ginther

Omnigraphics

615 Griswold Street • Detroit, MI 48226

Bibliographic Note

Because this page cannot legibly accommodate all the copyright notices, the Bibliographic Note portion of the Preface constitutes an extension of the copyright notice.

Edited by Catherine Ginther

Health Reference Series

Karen Bellenir, *Managing Editor*
David A. Cooke, M.D., *Medical Editor*
Elizabeth Barbour, *Permissions Associate*
Dawn Matthews, *Verification Assistant*
Laura Pleva Nielsen, *Index Editor*
EdIndex, Services for Publishers, *Indexers*

***

Omnigraphics, Inc.

Matthew P. Barbour, *Senior Vice President*
Kay Gill, *Vice President—Directories*
Kevin Hayes, *Operations Manager*
David P. Bianco, *Marketing Director*

***

Peter E. Ruffner, *Publisher*

Frederick G. Ruffner, Jr., *Chairman*

Copyright © 2004 Omnigraphics, Inc.

ISBN 0-7808-0740-5

Library of Congress Cataloging-in-Publication Data

Drug abuse sourcebook : basic consumer health information about illicit substances of abuse and the misuse of prescription and over-the-counter medications, including depressants, hallucinogens, inhalants, marijuana, stimulants, and anabolic steroids; along with facts about related health risks, treatment programs, prevention programs, a glossary of abuse and addiction terms, a glossary of drug-related street terms, and a directory of resources for more information / edited by Catherine Ginther.-- 2nd ed.
    p. cm.
Includes index.
ISBN 0-7808-0740-5 (hard cover : alk. paper)
1. Drug abuse--Prevention--Handbooks, manuals, etc. 2. Drug abuse--Treatment--Handbooks, manuals, etc. 3. Narcotic habit--Treatment--Handbooks, manuals, etc. I. Ginther, Catherine.
HV5801.D724 2004
362.29--dc22

2004016313

∞

This book is printed on acid-free paper meeting the ANSI Z39.48 Standard. The infinity symbol that appears above indicates that the paper in this book meets that standard.

Printed in the United States

Table of Contents

Visit www.healthreferenceseries.com to view *A Contents Guide to the Health Reference Series*, a listing of more than 10,000 topics and the volumes in which they are covered.

Part III: Drugs of Abuse

Part IV: Treating Drug Abuse

Part V: Health Risks Related to Drug Abuse

Part VI: Drug Abuse Prevention

Part VII: Additional Help and Information

Preface

About This Book

Drug abuse directly affects approximately 22 million Americans and cuts across all age groups, ethnicities, and gender lines. It can harm a person's physical and mental health. It impacts society by contributing to the spread of infectious diseases, such as hepatitis and HIV, and it has been linked to increased crime and violence and lost productivity and wages. Federal Bureau of Investigation (FBI) statistics indicate that more than 1.5 million arrests were made for drug abuse violations in 2002, and according to the National Institute on Drug Abuse, drug abuse costs the U.S. economy about $100 billion each year.

Drug Abuse Sourcebook, Second Edition presents information about the health risks and other effects of specific drugs of abuse, including depressants, hallucinogens, inhalants, marijuana, stimulants, anabolic steroids, and prescription and over-the-counter medications. It explains the processes involved as casual use turns to addiction and offers new information about prevention and treatment programs with successful track records. Glossaries of drug-related terms and a directory of resources able to offer assistance and information are also included.

How to Use This Book

This book is divided into parts and chapters. Parts focus on broad areas of interest. Chapters are devoted to single topics within a part.

Part I: An Introduction to Drug Abuse provides background information on drug abuse and addiction as well as a statistical overview of drug abuse in the United States and its trends in particular populations, such as women and minorities.

Part II: The Nature of Drug Addiction answers questions about how people use, abuse, and become addicted to drugs. It also explores the links between cigarette smoking, stress, eating disorders, and drug abuse.

Part III: Drugs of Abuse provides summary information about some of the most commonly abused substances, including cocaine, ecstasy, inhalants, marijuana, OxyContin, and steroids.

Part IV: Recognizing and Treating Drug Abuse describes how drug abuse can be identified and various treatment options, including methadone maintenance treatment, narcotic antagonist treatment, outpatient drug-free treatment, residential programs, and medical detoxification programs. Barriers to drug abuse treatment and ways to prevent relapse are also discussed.

Part V: Health Risks Related to Drug Abuse includes facts about hepatitis C, AIDS, and other infectious disease risks associated with drug abuse. It reports on mental and developmental concerns in prenatally exposed children and also discusses harmful drug-related behaviors, including drugged driving, risky sexual activity, and suicide.

Part VI: Drug Abuse Prevention offers information about how parents can prevent drug abuse at home and what schools can do. It describes steps employers can take to prevent drug abuse in the workplace and provides facts about drug testing.

Part VII: Additional Help and Information includes a glossary of drug abuse-related terms, a glossary of street terms, and a directory of national resources able to provide help and information related to drug abuse and addiction.

Bibliographic Note

This volume contains documents and excerpts from publications issued by the following U.S. government agencies: Bureau of Justice

Statistics (BJS); Consumer Product Safety Commission (CPSC); Drug Enforcement Administration (DEA); National Clearinghouse for Alcohol and Drug Information (NCADI); National Drug Intelligence Center (NDIC); National Institute on Drug Abuse (NIDA); Office of National Drug Control Policy (ONDCP); and Substance Abuse and Mental Health Services Administration (SAMHSA).

In addition, this volume contains documents from the following organizations: American Council for Drug Education (ACDE); American Medical Association (AMA); American Psychiatric Association (APA); Intervention Center; Kaiser Family Foundation; Marijuana Policy Project; NAMI, The Nation's Voice on Mental Illness; National Center on Addiction and Substance Abuse at Columbia University (CASA); National Organization for the Reform of Marijuana Laws (NORML); National Youth Anti-Drug Media Campaign/Freevibe.com; Nemours Foundation/KidsHealth.org; Society for Prevention Research; and University of Michigan.

Acknowledgements

Thanks go to the many organizations and agencies that have contributed materials for this Sourcebook and to medical consultant Dr. David A. Cooke, verification assistant Dawn Matthews, and document engineer Bruce Bellenir. Special thanks go to managing editor Karen Bellenir and permissions associate Elizabeth Barbour for their help and support.

About the Health Reference Series

The *Health Reference Series* is designed to provide basic medical information for patients, families, caregivers, and the general public. Each volume takes a particular topic and provides comprehensive coverage. This is especially important for people who may be dealing with a newly diagnosed disease or a chronic disorder in themselves or in a family member. People looking for preventive guidance, information about disease warning signs, medical statistics, and risk factors for health problems will also find answers to their questions in the *Health Reference Series*. The *Series*, however, is not intended to serve as a tool for diagnosing illness, in prescribing treatments, or as a substitute for the physician/patient relationship. All people concerned about medical symptoms or the possibility of disease are encouraged to seek professional care from an appropriate health care provider.

Locating Information within the Health Reference Series

The *Health Reference Series* contains a wealth of information about a wide variety of medical topics. Ensuring easy access to all the fact sheets, research reports, in-depth discussions, and other material contained within the individual books of the series remains one of our highest priorities. As the *Series* continues to grow in size and scope, however, locating the precise information needed by a reader may become more challenging.

A Contents Guide to the Health Reference Series was developed to direct readers to the specific volumes that address their concerns. It presents an extensive list of diseases, treatments, and other topics of general interest compiled from the Tables of Contents and major index headings. To access *A Contents Guide to the Health Reference Series*, visit www.healthreferenceseries.com.

Medical Consultant

Medical consultant services are provided to the *Health Reference Series* editors by David A. Cooke, M.D. Dr. Cooke is a graduate of Brandeis University, and he received his M.D. degree from the University of Michigan. He completed residency training at the University of Wisconsin Hospital and Clinics. He is board-certified in Internal Medicine. Dr. Cooke currently works as part of the University of Michigan Health System and practices in Brighton, MI. In his free time, he enjoys writing, science fiction, and spending time with his family.

Our Advisory Board

We would like to thank the following board members for providing guidance to the development of this *Series*:

Dr. Lynda Baker,
Associate Professor of Library and Information Science,
Wayne State University, Detroit, MI

Nancy Bulgarelli,
William Beaumont Hospital Library, Royal Oak, MI

Karen Imarisio,
Bloomfield Township Public Library, Bloomfield Township, MI

Karen Morgan,
Mardigian Library, University of Michigan-Dearborn,
Dearborn, MI

Rosemary Orlando,
St. Clair Shores Public Library, St. Clair Shores, MI

Health Reference Series *Update Policy*

The inaugural book in the *Health Reference Series* was the first edition of *Cancer Sourcebook* published in 1989. Since then, the *Series* has been enthusiastically received by librarians and in the medical community. In order to maintain the standard of providing high-quality health information for the layperson, the editorial staff at Omnigraphics felt it was necessary to implement a policy of updating volumes when warranted.

Medical researchers have been making tremendous strides, and it is the purpose of the *Health Reference Series* to stay current with the most recent advances. Each decision to update a volume will be made on an individual basis. Some of the considerations will include how much new information is available and the feedback we receive from people who use the books. If there is a topic you would like to see added to the update list, or an area of medical concern you feel has not been adequately addressed, please write to:

Editor
Health Reference Series
Omnigraphics, Inc.
615 Griswold Street
Detroit, MI 48226
E-mail: editorial@omnigraphics.com

Part One

An Introduction to Drug Abuse

Chapter 1

Understanding Drug Abuse and Addiction in the United States

What Is Drug Abuse?

Many people view drug abuse and addiction as strictly a social problem. Parents, teens, older adults, and other members of the community tend to characterize people who take drugs as morally weak or as having criminal tendencies. They believe that drug abusers and addicts should be able to stop taking drugs if they are willing to change their behavior.

These myths have not only stereotyped those with drug-related problems, but also their families, their communities, and the health care professionals who work with them. Drug abuse and addiction comprise a public health problem that affects many people and has wide-ranging social consequences. It is the National Institute on Drug Abuse (NIDA)'s goal to help the public replace its myths and long-held mistaken beliefs about drug abuse and addiction with scientific evidence that addiction is a chronic, relapsing, and treatable disease.

Addiction does begin with drug abuse when an individual makes a conscious choice to use drugs, but addiction is not just "a lot of drug use." Recent scientific research provides overwhelming evidence that not only do drugs interfere with normal brain functioning creating powerful feelings of pleasure, but they also have long-term effects on brain metabolism and activity. At some point, changes occur in the

---

"Understanding Drug Abuse and Addiction," National Institute on Drug Abuse (NIDA), June 2003; and "Nationwide Trends," NIDA, October 2002.

3

brain that can turn drug abuse into addiction, a chronic, relapsing illness. Those addicted to drugs suffer from a compulsive drug craving and usage and cannot quit by themselves. Treatment is necessary to end this compulsive behavior.

A variety of approaches are used in treatment programs to help patients deal with these cravings and possibly avoid drug relapse. NIDA research shows that addiction is clearly treatable. Through treatment that is tailored to individual needs, patients can learn to control their condition and live relatively normal lives.

Treatment can have a profound effect not only on drug abusers, but on society as a whole by significantly improving social and psychological functioning, decreasing related criminality and violence, and reducing the spread of AIDS. It can also dramatically reduce the costs to society of drug abuse.

Understanding drug abuse also helps in understanding how to prevent use in the first place. Results from NIDA-funded prevention research have shown that comprehensive prevention programs that involve the family, schools, communities, and the media are effective in reducing drug abuse. It is necessary to keep sending the message that it is better to not start at all than to enter rehabilitation if addiction occurs.

A tremendous opportunity exists to effectively change the ways in which the public understands drug abuse and addiction because of the wealth of scientific data NIDA has amassed. Overcoming misconceptions and replacing ideology with scientific knowledge is the best hope for bridging the "great disconnect"—the gap between the public perception of drug abuse and addiction and the scientific facts.

Nationwide Trends

This fact sheet highlights information from the latest published proceedings of NIDA's Community Epidemiology Work Group (CEWG). The information covers current and emerging trends in drug abuse for 21 major U.S. metropolitan areas, as shared at CEWG's December 2001 meeting. The findings are intended to alert the general public, policy makers, and authorities at the local, State, regional, and national levels to the latest trends in drug abuse.

The CEWG is a network of researchers from Atlanta, Baltimore, Boston, Chicago, Denver, Detroit, Honolulu, Los Angeles, Miami, Minneapolis/St. Paul, Newark, New Orleans, New York, Philadelphia, Phoenix, St. Louis, San Diego, San Francisco, Seattle, Texas, and Washington, D.C.

CEWG members (epidemiologists and researchers) assess drug abuse patterns and trends from the health and other drug abuse indicator sources below. These data are enhanced with qualitative information from ethnographic research, focus groups, and other community-based sources:

- the Treatment Episode Data Set (data from treatment facilities) and the Drug Abuse Warning Network (emergency room mentions and medical examiner deaths involving illicit drugs), both funded by the Substance Abuse and Mental Health Services Administration;

- the Arrestee Drug Abuse Monitoring program, funded by the National Institute of Justice;

- the System to Retrieve Information on Drug Evidence and other information on drug seizures, price, and purity, from the Drug Enforcement Administration;

- drug seizure data from the United States Customs Service; and

- the Uniform Crime Reports, maintained by the Federal Bureau of Investigation.

Findings presented at the December 2001 CEWG meeting are based on comparisons of 1999 and 2000 data from these sources. The findings also may be supplemented by data from earlier periods and from the first half of 2001.

Trends of Use

Cocaine/Crack: Although still at high levels, cocaine/crack indicators decreased in 10 CEWG sites, remained stable or mixed in nine, and increased in two (Atlanta and Seattle). In 2000, rates of emergency room cocaine mentions were higher than those for heroin/morphine in 16 sites, and were higher in all CEWG sites than rates for marijuana and methamphetamine. Adult arrestees were more likely to test positive for cocaine than opiates in 2000; in the sites where both men and women were tested, women were more likely to test positive for cocaine than marijuana. Year 2000 treatment admissions indicated that crack accounted for a substantially greater percentage of primary admissions than powder cocaine in all CEWG sites. However, indicators suggest that crack use has decreased as powder cocaine has become more available in Denver, Miami/South Florida, Phoenix, the Texas border, and Washington, D.C.

Heroin: CEWG indicators for heroin/morphine abuse increased in 2000 in 15 CEWG sites, remained stable in two, and decreased in four. The decreases were reported in Honolulu, Los Angeles, San Francisco, and Seattle—areas where Mexican black tar heroin is the primary type available. Boston, New York, Newark, and Philadelphia report that heroin is relatively cheap, widely available, and of high purity. In 2000, heroin/ morphine emergency room mentions were higher than those for cocaine in Baltimore, Newark, San Diego, and San Francisco and higher than rates for marijuana and methamphetamine in eight other CEWG sites. Heroin treatment admissions were especially high in Baltimore (64.3%), Boston (69.1%), and Newark (83.8%), and were more than half of the primary illicit drug admissions in Los Angeles and San Francisco. Among adult arrestees, particularly high rates of opiate-positive tests occurred in Chicago, New York, and Philadelphia. Heroin purity levels are highest east of the Mississippi, where South American heroin dominates.

Misuse of Prescription Opiates: Indicators of the illicit use of prescription narcotics, particularly oxycodone and hydrocodone, increased in all 14 of the CEWG sites that report on these drugs. Emergency room mentions of oxycodone combinations were highest in Philadelphia, Boston, and Phoenix. Mentions for hydrocodone combinations were highest in Los Angeles and Detroit. Deaths involving hydrocodone, oxycodone, or both were reported in Atlanta, Detroit, Miami, Philadelphia, and Texas. Abuse of codeine (in pill and cough syrup forms) was reported as a problem in six CEWG sites, particularly in Detroit.

Marijuana: Marijuana use indicators increased in 12 CEWG sites, remained stable or mixed in eight, and decreased in one (Atlanta). Marijuana emergency room mentions, arrests, and treatment admissions have been increasing. In 2000, emergency room mentions for marijuana increased significantly in seven CEWG sites. In Minneapolis, 49% of treatment admissions in 2000 were for primary abuse of marijuana; in Miami, New Orleans, St. Louis, and Seattle, marijuana admissions ranged from 31 to 37%. Among adult arrestees, the percentage of males testing marijuana-positive was higher than those testing cocaine-positive in 13 CEWG sites.

Methamphetamine: Methamphetamine use indicators increased in six of the seven CEWG areas that typically have high rates of emergency room methamphetamine mentions and/or high percentages of methamphetamine treatment admissions. These are: Denver, Hawaii, Los Angeles, Phoenix, San Diego, and Seattle. Increases in indicators were also reported in Atlanta, Minneapolis/St. Paul, St. Louis, and cities in Texas. San Francisco was the only CEWG site reporting a decrease in methamphetamine indicators in 2000. Sites reporting increases in methamphetamine availability and use, but still at low levels, were New York, Chicago, Detroit, Philadelphia, and Washington, D.C. Methamphetamine treatment admissions were especially high in Hawaii (46.6%) and San Diego (45.3%). Among adult arrestees in 2000, the highest methamphetamine-positive rates were among men and women in Honolulu, San Diego, Phoenix, Los Angeles, and Seattle. Availability of methamphetamine decreased in Chicago and San Francisco. Purity levels were close to 100% in Honolulu and Phoenix.

MDMA: MDMA (methylenedioxymethamphetamine; often called ecstasy) indicators increased in 19 CEWG sites in 2000 and remained stable in two (New Orleans and Newark). Emergency room mentions increased significantly for MDMA in 14 CEWG sites. Although still small, the number of persons being admitted for treatment of primary MDMA abuse is increasing in Denver, Minneapolis/St. Paul, and Texas. Deaths associated with MDMA were reported in seven CEWG sites. Most MDMA pills are produced in Belgium and the Netherlands, but there have been reports of attempts to establish clandestine MDMA labs in CEWG sites such as Minneapolis, San Diego, and areas of Michigan and South Florida.

Emerging Drugs—PCP: Although PCP indicators suggest abuse of this drug was not widespread in 2000, there was evidence of increased abuse in some CEWG areas. Rates of emergency room PCP mentions increased significantly between 1999 and 2000 in eight CEWG sites. Sites with the highest emergency room PCP mentions were Chicago, Philadelphia, Los Angeles, Seattle, and Washington, D.C. Los Angeles reported 50 PCP-related deaths in 2000 and Philadelphia reported 22.

Treatment admissions for primary PCP abuse accounted for less than 1% of admissions in most CEWG sites, but did increase in Newark and Los Angeles. Only small percentages of arrestees tested PCP-positive in 2000, with the highest (4.8%) among adult male arrestees in Houston.

For Further Information

For national and state use data, please visit www.samhsa.gov/oas/nhsda.htm, which is the website for the *National Household Survey on Drug Abuse (NHSDA)*, funded by the Substance Abuse and Mental

Health Services Administration, U.S. Department of Health and Human Services. NHSDA is an annual survey on the nationwide prevalence and incidence of illicit drug, alcohol, and tobacco use among Americans age 12 and older. You can also order a free copy of the latest NHSDA summaries from the National Clearinghouse for Alcohol and Drug Information by calling (800) 729-6686.

Chapter 2

Trends in Adolescent Drug Abuse

The proportion of American 10th- and 12th-grade students who reported using the drug ecstasy in the prior 12 months has fallen by more than half just since 2001. The usage rate among eighth-graders is down considerably, as well, over the same two-year interval. That is just some of the encouraging news to emerge from the 2003 Monitoring the Future (MTF) survey of nearly 50,000 students in 392 secondary schools across the country.

Ecstasy rose rapidly in popularity from 1998 through 2001, but in 2001 the study's investigators detected the beginning of an increase in the proportion of students coming to see ecstasy as a dangerous drug (see Figure 2.1). That perception strengthened further in 2002 as use began to decline, and use dropped more sharply in 2003 as the perceived dangers of ecstasy continued to increase. "We have been saying for several years that use of this newly popular drug was not going to diminish until young people began to perceive its use as dangerous," states Lloyd Johnston, the study's principal investigator. "It now appears that teens are finally getting the word about ecstasy's potential consequences, probably due to extensive media coverage of the issue and concerted efforts by several organizations active in educating young people about the dangers of ecstasy." These organizations

Johnston, L.D., O'Malley, P.M., & Bachman, J.G. (2003, December 19). National press release, "Ecstasy use falls for second year in a row, overall teen drug use drops." Monitoring the Future Study, Institute for Social Research, University of Michigan, Ann Arbor, 44 pp.

include the National Institute on Drug Abuse, the White House Office on National Drug Control Policy, and the Partnership for a Drug-Free America. The latter two organizations launched an anti-ecstasy ad campaign in January 2002.

The availability of ecstasy, as reported by the students in the survey, rose sharply during the 1990s, peaked in 2001, and has fallen back a bit since then (see Figure 2.1). But the proportional decline in availability has been much smaller than the proportional decline in use, suggesting that reduced availability did not play a key role in the recent downturn in use.

The 2003 survey is the 29th in the annual series of surveys of American 12th-graders, and the 13th in the series of eighth- and 10th-graders, who were added to the study in 1991. The MTF study, funded by the National Institute on Drug Abuse through investigator-initiated research grants, was designed and conducted by scientists at the University of Michigan Institute for Social Research. The authors of the forthcoming report are Lloyd Johnston, Patrick O'Malley, Jerald Bachman, and John Schulenberg—all research professors at the University of Michigan.

Earlier surveys in this series showed that illicit drug use reached its recent peak among teens in 1996 or 1997, depending on grade. Since then, only the eighth-graders have exhibited a gradual, ongoing decline. Use in the upper grades held fairly constant until 2002, when all three grades finally began to show some decline. That decline continued into 2003, with statistically significant drops observed in annual prevalence in eighth and 10th grades and a nearly significant drop in 12th grade (see Figure 2.2). In addition, fewer young people in each grade say that they have ever used an illicit drug (see Table 2.1).

Because marijuana is by far the most widely used of the illicit drugs, trends in its use tend to drive the index of any illicit drug use. In 2003, marijuana use exhibited its second year of decline in the upper grades and its seventh year of decline among eighth-graders. Its use has now fallen by three-tenths among eighth-graders since their peak in 1996 and by about two-tenths and one-tenth, respectively, among the 10th- and 12th-graders since their recent peaks in 1997. In 2003, 13%, 28%, and 35% of the eighth-, 10th-, and 12th-graders indicated having smoked marijuana in the prior 12 months.

All three grades showed significant increases in perceived risk of marijuana use this year, for the first time in some years, a fact that may well help to explain this year's declines in use. "It is quite possible that the National Youth Anti-Drug Media Campaign by the Office of

National Drug Control Policy and the Partnership for a Drug-Free America, which communicates the dangers of marijuana use, has had its intended effect," states Johnston. "We have definitely seen a change in that direction." That campaign began to air in October 2002.

The proportions of students using any illicit drug other than marijuana also declined in 2003 among 10th-grade students (significantly) and 12th-grade students (not significantly; see Table 2.2). However, use among the eighth-graders—which had fallen by a third in earlier years from the recent peak in 1996—showed no further decline this year. Among the drugs in this general category that help to account for the overall decline in the upper grades are LSD, amphetamines, tranquilizers, and sedatives.

LSD use has been declining in all three grades since 1996, but the decline has been particularly sharp in the past two years (see Figure 2.3). Since 2001, the annual prevalence of LSD use has declined by about four-tenths among eighth-graders (who showed no further improvement this year), six-tenths among 10th-graders, and seven-tenths among 12th-graders. Perceived risk and personal disapproval of LSD use generally have not moved in ways that would explain this downturn in use. Reported availability, however, has declined considerably.

In 2003 overall amphetamine use showed its first decline in recent years in the two upper grades (see Figure 2.4). Among eighth-graders amphetamine use, which had been declining steadily since 1996, showed no further decline this year. Perceived risk associated with amphetamine use has been rising some among 12th-graders (the only ones asked the question) in recent years, perhaps helping to explain the decline in use in the upper grades in 2003. The use of the specific amphetamine Ritalin showed some decline in the lower two grades in 2003, though none of this year's changes reached statistical significance. Ritalin use is now below recent peak levels in all three grades. Methamphetamine use has been showing a gradual decline over the past several years in all three grades (see Figure 2.5).

The use of tranquilizers also declined in both 10th and 12th grades this year (see Figure 2.6). This is the first year of decline for the 12th-graders, following a decade of gradual increase in tranquilizer use. Among 10th-graders it is the second year of decline. By way of contrast, there has been very little change in the considerably lower rates of tranquilizer use among eighth-graders since 1995.

Sedatives (including barbiturates) constitute another class of psychotherapeutic drugs that, like tranquilizers, act as central nervous system depressants. (Data for this class of drug are reported only for

12th-graders.) As was true for tranquilizers, sedatives had shown a decade-long rise among 12th-graders before leveling and possibly beginning to decline for the first time in 2003 (see Figure 2.7).

Use of Some Illicit Drugs Held Steady

Several classes of drugs showed little systematic change this year, though in most cases they have shown some decline in recent years. These include several "club drugs," hallucinogens other than LSD (taken as a class), cocaine, crack, heroin, and other narcotics other than heroin (taken as a class).

Rohypnol, GHB (gamma hydroxybutyrate), and ketamine are three of the so-called club drugs. All have relatively low prevalence rates among secondary school students. There were no statistically significant changes in the annual prevalence of use for any of them in 2003. Use of each tends to be at or, for the most part, below their recent peak levels (see Table 2.2).

There was no significant change in 2003 in the annual prevalence of hallucinogens other than LSD, taken as a class (see Figure 2.8). The current rates are below recent peak levels for this class of drugs.

Annual prevalence rates for the use of powdered cocaine and of crack cocaine also are both below their recent peak levels in all three grades. While both forms of the drug exhibited some decline in all grades in 2003, most of these changes are not significant.

Current levels of heroin use are on the order of half what they were at their recent peaks in the mid-1990s; however, little further improvement was observed this year (see Figure 2.9).

The use of narcotic drugs other than heroin, taken as a class, is reported only for 12th-graders.

Like most of the other psychotherapeutic drugs discussed earlier (amphetamines, tranquilizers, and sedatives), the illicit use of these analgesic drugs had risen considerably over a decade among 12th-graders. This long-term trend made even the leveling in use in 2003 (at 9.3%) a welcome development (see Table 2.2). Two drugs in this class, however, are showing signs of increase in use, as is discussed next.

A Few Illicit Drugs Showed Signs of Increasing Use

Use of the drug OxyContin (a time-released tablet containing oxycodone) was added to the study in 2002 because of rising concerns about its use outside of medical regimen. It is a powerful, long-acting, synthetic narcotic prescribed for its analgesic effects. The annual prevalence rates for OxyContin use without a doctor's orders in 2003 are 1.7%, 3.6%, and 4.5% for eighth-, 10th-, and 12th-grade students. All three grades showed some increase over the rate of use in 2002, though none reached statistical significance (see Table 2.2). "Considering the addictive potential of this drug, these are disturbingly high rates of use," observes Johnston, "and they contrast with heroin's annual prevalence rate of less than 1% at all three grades, for instance."

Vicodin is another synthetic narcotic drug used for pain control (it contains the generic drug hydrocodone) and is some times prescribed in dental practice. Its prevalence rate is considerably higher than OxyContin, at 2.8%, 7.2%, and 10.5% in grades eight, 10, and 12, respectively. It, too, showed some increase in all three grades in 2003, though none of them reached statistical significance.

Inhalants are a class of drugs defined by form (fumes) and mode of administration (inhalation), rather than by their chemical or psychoactive properties. They encompass a range of substances, including glues, aerosols, butane, paint thinner, and nail polish remover. Use of inhalants has consistently been highest among eighth-graders, probably because these types of products are cheap and easy to obtain. Following a long and substantial decline in the use of inhalants by students in all three grades, use by eighth-graders increased significantly this year (see Figure 2.10). Between 1995 and 2002, eighth-graders' annual prevalence fell by four-tenths, from 12.8% to 7.7%, as an increasing proportion of students came to see inhalant use as dangerous. However, eighth-graders' use rose to 8.7% in 2003. While not a major turnaround, this increase could suggest the need for renewed attention to this class of substances. Perceptions of the dangers of inhalant use have declined over the past two years among both eighth- and 10th-graders, quite possibly explaining the reversal in their use.

Alcohol Use Changed Little

Last year, the survey results from 2002 showed a decline in the 30-day prevalence of alcohol use, as well as a decline in occasions of heavy drinking, in all three grades. This year, only the 12th-graders showed any further decline in 30-day prevalence of drinking (not statistically significant). Occasions of heavy drinking (having five or more drinks in a row sometime in the past two weeks) continued to decline slightly in all three grades, though none reached statistical significance.

13

Interpreting the Results from Eighth-Graders

This year's halting of declines in eighth-graders' use of several substances is of some concern. "The eighth-graders have been the harbingers of change observed later in the upper grades," observes Johnston, "So, the fact that they are no longer showing declines in their use of a number of drugs could mean that the declines now being observed in the upper grades also will come to an end soon."

In the past, the eighth-graders have been the first to show change in their use of marijuana, hallucinogens other than LSD, crack, cocaine powder, amphetamines, tranquilizers, and even cigarettes. (See the relevant figures for these drugs.) Thus, their turnaround in inhalant use this year and the leveling in their use of hallucinogens other than LSD, amphetamines and methamphetamine, tranquilizers, and 30-day alcohol use are a bit troubling. (The decline in their use of cigarettes has also decelerated this year, as is discussed in a separate release.)

"One concept that we have offered to the understanding of drug epidemics is that of 'generational forgetting'," notes Johnston. "By this we mean that even though one generation or cohort of young people may come to appreciate the hazards of a drug, those young people who follow after them may not possess that knowledge. They may not have lived through the series of events in a particular historical period that gave rise to that knowledge in previous cohorts, and therefore they may be less deterred from using that drug. It is possible that what we are observing with today's eighth-graders is an early signal that generational forgetting is about to take place again, as it did in the early 1990s. Therefore, while most of the news from the survey this year is good news, it is worth attending to early warning signs of possible trouble ahead."

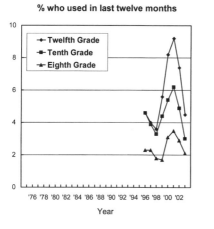

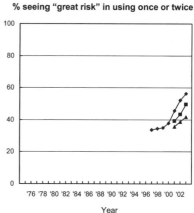

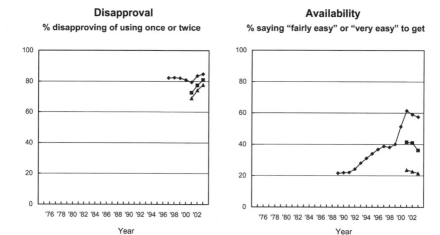

Figure 2.1. *MDMA (Ecstasy): Trends in Annual Use, Risk, Disapproval, and Availability*

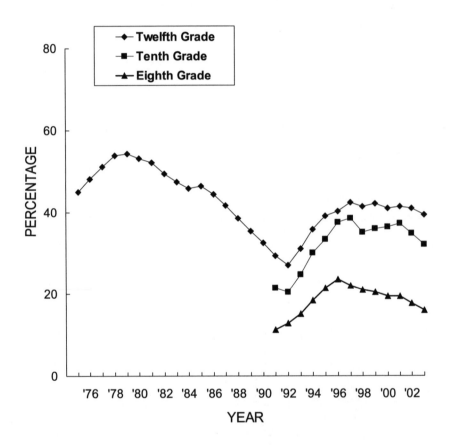

Figure 2.2. *Trends in Annual Prevalence of an Illicit Drug Use Index*

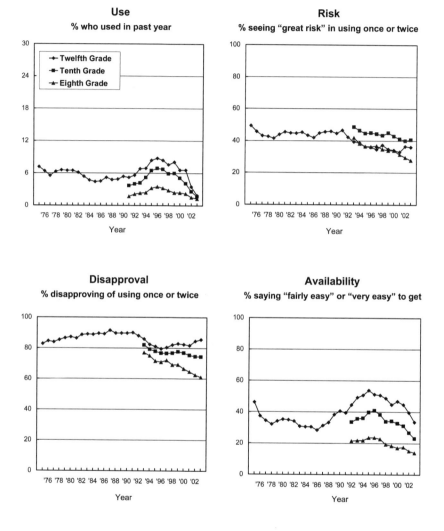

Figure 2.3. LSD: Trends in Annual Use, Risk, Disapproval, and Availability

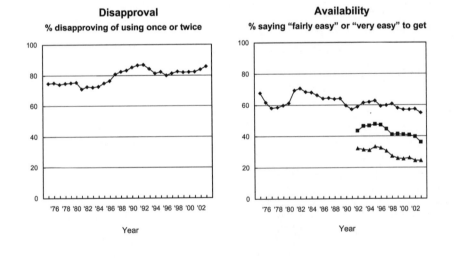
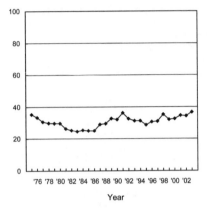
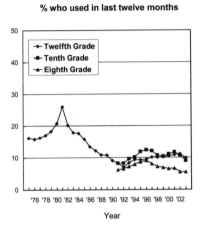

Figure 2.4. *Amphetamines: Trends in Annual Use, Risk, Disapproval, and Availability*

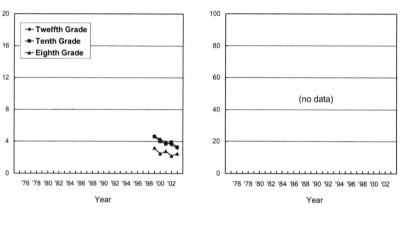

Use
% who used in last twelve months

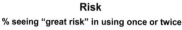

Risk
% seeing "great risk" in using once or twice

(no data)

Disapproval
% disapproving of using once or twice

(no data)

Availability
% saying "fairly easy" or "very easy" to get

(no data)

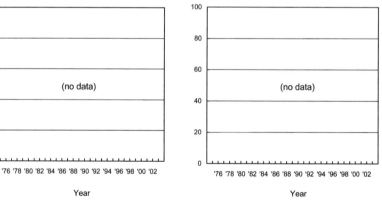

Figure 2.5. *Methamphetamine: Trends in Annual Use, Risk, Disapproval, and Availability*

19

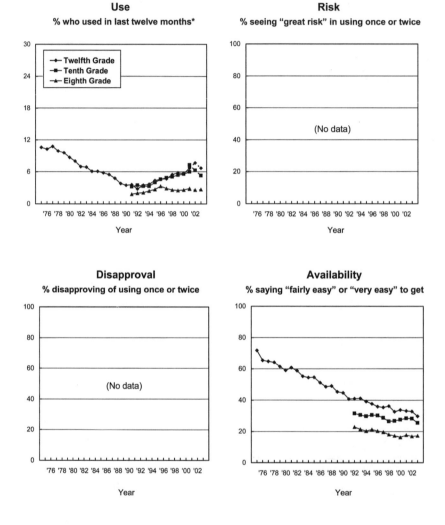

Figure 2.6. Tranquilizers: Trends in Annual Use, Risk, Disapproval, and Availability

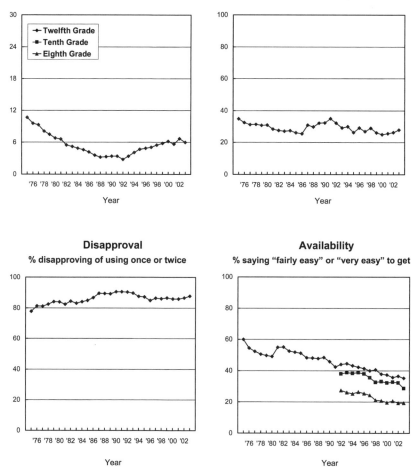

Figure 2.7. Sedatives (Barbiturates): Trends in Annual Use, Risk, Disapproval, and Availability

Use
% who used in last twelve months*

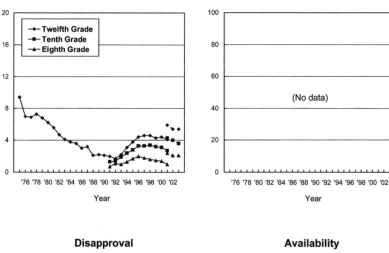

Risk
% seeing "great risk" in using once or twice

(No data)

Disapproval
% disapproving of using once or twice

(No data)

Availability
% saying "fairly easy" or "very easy" to get**

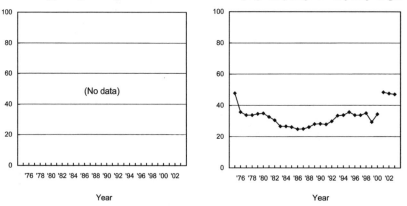

Figure 2.8. *Hallucinogens Other than LSD: Trends in Annual Use, Risk, Disapproval, and Availability*

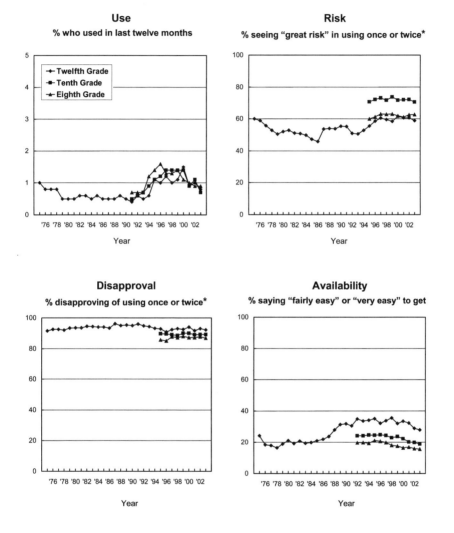

Figure 2.9. Heroin: Trends in Annual Use, Risk, Disapproval, and Availability

23

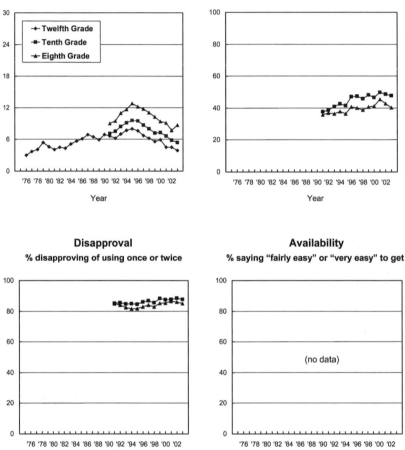

Use
% who used in last twelve months

- Twelfth Grade
- Tenth Grade
- Eighth Grade

Year

Risk
% seeing "great risk" in using once or twice

Year

Disapproval
% disapproving of using once or twice

Year

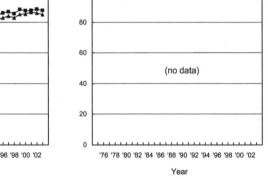

Availability
% saying "fairly easy" or "very easy" to get

(no data)

Year

Figure 2.10. Inhalants: Trends in Annual Use, Risk, Disapproval, and Availability

Table 2.1. Trends in Lifetime Prevalence of Use of Various Drugs for Eighth, 10th, and 12th Graders, continued on next pages.

	Lifetime													'02–'03
	1991	1992	1993	1994	1995	1996	1997	1998	1999	2000	2001	2002	2003	change
Any Illicit Drug[a]														
8th Grade	18.7	20.6	22.5	25.7	28.5	31.2	29.4	29.0	28.3	26.8	26.8	24.5	22.8	-1.7
10th Grade	30.6	29.8	32.8	37.4	40.9	45.4	47.3	44.9	46.2	45.6	45.6	44.6	41.4	-3.2s
12th Grade	44.1	40.7	42.9	45.6	48.4	50.8	54.3	54.1	54.7	54.0	53.9	53.0	51.1	-2.0
Any Illicit Drug Other Than Marijuana[a,b]														
8th Grade	14.3	15.6	16.8	17.5	18.8	19.2	17.7	16.9	16.3	15.8‡	17.0	13.7	13.6	-0.2
10th Grade	19.1	19.2	20.9	21.7	24.3	25.5	25.0	23.6	24.0	23.1‡	23.6	22.1	19.7	-2.4s
12th Grade	26.9	25.1	26.7	27.6	28.1	28.5	30.0	29.4	29.4	29.0‡	30.7	29.5	27.7	-1.8
Any Illicit Drug Including Inhalants[a,c]														
8th Grade	28.5	29.6	32.3	35.1	38.1	39.4	38.1	37.8	37.2	35.1	34.5	31.6	30.3	-1.4
10th Grade	36.1	36.2	38.7	42.7	45.9	49.8	50.9	49.3	49.9	49.3	48.8	47.7	44.9	-2.8s
12th Grade	47.6	44.4	46.6	49.1	51.5	53.5	56.3	56.1	56.3	57.0	56.0	54.6	52.8	-1.8
Marijuana/Hashish														
8th Grade	10.2	11.2	12.6	16.7	19.9	23.1	22.6	22.2	22.0	20.3	20.4	19.2	17.5	-1.7
10th Grade	23.4	21.4	24.4	30.4	34.1	39.8	42.3	39.6	40.9	40.3	40.1	38.7	36.4	-2.3
12th Grade	36.7	32.6	35.3	38.2	41.7	44.9	49.6	49.1	49.7	48.8	49.0	47.8	46.1	-1.7
Inhalants[c,d]														
8th Grade	17.6	17.4	19.4	19.9	21.6	21.2	21.0	20.5	19.7	17.9	17.1	15.2	15.8	+0.6
10th Grade	15.7	16.6	17.5	18.0	19.0	19.3	18.3	18.3	17.0	16.6	15.2	13.5	12.7	-0.8
12th Grade	17.6	16.6	17.4	17.7	17.4	16.6	16.1	15.2	15.4	14.2	13.0	11.7	11.2	-0.5
Nitrites[e]														
8th Grade	—	—	—	—	—	—	—	—	—	—	—	—	—	—
10th Grade	—	—	—	—	—	—	—	—	—	—	—	—	—	—
12th Grade	1.6	1.5	1.4	1.7	1.5	1.8	2.0	2.7	1.7	0.8	1.9	1.5	1.6	+0.1
Hallucinogens[b,f]														
8th Grade	3.2	3.8	3.9	4.3	5.2	5.9	5.4	4.9	4.8	4.6‡	5.2	4.1	4.0	-0.1
10th Grade	6.1	6.4	6.8	8.1	9.3	10.5	10.5	9.8	9.7	8.9‡	8.9	7.8	6.9	-0.9
12th Grade	9.6	9.2	10.9	11.4	12.7	14.0	15.1	14.1	13.7	13.0‡	14.7	12.0	10.6	-1.5
LSD														
8th Grade	2.7	3.2	3.5	3.7	4.4	5.1	4.7	4.1	4.1	3.9	3.4	2.5	2.1	-0.3
10th Grade	5.6	5.8	6.2	7.2	8.4	9.4	9.5	8.5	8.5	7.6	6.3	5.0	3.5	-1.4ss
12th Grade	8.8	8.6	10.3	10.5	11.7	12.6	13.6	12.6	12.2	11.1	10.9	8.4	5.9	-2.5sss
Hallucinogens Other Than LSD[b]														
8th Grade	1.4	1.7	1.7	2.2	2.5	3.0	2.6	2.5	2.4	2.3‡	3.9	3.3	3.2	0.0
10th Grade	2.2	2.5	2.8	3.8	3.9	4.7	4.8	5.0	4.7	4.8‡	6.6	6.3	5.9	-0.4
12th Grade	3.7	3.3	3.9	4.9	5.4	6.8	7.5	7.1	6.7	6.9‡	10.4	9.2	9.0	-0.2
PCP[e]														
8th Grade	—	—	—	—	—	—	—	—	—	—	—	—	—	—
10th Grade	—	—	—	—	—	—	—	—	—	—	—	—	—	—
12th Grade	2.9	2.4	2.9	2.8	2.7	4.0	3.9	3.9	3.4	3.4	3.5	3.1	2.5	-0.6

(Table continued on next page)

25

Table 2.1. Trends in Lifetime Prevalence of Use of Various Drugs for Eighth, 10th, and 12th Graders, continued.

						Lifetime								'02–'03
	1991	1992	1993	1994	1995	1996	1997	1998	1999	2000	2001	2002	2003	change
MDMA (Ecstasy)[g]														
8th Grade	—	—	—	—	—	3.4	3.2	2.7	2.7	4.3	5.2	4.3	3.2	-1.1s
10th Grade	—	—	—	—	—	5.6	5.7	5.1	6.0	7.3	8.0	6.6	5.4	-1.2
12th Grade	—	—	—	—	—	6.1	6.9	5.8	8.0	11.0	11.7	10.5	8.3	-2.2s
Cocaine														
8th Grade	2.3	2.9	2.9	3.6	4.2	4.5	4.4	4.6	4.7	4.5	4.3	3.6	3.6	0.0
10th Grade	4.1	3.3	3.6	4.3	5.0	6.5	7.1	7.2	7.7	6.9	5.7	6.1	5.1	-1.1
12th Grade	7.8	6.1	6.1	5.9	6.0	7.1	8.7	9.3	9.8	8.6	8.2	7.8	7.7	-0.1
Crack														
8th Grade	1.3	1.6	1.7	2.4	2.7	2.9	2.7	3.2	3.1	3.1	3.0	2.5	2.5	0.0
10th Grade	1.7	1.5	1.8	2.1	2.8	3.3	3.6	3.9	4.0	3.7	3.1	3.6	2.7	-0.9ss
12th Grade	3.1	2.6	2.6	3.0	3.0	3.3	3.9	4.4	4.6	3.9	3.7	3.8	3.6	-0.2
Other Cocaine[h]														
8th Grade	2.0	2.4	2.4	3.0	3.4	3.8	3.5	3.7	3.8	3.5	3.3	2.8	2.7	-0.1
10th Grade	3.8	3.0	3.3	3.8	4.4	5.5	6.1	6.4	6.8	6.0	5.0	5.2	4.5	-0.7
12th Grade	7.0	5.3	5.4	5.2	5.1	6.4	8.2	8.4	8.8	7.7	7.4	7.0	6.7	-0.2
Heroin[i]														
8th Grade	1.2	1.4	1.4	2.0	2.3	2.4	2.1	2.3	2.3	1.9	1.7	1.6	1.6	0.0
10th Grade	1.2	1.2	1.3	1.5	1.7	2.1	2.1	2.3	2.3	2.2	1.7	1.8	1.5	-0.3
12th Grade	0.9	1.2	1.1	1.2	1.6	1.8	2.1	2.0	2.0	2.4	1.8	1.7	1.5	-0.2
With a needle[j]														
8th Grade	—	—	—	—	1.5	1.6	1.3	1.4	1.6	1.1	1.2	1.0	1.0	-0.1
10th Grade	—	—	—	—	1.0	1.1	1.1	1.2	1.3	1.0	0.8	1.0	0.9	-0.1
12th Grade	—	—	—	—	0.7	0.8	0.9	0.8	0.9	0.8	0.7	0.8	0.7	-0.1
Without a needle[j]														
8th Grade	—	—	—	—	1.5	1.6	1.4	1.5	1.4	1.3	1.1	1.0	1.1	+0.1
10th Grade	—	—	—	—	1.1	1.7	1.7	1.7	1.6	1.7	1.3	1.3	1.0	-0.3
12th Grade	—	—	—	—	1.4	1.7	2.1	1.6	1.8	2.4	1.5	1.6	1.8	+0.2
Other Narcotics[k,l]														
8th Grade	—	—	—	—	—	—	—	—	—	—	—	—	—	—
10th Grade	—	—	—	—	—	—	—	—	—	—	—	—	—	—
12th Grade	6.6	6.1	6.4	6.6	7.2	8.2	9.7	9.8	10.2	10.6	9.9‡	13.5	13.2	-0.4
Amphetamines[k]														
8th Grade	10.5	10.8	11.8	12.3	13.1	13.5	12.3	11.3	10.7	9.9	10.2	8.7	8.4	-0.4
10th Grade	13.2	13.1	14.9	15.1	17.4	17.7	17.0	16.0	15.7	15.7	16.0	14.9	13.1	-1.8s
12th Grade	15.4	13.9	15.1	15.7	15.3	15.3	16.5	16.4	16.3	15.6	16.2	16.8	14.4	-2.4ss
Methamphetamine[m,n]														
8th Grade	—	—	—	—	—	—	—	—	4.5	4.2	4.4	3.5	3.9	+0.4
10th Grade	—	—	—	—	—	—	—	—	7.3	6.9	6.4	6.1	5.2	-0.9
12th Grade	—	—	—	—	—	—	—	—	8.2	7.9	6.9	6.7	6.2	-0.5
Ice[n]														
8th Grade	—	—	—	—	—	—	—	—	—	—	—	—	—	—
10th Grade	—	—	—	—	—	—	—	—	—	—	—	—	—	—
12th Grade	3.3	2.9	3.1	3.4	3.9	4.4	4.4	5.3	4.8	4.0	4.1	4.7	3.9	-0.8

(Table continued on next page)

Table 2.1. Trends in Lifetime Prevalence of Use of Various Drugs for Eighth, 10th, and 12th Graders, continued from previous pages.

Lifetime

	1991	1992	1993	1994	1995	1996	1997	1998	1999	2000	2001	2002	2003	'02–'03 change
Sedatives (Barbiturates)[k]														
8th Grade	—	—	—	—	—	—	—	—	—	—	—	—	—	—
10th Grade	—	—	—	—	—	—	—	—	—	—	—	—	—	—
12th Grade	6.2	5.5	6.3	7.0	7.4	7.6	8.1	8.7	8.9	9.2	8.7	9.5	8.8	-0.7
Methaqualone[e,k]														
8th Grade	—	—	—	—	—	—	—	—	—	—	—	—	—	—
10th Grade	—	—	—	—	—	—	—	—	—	—	—	—	—	—
12th Grade	1.3	1.6	0.8	1.4	1.2	2.0	1.7	1.6	1.8	0.8	1.1	1.5	1.0	-0.5
Tranquilizers[b,k]														
8th Grade	3.8	4.1	4.4	4.6	4.5	5.3	4.8	4.6	4.4	4.4‡	5.0	4.3	4.4	+0.1
10th Grade	5.8	5.9	5.7	5.4	6.0	7.1	7.3	7.8	7.9	8.0‡	9.2	8.8	7.8	-1.1s
12th Grade	7.2	6.0	6.4	6.6	7.1	7.2	7.8	8.5	9.3	8.9‡	10.3	11.4	10.2	-1.2s
Rohypnol[e,o,p]														
8th Grade	—	—	—	—	—	1.5	1.1	1.4	1.3	1.0	1.1	0.8	1.0	+0.1
10th Grade	—	—	—	—	—	1.5	1.7	2.0	1.8	1.3	1.5	1.3	1.0	-0.2
12th Grade	—	—	—	—	—	1.2	1.8	3.0	2.0	1.5	1.7	—	—	—
Alcohol[q]														
Any use														
8th Grade	70.1	69.3‡	55.7	55.8	54.5	55.3	53.8	52.5	52.1	51.7	50.5	47.0	45.6	-1.5
10th Grade	83.8	82.3‡	71.6	71.1	70.5	71.8	72.0	69.8	70.6	71.4	70.1	66.9	66.0	-0.9
12th Grade	88.0	87.5‡	80.0	80.4	80.7	79.2	81.7	81.4	80.0	80.3	79.7	78.4	76.6	-1.8
Been Drunk[n]														
8th Grade	26.7	26.8	26.4	25.9	25.3	26.8	25.2	24.8	24.8	25.1	23.4	21.3	20.3	-1.0
10th Grade	50.0	47.7	47.9	47.2	46.9	48.5	49.4	46.7	48.9	49.3	48.2	44.0	42.4	-1.6
12th Grade	65.4	63.4	62.5	62.9	63.2	61.8	64.2	62.4	62.3	62.3	63.9	61.6	58.1	-3.5
Cigarettes														
Any use														
8th Grade	44.0	45.2	45.3	46.1	46.4	49.2	47.3	45.7	44.1	40.5	36.6	31.4	28.4	-3.0ss
10th Grade	55.1	53.5	56.3	56.9	57.6	61.2	60.2	57.7	57.6	55.1	52.8	47.4	43.0	-4.4sss
12th Grade	63.1	61.8	61.9	62.0	64.2	63.5	65.4	65.3	64.6	62.5	61.0	57.2	53.7	-3.5ss
Smokeless Tobacco[e,r]														
8th Grade	22.2	20.7	18.7	19.9	20.0	20.4	16.8	15.0	14.4	12.8	11.7	11.2	11.3	+0.1
10th Grade	28.2	26.6	28.1	29.2	27.6	27.4	26.3	22.7	20.4	19.1	19.5	16.9	14.6	-2.4s
12th Grade	—	32.4	31.0	30.7	30.9	29.8	25.3	26.2	23.4	23.1	19.7	18.3	17.0	-1.3
Steroids[n]														
8th Grade	1.9	1.7	1.6	2.0	2.0	1.8	1.8	2.3	2.7	3.0	2.8	2.5	2.5	0.0
10th Grade	1.8	1.7	1.7	1.8	2.0	1.8	2.0	2.0	2.7	3.5	3.5	3.5	3.0	-0.5
12th Grade	2.1	2.1	2.0	2.4	2.3	1.9	2.4	2.7	2.9	2.5	3.7	4.0	3.5	-0.5

NOTES: Level of significance of difference between the two most recent classes: s = .05, ss = .01, sss = .001.
'—' indicates data not available.
'‡' indicates some change in the question. See relevant footnote for that drug.
Any apparent inconsistency between the change estimate and the prevalence of use estimates for the two most recent classes is due to rounding error.
SOURCE: The Monitoring the Future Study, the University of Michigan.

27

Table 2.2. Trends in Annual and 30-Day Prevalence of Use of Various Drugs for Eighth, 10th, and 12th Graders, continued on next pages.

Annual

	1991	1992	1993	1994	1995	1996	1997	1998	1999	2000	2001	2002	2003	'02–'03 change
Any Illicit Drug[a]														
8th Grade	11.3	12.9	15.1	18.5	21.4	23.6	22.1	21.0	20.5	19.5	19.5	17.7	16.1	-1.7s
10th Grade	21.4	20.4	24.7	30.0	33.3	37.5	38.5	35.0	35.9	36.4	37.2	34.8	32.0	-2.8s
12th Grade	29.4	27.1	31.0	35.8	39.0	40.2	42.4	41.4	42.1	40.9	41.4	41.0	39.3	-1.7
Any Illicit Drug Other Than Marijuana[a,b]														
8th Grade	8.4	9.3	10.4	11.3	12.6	13.1	11.8	11.0	10.5	10.2‡	10.8	8.8	8.8	0.0
10th Grade	12.2	12.3	13.9	15.2	17.5	18.4	18.2	16.6	16.7	16.7‡	17.9	15.7	13.8	-2.0ss
12th Grade	16.2	14.9	17.1	18.0	19.4	19.8	20.7	20.2	20.7	20.4‡	21.6	20.9	19.8	-1.1
Any Illicit Drug Including Inhalants[a,c]														
8th Grade	16.7	18.2	21.1	24.2	27.1	28.7	27.2	26.2	25.3	24.0	23.9	21.4	20.4	-0.9
10th Grade	23.9	23.5	27.4	32.5	35.6	39.6	40.3	37.1	37.7	38.0	38.7	36.1	33.5	-2.7s
12th Grade	31.2	28.8	32.5	37.6	40.2	41.9	42.4	42.4	42.4	40.5	42.1	42.1	41.4	-1.3
Marijuana/Hashish														
8th Grade	6.2	7.2	9.2	13.0	15.8	18.3	17.7	16.9	16.5	15.6	15.4	14.6	12.8	-1.9ss
10th Grade	16.5	15.2	19.2	25.2	28.7	33.6	34.8	31.1	32.1	32.2	32.7	30.3	28.2	-2.1
12th Grade	23.9	21.9	26.0	30.7	34.7	35.8	38.5	37.5	37.8	36.5	37.0	36.2	34.9	-1.4
Inhalants[c,d]														
8th Grade	9.0	9.5	11.0	11.7	12.8	12.2	11.8	11.1	10.3	9.4	9.1	7.7	8.7	+1.1s
10th Grade	7.1	7.5	8.4	9.1	9.6	9.5	8.7	8.0	7.2	7.3	6.6	5.8	5.4	-0.3
12th Grade	6.6	6.2	7.0	7.7	8.0	7.6	6.7	6.2	5.6	5.9	4.5	4.5	3.9	-0.6
Nitrites[e]														
8th Grade	—	—	—	—	—	—	—	—	—	—	—	—	—	—
10th Grade	—	—	—	—	—	—	—	—	—	—	—	—	—	—
12th Grade	0.9	0.5	0.9	1.1	1.1	1.6	1.2	1.4	0.9	0.6	0.6	1.1	0.9	-0.1
Hallucinogens[d,f]														
8th Grade	1.9	2.5	2.6	2.7	3.6	4.1	3.7	3.4	2.9	2.8‡	3.4	2.6	2.6	0.0
10th Grade	4.0	4.3	4.7	5.8	7.2	7.8	7.6	6.9	6.9	6.1‡	6.2	4.7	4.1	-0.6
12th Grade	5.8	5.9	7.4	7.6	9.3	10.1	9.8	9.0	9.4	8.1‡	9.1	6.6	5.9	-0.7
LSD[b]														
8th Grade	1.7	2.1	2.3	2.4	3.2	3.5	3.2	3.2	2.4	2.2	2.2	1.5	1.3	-0.2
10th Grade	3.7	4.0	4.2	5.2	6.5	6.9	6.7	6.0	6.0	4.1	4.1	2.6	1.7	-0.9ss
12th Grade	5.2	5.6	6.8	6.9	8.4	8.8	8.4	7.6	8.1	6.6	6.6	3.5	1.9	-1.6ss
Hallucinogens Other Than LSD[b]														
8th Grade	0.7	1.1	1.0	1.3	1.7	2.0	1.8	1.6	1.5	1.4‡	2.4	2.1	2.1	+0.1
10th Grade	1.3	1.4	1.9	2.4	2.8	3.3	3.3	3.4	3.2	3.1‡	4.3	4.0	3.6	-0.5
12th Grade	2.0	1.7	2.2	3.1	3.8	4.4	4.6	4.6	4.3	4.4‡	5.9	5.4	5.4	-0.1ss

30-Day

	1991	1992	1993	1994	1995	1996	1997	1998	1999	2000	2001	2002	2003	'02–'03 change
Any Illicit Drug[a]														
8th Grade	5.7	6.8	8.4	10.9	12.4	14.6	12.9	12.1	12.2	11.9	11.7	10.4	9.7	-0.7
10th Grade	11.6	11.0	14.0	18.5	20.2	23.2	23.0	21.5	22.1	22.5	22.7	20.8	19.5	-1.3
12th Grade	16.4	14.4	18.3	21.9	23.8	24.6	26.2	25.6	25.9	24.9	25.7	25.4	24.1	-1.2
Any Illicit Drug Other Than Marijuana[a,b]														
8th Grade	3.8	4.7	5.3	5.6	6.5	6.9	6.0	5.5	5.5	5.6‡	5.5	4.7	4.7	0.0
10th Grade	5.5	5.7	6.5	7.1	8.9	8.9	8.8	8.6	8.6	8.5‡	8.7	8.1	6.9	-1.2s
12th Grade	7.1	6.3	7.9	8.8	10.0	9.5	10.7	10.7	10.4	10.4‡	11.0	11.3	10.4	-1.0
Any Illicit Drug Including Inhalants[a,c]														
8th Grade	8.8	10.0	12.0	14.3	16.1	17.5	16.0	14.9	15.1	14.4	14.0	12.6	12.1	-0.6
10th Grade	13.1	12.6	15.5	20.0	21.6	24.5	24.1	22.5	23.1	23.6	23.6	21.7	20.5	-1.2
12th Grade	17.8	15.5	19.3	23.0	24.8	25.5	26.6	26.6	26.4	26.5	26.5	25.9	24.6	-1.3
Marijuana/Hashish														
8th Grade	3.2	3.7	5.1	7.8	9.1	11.3	10.2	9.7	9.1	9.1	9.2	8.3	7.5	-0.8
10th Grade	8.7	8.1	10.9	15.8	17.2	20.4	20.5	18.7	19.4	19.7	19.8	17.8	17.0	-0.8
12th Grade	13.8	11.9	15.5	19.0	21.2	21.9	23.7	22.8	23.1	21.6	22.4	21.5	21.2	-0.3
Inhalants[c,d]														
8th Grade	4.4	4.7	5.4	5.6	6.1	5.8	5.6	4.8	5.0	4.5	4.0	3.8	4.1	+0.3
10th Grade	2.7	2.7	3.3	3.6	3.5	3.3	3.6	2.9	2.6	2.4	2.4	2.4	2.2	-0.1
12th Grade	2.4	2.3	2.5	2.7	3.2	2.5	2.5	2.3	2.0	2.2	1.7	1.5	1.5	+0.1
Nitrites[e]														
8th Grade	—	—	—	—	—	—	—	—	—	—	—	—	—	—
10th Grade	—	—	—	—	—	—	—	—	—	—	—	—	—	—
12th Grade	0.4	0.3	0.6	0.4	0.4	0.7	0.7	1.0	0.4	0.3	0.5	0.6	0.7	+0.1
Hallucinogens[d,f]														
8th Grade	0.8	1.1	1.2	1.3	1.7	1.9	1.8	1.4	1.3	1.2‡	1.6	1.2	1.2	-0.1
10th Grade	1.6	1.8	1.9	2.4	3.3	2.8	3.3	3.2	2.9	2.3‡	2.1	1.6	1.5	-0.2
12th Grade	2.2	2.1	2.7	3.1	4.4	3.5	3.9	3.8	3.5	2.6‡	3.3	2.3	1.8	-0.5
LSD[b]														
8th Grade	0.6	0.9	1.0	1.1	1.1	1.5	1.5	1.1	1.1	1.0	1.0	0.7	0.6	-0.1
10th Grade	1.5	1.6	1.6	2.0	3.0	2.4	2.8	2.7	1.5	1.6	1.5	0.7	0.6	-0.1
12th Grade	1.9	2.0	2.4	2.6	4.0	2.5	3.1	3.2	2.7	1.6	2.3	0.7	0.6	-0.1
Hallucinogens Other Than LSD[b]														
8th Grade	0.3	0.4	0.5	0.7	0.8	0.9	0.7	0.7	0.6	0.6‡	1.1	1.0	1.0	0.0
10th Grade	0.4	0.5	0.7	1.0	1.0	1.0	1.2	1.4	1.2	1.2‡	1.4	1.4	1.2	-0.2
12th Grade	0.7	0.5	0.8	1.2	1.3	1.6	1.7	1.6	1.6	1.7‡	1.9	2.0	1.5	-0.5ss

(Table continued on next page)

Table 2.2. Trends in Annual and 30-Day Prevalence of Use of Various Drugs for Eighth, 10th, and 12th Graders, continued.

Annual

	1991	1992	1993	1994	1995	1996	1997	1998	1999	2000	2001	2002	2003	'02–'03 change
PCP[a]														
8th Grade	—	—	—	—	—	—	—	—	—	—	—	—	—	—
10th Grade	—	—	—	—	—	—	—	—	—	—	—	—	—	—
12th Grade	1.4	1.4	1.4	1.6	1.8	2.6	2.3	2.1	1.8	2.3	1.8	1.1	1.3	+0.2
MDMA (Ecstasy)[g]														
8th Grade	—	—	—	—	—	2.3	2.3	1.8	1.7	3.1	3.5	2.9	2.1	-0.8s
10th Grade	—	—	—	—	—	4.6	3.9	3.3	4.4	5.4	6.2	4.9	3.0	-1.8sss
12th Grade	—	—	—	—	—	4.6	4.0	3.6	5.6	8.2	9.2	7.4	4.5	-2.9sss
Cocaine														
8th Grade	1.1	1.5	1.7	2.1	2.6	3.0	2.8	3.1	2.7	2.6	2.5	2.3	2.2	-0.1
10th Grade	2.2	1.9	2.1	2.8	3.5	4.2	4.7	4.7	4.9	4.4	3.6	4.0	3.3	-0.8
12th Grade	3.5	3.1	3.3	3.6	4.0	4.9	5.5	5.7	6.2	5.0	4.8	5.0	4.8	-0.1
Crack														
8th Grade	0.7	0.9	1.0	1.3	1.6	1.8	1.7	2.1	1.8	1.8	1.7	1.6	1.6	-0.1
10th Grade	0.9	0.9	1.1	1.4	1.8	2.1	2.2	2.5	2.4	2.2	1.8	1.6	1.6	-0.1
12th Grade	1.5	1.5	1.5	1.9	2.1	2.1	2.4	2.5	2.7	2.2	2.1	2.3	2.2	-0.7sss
Other Cocaine[h]														
8th Grade	1.0	1.2	1.3	1.7	2.1	2.5	2.2	2.4	2.3	1.9	1.9	1.8	1.6	-0.2
10th Grade	2.1	1.7	1.8	2.4	3.0	3.5	4.1	4.0	4.4	3.8	3.0	3.4	2.8	-0.6
12th Grade	3.2	2.6	2.9	3.0	3.4	4.2	5.0	4.9	5.8	4.5	4.4	4.4	4.2	-0.1
Heroin[i]														
8th Grade	0.7	0.7	0.7	1.2	1.4	1.6	1.3	1.3	1.4	1.1	1.0	0.9	0.9	0.0
10th Grade	0.5	0.6	0.7	0.9	1.1	1.2	1.4	1.4	1.4	1.4	0.9	1.1	0.7	-0.3ss
12th Grade	0.4	0.6	0.5	0.6	1.1	1.0	1.2	1.0	1.5	1.5	0.9	1.0	0.8	-0.2
With a needle[j]														
8th Grade	—	—	—	—	0.9	1.0	0.8	0.8	0.9	0.6	0.7	0.6	0.6	0.0
10th Grade	—	—	—	—	0.6	0.7	0.7	0.8	0.6	0.5	0.4	0.6	0.5	-0.1
12th Grade	—	—	—	—	0.5	0.5	0.5	0.4	0.4	0.4	0.3	0.4	0.4	+0.1
Without a needle[j]														
8th Grade	—	—	—	—	0.8	1.0	0.8	0.8	0.9	0.7	0.6	0.6	0.6	0.0
10th Grade	—	—	—	—	0.8	0.9	0.7	1.0	1.1	1.1	0.7	0.8	0.5	-0.3s
12th Grade	—	—	—	—	1.0	1.0	1.2	0.8	1.0	1.6	0.8	0.8	0.8	-0.1
Other Narcotics[k,l]														
8th Grade	—	—	—	—	—	—	—	—	—	—	—	—	—	—
10th Grade	—	—	—	—	—	—	—	—	—	—	—	—	—	—
12th Grade	3.5	3.3	3.6	3.8	4.7	5.4	6.2	6.3	6.7	7.0	6.7‡	9.4	9.3	-0.2
OxyContin[m,n]														
8th Grade	—	—	—	—	—	—	—	—	—	—	—	1.3	1.7	+0.4
10th Grade	—	—	—	—	—	—	—	—	—	—	—	3.0	3.6	+0.6
12th Grade	—	—	—	—	—	—	—	—	—	—	—	4.0	4.5	+0.5

30-Day

	1991	1992	1993	1994	1995	1996	1997	1998	1999	2000	2001	2002	2003	'02–'03 change
PCP[a]														
8th Grade	—	—	—	—	—	—	—	—	—	—	—	—	—	—
10th Grade	—	—	—	—	—	—	—	—	—	—	—	—	—	—
12th Grade	0.5	0.6	1.0	0.7	0.6	1.3	0.7	1.0	0.8	0.9	0.5	0.4	0.6	+0.2
MDMA (Ecstasy)[g]														
8th Grade	—	—	—	—	—	0.8	1.0	0.9	0.8	1.4	1.8	1.4	0.7	-0.7sss
10th Grade	—	—	—	—	—	1.8	1.3	1.5	1.8	2.6	2.6	1.8	1.1	-0.7ss
12th Grade	—	—	—	—	—	2.0	1.6	1.5	2.5	3.6	2.8	2.4	1.3	-1.1sss
Cocaine														
8th Grade	0.5	0.7	0.7	1.0	1.2	1.3	1.1	1.4	1.3	1.2	1.2	1.1	0.9	-0.2
10th Grade	0.7	0.7	0.9	1.2	1.7	1.7	2.0	2.1	1.8	1.8	1.3	1.6	1.3	-0.3
12th Grade	1.4	1.3	1.3	1.5	1.8	2.0	2.3	2.4	2.6	2.1	2.1	2.3	2.1	-0.2
Crack														
8th Grade	0.3	0.5	0.4	0.7	0.7	0.8	0.7	0.9	0.8	0.8	0.8	0.8	0.7	-0.1
10th Grade	0.3	0.4	0.5	0.6	0.9	0.8	0.9	1.1	0.8	0.9	0.7	1.0	0.7	-0.2s
12th Grade	0.7	0.6	0.7	0.8	1.0	1.0	0.9	1.0	1.1	1.0	1.1	1.2	0.9	-0.3
Other Cocaine[h]														
8th Grade	0.5	0.5	0.6	0.9	1.0	1.0	0.8	1.0	1.1	0.9	0.8	0.8	0.7	-0.2
10th Grade	0.6	0.6	0.7	1.0	1.4	1.3	1.6	1.8	1.6	1.6	1.2	1.3	1.1	-0.3
12th Grade	1.2	1.0	1.2	1.3	1.3	1.6	2.0	2.0	2.5	1.7	1.8	1.9	1.8	-0.1
Heroin[i]														
8th Grade	0.3	0.4	0.4	0.6	0.6	0.6	0.6	0.6	0.6	0.5	0.6	0.5	0.4	0.0
10th Grade	0.2	0.2	0.3	0.4	0.6	0.5	0.6	0.7	0.7	0.5	0.5	0.5	0.3	-0.2
12th Grade	0.2	0.3	0.2	0.3	0.6	0.5	0.6	0.5	0.5	0.7	0.4	0.5	0.4	-0.1
With a needle[j]														
8th Grade	—	—	—	—	0.4	0.5	0.4	0.5	0.4	0.3	0.4	0.3	0.5	0.0
10th Grade	—	—	—	—	0.3	0.3	0.3	0.4	0.3	0.3	0.2	0.2	0.2	-0.2
12th Grade	—	—	—	—	0.3	0.4	0.3	0.2	0.2	0.2	0.3	0.3	0.3	-0.1
Without a needle[j]														
8th Grade	—	—	—	—	0.3	0.3	0.4	0.5	0.4	0.3	0.4	0.3	0.6	0.0
10th Grade	—	—	—	—	0.3	0.3	0.3	0.5	0.5	0.2	0.2	0.4	0.5	-0.1
12th Grade	—	—	—	—	0.6	0.4	0.6	0.4	0.4	0.7	0.3	0.5	0.4	0.0
Other Narcotics[k,l]														
8th Grade	—	—	—	—	—	—	—	—	—	—	—	—	—	—
10th Grade	—	—	—	—	—	—	—	—	—	—	—	—	—	—
12th Grade	1.1	1.2	1.3	1.5	1.8	2.0	2.3	2.4	2.6	2.9	3.0‡	4.0	4.1	+0.2
OxyContin[m,n]														
8th Grade	—	—	—	—	—	—	—	—	—	—	—	—	—	—
10th Grade	—	—	—	—	—	—	—	—	—	—	—	—	—	—
12th Grade	—	—	—	—	—	—	—	—	—	—	—	—	—	—

(Table continued on next page)

29

Table 2.2. Trends in Annual and 30-Day Prevalence of Use of Various Drugs for Eighth, 10th, and 12th Graders, continued.

Annual

Drug / Grade	1991	1992	1993	1994	1995	1996	1997	1998	1999	2000	2001	2002	2003	'02–'03 change
Vicodin[m,n]														
8th Grade	—	—	—	—	—	—	—	—	—	—	—	2.5	2.8	+0.2
10th Grade	—	—	—	—	—	—	—	—	—	—	—	6.9	7.2	+0.3
12th Grade	—	—	—	—	—	—	—	—	—	—	—	9.6	10.5	+0.9
Amphetamines[k]														
8th Grade	6.2	6.5	7.2	7.9	8.7	9.1	8.1	7.2	6.9	6.5	6.7	5.5	5.5	0.0
10th Grade	8.2	8.2	9.6	10.2	11.9	12.4	12.1	10.7	10.4	11.1	11.7	10.7	9.0	-1.7ss
12th Grade	8.2	7.1	8.4	9.4	9.3	9.5	10.2	10.1	10.2	10.5	10.9	11.1	9.9	-1.3ss
Ritalin[m,n]														
8th Grade	—	—	—	—	—	—	—	—	—	—	2.9	2.8	2.6	-0.2
10th Grade	—	—	—	—	—	—	—	—	—	—	4.8	4.8	4.1	-0.8
12th Grade	—	—	—	—	—	—	—	—	—	—	5.1	4.0	4.0	0.0
Methamphetamine[m,n]														
8th Grade	—	—	—	—	—	—	—	—	3.2	2.5	2.8	2.2	2.5	+0.4
10th Grade	—	—	—	—	—	—	—	—	4.6	4.0	3.7	3.9	3.3	-0.6
12th Grade	—	—	—	—	—	—	—	—	4.7	4.3	3.9	3.6	3.2	-0.5
Ice[n]														
8th Grade	—	—	—	—	—	—	—	—	—	—	—	—	—	—
10th Grade	—	—	—	—	—	—	—	—	—	—	—	—	—	—
12th Grade	1.4	1.3	1.7	1.8	2.4	2.8	2.3	3.0	1.9	2.2	2.5	3.0	2.0	-1.1ss
Sedatives (Barbiturates)[k]														
8th Grade	—	—	—	—	—	—	—	—	—	—	—	—	—	—
10th Grade	—	—	—	—	—	—	—	—	—	—	—	—	—	—
12th Grade	3.4	2.8	3.4	4.1	4.7	4.9	5.1	5.5	5.8	6.2	5.7	6.7	6.0	-0.7
Methaqualone[a,k]														
8th Grade	—	—	—	—	—	—	—	—	—	—	—	—	—	—
10th Grade	—	—	—	—	—	—	—	—	—	—	—	—	—	—
12th Grade	0.5	0.6	0.2	0.8	0.7	1.1	1.0	1.1	1.1	0.3	0.8	0.9	0.6	-0.3
Tranquilizers[k,k]														
8th Grade	1.8	2.0	2.1	2.4	2.7	3.3	2.9	2.6	2.5	2.6†	2.8	2.6	2.7	+0.1
10th Grade	3.2	3.5	3.3	3.3	4.0	4.6	4.9	5.1	5.4	5.6†	7.3	6.3	5.3	-1.0s
12th Grade	3.6	2.8	3.5	3.7	4.4	4.6	4.7	5.5	5.8	5.7†	6.9	7.7	6.7	-1.0s
Rohypnol[m,o,p]														
8th Grade	—	—	—	—	—	0.5	0.8	0.8	0.5	0.5	0.7	0.3	0.5	+0.2
10th Grade	—	—	—	—	—	1.0	1.3	1.2	1.0	0.8	1.0	0.7	0.6	-0.1
12th Grade	—	—	—	—	—	1.1	1.3	1.0	0.9‡	0.8	1.0	1.6	1.3	-0.3
GHB[m,a]														
8th Grade	—	—	—	—	—	—	—	—	—	1.2	1.1	0.8	0.9	+0.1
10th Grade	—	—	—	—	—	—	—	—	—	1.1	1.0	1.4	1.4	0.0
12th Grade	—	—	—	—	—	—	—	—	—	1.9	1.6	1.5	1.4	-0.1
Ketamine[m,i]														
8th Grade	—	—	—	—	—	—	—	—	—	1.6	1.3	1.3	1.1	-0.2
10th Grade	—	—	—	—	—	—	—	—	—	2.1	2.1	2.2	1.9	-0.2
12th Grade	—	—	—	—	—	—	—	—	—	2.5	2.5	2.6	2.1	-0.6

30-Day

Drug / Grade	1991	1992	1993	1994	1995	1996	1997	1998	1999	2000	2001	2002	2003	'02–'03 change
Vicodin														
8th Grade	—	—	—	—	—	—	—	—	—	—	—	—	—	—
10th Grade	—	—	—	—	—	—	—	—	—	—	—	—	—	—
12th Grade	—	—	—	—	—	—	—	—	—	—	—	—	—	—
Amphetamines														
8th Grade	2.6	3.3	3.6	3.6	4.2	4.6	3.8	3.3	3.4	3.4	3.2	2.8	2.7	-0.1
10th Grade	3.3	3.6	4.3	4.5	5.3	5.5	5.1	5.1	5.0	5.4	5.6	5.2	4.3	-0.9ss
12th Grade	3.2	2.8	3.7	4.0	4.0	4.1	4.8	4.6	4.5	5.0	5.6	5.5	5.0	-0.5
Ritalin														
8th Grade	—	—	—	—	—	—	—	—	—	—	—	—	—	—
10th Grade	—	—	—	—	—	—	—	—	—	—	—	—	—	—
12th Grade	—	—	—	—	—	—	—	—	—	—	—	—	—	—
Methamphetamine														
8th Grade	—	—	—	—	—	—	—	—	1.1	0.8	1.3	1.1	1.2	+0.1
10th Grade	—	—	—	—	—	—	—	—	1.8	1.5	1.5	1.8	1.4	-0.4
12th Grade	—	—	—	—	—	—	—	—	1.7	1.9	1.5	1.7	1.7	+0.1
Ice														
8th Grade	—	—	—	—	—	—	—	—	—	—	—	—	—	—
10th Grade	—	—	—	—	—	—	—	—	—	—	—	—	—	—
12th Grade	0.6	0.5	0.6	0.7	1.1	1.1	0.8	1.2	0.8	1.0	1.1	1.2	0.8	-0.4
Sedatives (Barbiturates)														
8th Grade	—	—	—	—	—	—	—	—	—	—	—	—	—	—
10th Grade	—	—	—	—	—	—	—	—	—	—	—	—	—	—
12th Grade	1.4	1.1	1.3	1.7	2.2	2.1	2.1	2.6	2.6	3.0	2.8	3.2	2.9	-0.3
Methaqualone														
8th Grade	—	—	—	—	—	—	—	—	—	—	—	—	—	—
10th Grade	—	—	—	—	—	—	—	—	—	—	—	—	—	—
12th Grade	0.2	0.4	0.1	0.4	0.4	0.6	0.3	0.6	0.4	0.2	0.5	0.3	0.4	0.0
Tranquilizers														
8th Grade	0.8	0.8	0.9	1.1	1.2	1.5	1.2	1.2	1.1	1.4†	1.2	1.2	1.4	+0.3
10th Grade	1.2	1.5	1.1	1.5	1.7	1.7	2.2	2.2	2.2	2.5†	2.9	2.9	2.4	-0.5s
12th Grade	1.4	1.0	1.2	1.4	1.8	2.0	1.8	2.4	2.5	2.6†	2.9	3.3	2.8	-0.5s
Rohypnol														
8th Grade	—	—	—	—	—	0.3	0.5	0.3	0.3	0.4	0.3	0.2	0.1	-0.1
10th Grade	—	—	—	—	—	0.5	0.5	0.5	0.3	0.4	0.4	0.3	0.4	-0.1
12th Grade	—	—	—	—	—	—	—	—	—	—	—	—	—	—
GHB														
8th Grade	—	—	—	—	—	—	—	—	—	—	—	—	—	—
10th Grade	—	—	—	—	—	—	—	—	—	—	—	—	—	—
12th Grade	—	—	—	—	—	—	—	—	—	—	—	—	—	—
Ketamine														
8th Grade	—	—	—	—	—	—	—	—	—	—	—	—	—	—
10th Grade	—	—	—	—	—	—	—	—	—	—	—	—	—	—
12th Grade	—	—	—	—	—	—	—	—	—	—	—	—	—	—

(Table continued on next page)

Table 2.2. Trends in Annual and 30-Day Prevalence of Use of Various Drugs for Eighth, 10th, and 12th Graders, continued from previous pages.

Annual

	1991	1992	1993	1994	1995	1996	1997	1998	1999	2000	2001	2002	2003	'02–'03 change
Alcohol[f]														
Any use														
8th Grade	54.0	53.7‡	45.4	46.8	45.3	46.5	45.5	43.7	43.5	43.1	41.9	38.7	37.2	-1.6
10th Grade	72.3	70.2‡	63.4	63.9	63.5	65.0	65.2	62.7	63.7	65.3	63.5	60.0	59.3	-0.7
12th Grade	77.7	76.8‡	72.7	73.0	73.7	72.5	74.8	74.3	73.8	73.2	73.3	71.5	70.1	-1.4
Flavored alcoholic beverages ("alcopops")														
8th Grade	—	—	—	—	—	—	—	—	—	—	—	—	—	—
10th Grade	—	—	—	—	—	—	—	—	—	—	—	—	—	—
12th Grade	—	—	—	—	—	—	—	—	—	—	—	—	55.6	—
Been Drunk[a]														
8th Grade	17.5	18.3	18.2	18.2	18.4	19.8	18.4	17.9	18.5	18.5	16.6	15.0	14.5	-0.5
10th Grade	40.1	37.0	37.8	38.0	38.5	40.1	40.7	38.3	40.9	41.6	39.9	35.4	34.7	-0.8
12th Grade	52.7	50.3	49.6	51.7	52.5	51.9	53.2	52.0	53.2	51.8	53.2	50.4	48.0	-2.4
Cigarettes														
Any use														
8th Grade	—	—	—	—	—	—	—	—	—	—	—	—	—	—
10th Grade	—	—	—	—	—	—	—	—	—	—	—	—	—	—
12th Grade	—	—	—	—	—	—	—	—	—	—	—	—	—	—
Bidis[m,n]														
8th Grade	—	—	—	—	—	—	—	—	—	3.9	2.7	2.7	2.0	-0.7
10th Grade	—	—	—	—	—	—	—	—	—	6.4	4.9	3.1	2.8	-0.3
12th Grade	—	—	—	—	—	—	—	—	—	9.2	7.0	5.9	4.0	-1.8ss
Kreteks[m,n]														
8th Grade	—	—	—	—	—	—	—	—	—	—	2.6	2.6	2.0	-0.5
10th Grade	—	—	—	—	—	—	—	—	—	—	6.0	4.9	3.8	-1.0
12th Grade	—	—	—	—	—	—	—	—	—	—	10.1	8.4	6.7	-1.8s
Smokeless Tobacco[e,r]														
8th Grade	—	—	—	—	—	—	—	—	—	—	—	—	—	—
10th Grade	—	—	—	—	—	—	—	—	—	—	—	—	—	—
12th Grade	—	—	—	—	—	—	—	—	—	—	—	—	—	—
Steroids[h]														
8th Grade	1.0	1.1	0.9	1.2	1.0	0.9	1.0	1.2	1.7	1.7	1.6	1.5	1.4	-0.1
10th Grade	1.1	1.1	1.0	1.1	1.2	1.2	1.2	1.2	1.7	2.2	2.1	2.2	1.7	-0.5ss
12th Grade	1.4	1.1	1.2	1.3	1.5	1.4	1.4	1.7	1.8	1.7	2.4	2.5	2.1	-0.4

30-Day

	1991	1992	1993	1994	1995	1996	1997	1998	1999	2000	2001	2002	2003	'02–'03 change
Alcohol[f]														
Any use														
8th Grade	25.1	26.1‡	24.3	25.5	24.6	26.2	24.5	23.0	24.0	22.4	21.5	19.6	19.7	+0.1
10th Grade	42.8	39.9‡	38.2	39.2	38.8	40.4	40.1	38.8	40.0	41.0	39.0	35.4	35.4	0.0
12th Grade	54.0	51.3‡	48.6	50.1	51.3	50.8	52.7	52.0	51.0	50.0	49.8	48.6	47.5	-1.0
Flavored alcoholic beverages ("alcopops")														
8th Grade	—	—	—	—	—	—	—	—	—	—	—	—	—	—
10th Grade	—	—	—	—	—	—	—	—	—	—	—	—	—	—
12th Grade	—	—	—	—	—	—	—	—	—	—	—	—	—	—
Been Drunk[a]														
8th Grade	7.6	7.5	7.8	8.7	8.3	9.6	8.2	8.4	9.4	8.3	7.7	6.7	6.7	+0.1
10th Grade	20.5	18.1	19.8	20.3	20.8	21.3	22.4	24.1	22.5	23.5	21.9	18.3	18.2	-0.1
12th Grade	31.6	29.9	28.9	30.8	33.2	31.3	34.2	32.9	32.9	32.3	32.7	30.3	30.9	+0.6
Cigarettes														
Any use														
8th Grade	14.3	15.5	16.7	18.6	19.1	21.0	19.4	19.1	17.5	14.6	12.2	10.7	10.2	-0.5
10th Grade	20.8	21.5	24.7	25.4	27.9	30.4	29.8	27.6	25.7	23.9	21.3	17.7	16.7	-1.0
12th Grade	28.3	27.8	29.9	31.2	33.5	34.0	36.5	35.1	34.6	31.4	29.5	26.7	24.4	-2.3s
Bidis[m,n]														
8th Grade	—	—	—	—	—	—	—	—	—	—	—	—	—	—
10th Grade	—	—	—	—	—	—	—	—	—	—	—	—	—	—
12th Grade	—	—	—	—	—	—	—	—	—	—	—	—	—	—
Kreteks[m,n]														
8th Grade	—	—	—	—	—	—	—	—	—	—	—	—	—	—
10th Grade	—	—	—	—	—	—	—	—	—	—	—	—	—	—
12th Grade	—	—	—	—	—	—	—	—	—	—	—	—	—	—
Smokeless Tobacco[e,r]														
8th Grade	6.9	7.0	6.6	7.7	7.1	7.1	5.5	4.8	4.5	4.2	4.0	3.3	4.1	+0.9
10th Grade	10.0	9.6	10.4	10.5	9.7	8.6	8.9	7.5	6.5	6.1	6.9	6.1	5.3	-0.8
12th Grade	—	11.4	10.7	11.1	12.2	9.8	9.7	8.8	8.4	7.6	7.8	6.5	6.7	+0.2
Steroids[h]														
8th Grade	0.4	0.5	0.5	0.5	0.6	0.4	0.5	0.5	0.7	0.8	0.7	0.8	0.7	-0.1
10th Grade	0.6	0.6	0.5	0.6	0.6	0.5	0.7	0.6	0.9	1.0	0.9	1.0	0.8	-0.3s
12th Grade	0.8	0.6	0.7	0.9	0.7	0.7	1.0	1.1	0.9	0.8	1.3	1.4	1.3	-0.1

NOTES: Level of significance of difference between the two most recent classes: s = .05, ss = .01, sss = .001.
'—' indicates data not available.
‡ indicates some change in the question. See relevant footnote for that drug.
Any apparent inconsistency between the change estimate and the prevalence of use estimates for the two most recent classes is due to rounding error.
SOURCE: The Monitoring the Future Study, the University of Michigan.

Notes for Tables 2.1 and 2.2

a. For 12th graders only: Use of "any illicit drug" includes any use of marijuana, LSD, other hallucinogens, crack, other cocaine, or heroin, or any use of other narcotics, amphetamines, sedatives (barbiturates), or tranquilizers not under a doctor's orders. For 8th and 10th graders: The use of other narcotics and barbiturates has been excluded, because these younger respondents appear to overreport use (perhaps because they include the use of nonprescription drugs in their answers).

b. In 2001 the question text was changed on half of the questionnaire forms for each grade. "Other psychedelics" was changed to "other hallucinogens" and "shrooms" was added to the list of examples. For the tranquilizer list of examples, Miltown was replaced with Xanax. The 2001 data presented here are based on the changed forms only; N is one-half of N indicated. In 2002 the remaining forms were changed to the new wording. The data are based on all forms beginning in 2002. Data for "any illicit drug other than marijuana" and "hallucinogens" are also affected by these changes and have been handled in a parallel manner.

c. For 12th graders only: Data based on five of six forms in 1991–98; N is five-sixths of N indicated. Beginning in 1999, data based on three of six forms; N is one-half of N indicated.

d. Inhalants are unadjusted for underreporting of amyl and butyl nitrites.

e. For 12th graders only: Data based on one of six forms; N is one-sixth of N indicated.

f. Hallucinogens are unadjusted for underreporting of PCP.

g. For 8th and 10th graders only: Data based on one of two forms in 1996; N is one-half of N indicated. In 1997–2001, data based on one-third of N indicated due to changes on the questionnaire forms. Data based on two of four forms beginning in 2002; N is one-half of N indicated. For 12th graders only: Data based on one of six forms in 1996–2001; N is one-sixth of N indicated. Data based on two of six forms beginning in 2002; N is two-sixths of N indicated.

h. For 12th graders only: Data based on four of six forms; N is four-sixths of N indicated.

i. In 1995, the heroin question was changed in three of six forms for 12th graders and in one of two forms for 8th and 10th graders. Separate questions were asked for use with injection and without injection. Data presented here represent the combined data from all forms. In 1996, the heroin question was changed in all remaining 8th and 10th grade forms.

j. For 8th and 10th graders only: Data based on one of two forms in 1995; N is one-half of N indicated. Data based on all forms beginning in 1996. For 12th graders only: Data based on three of six forms; N is one-half of N indicated.

k. Only drug use not under a doctor's orders is included here.

l. In 2002 the question text was changed in half of the questionnaire forms. The list of examples of narcotics other than heroin was updated: Talwin, laudanum, and paregoric—all of which had negligible rates of use by 2001—were replaced with Vicodin, OxyContin, and Percocet. The 2002 data presented here are based on the changed forms only; N is one-half of N indicated. In 2003, the remaining forms were changed to the new wording. The data are based on all forms in 2003.

m. For 8th and 10th graders only: Data based on one of four forms; N is one-third of N indicated.

n. For 12th graders only: Data based on two of six forms; N is two-sixths of N indicated.

o. For 8th and 10th graders only: Data based on one of two forms in 1996; N is one-half of N indicated. Data based on three of four forms in 1997–98; N is two-thirds of N indicated. Data based on two of four forms in 1999–2001; N is one-third of N indicated. Data based on one of four forms beginning in 2002; N is one-sixth of N indicated.

p. For 12th graders only: Data for Rohypnol for 2001 and 2002 are not comparable due to changes in the questionnaire forms.

q. In 1993, the question text was changed slightly in half of the forms to indicate that a "drink" meant "more than a few sips." The 1993 data are based on the changed forms only; N is one-half of N indicated. In 1994 the remaining forms were changed to the new wording. Beginning in 1994, the data are based on all forms.

r.   For 8th and 10th graders only: Data based on one of two forms for 1991–96 and on two of four forms beginning in 1997; N is one-half of N indicated.

s.   For 12th graders only: Data based on two of six forms in 2000; N is two-sixths of N indicated. Data based on three of six forms in 2001; N is one-half of N indicated. Data based on one of six forms beginning in 2002; N is one-sixth of N indicated.

t.   For 12th graders only: Data based on two of six forms in 2000; N is two-sixths of N indicated. Data based on three of six forms beginning in 2001; N is one-half of N indicated.

u.   Daily use is defined as use on twenty or more occasions in the past thirty days except for cigarettes and smokeless tobacco, for which actual daily use is measured, and for 5+ drinks, for which the prevalence or having five or more drinks in a row in the last two weeks is measured.

About the Survey

Monitoring the Future has been funded under a series of competing, investigator-initiated research grants from the National Institute on Drug Abuse. Surveys of nationally representative samples of American high school seniors were begun in 1975, making the class of 2003 the 29th such class surveyed. Surveys of eighth- and 10th-graders were added to the design in 1991, making the 2003 nationally representative samples the 13th such classes surveyed. The sample sizes in 2003 are 17,000 eighth-graders located in 141 schools, 16,200 10th-graders located in 129 schools, and 15,200 12th-graders located in 122 schools, for a total of 48,500 students in 392 schools overall. The samples are drawn to be representative of students in private and public secondary schools across the coterminous United States, selected with probability proportionate to estimated class size, to yield separate, nationally representative samples of students from each of the three grade levels.

The findings summarized here are published in the volume: Johnston, L. D., O'Malley, P. M., Bachman, J. G., & Schulenberg, J. E. (2004). *Monitoring the Future national results on adolescent drug use: Overview of key findings, 2003.* (NIH Publication No. 04-5506.) Bethesda, MD: National Institute on Drug Abuse. It and many other publications from the study may be found on the study's website, www.monitoring thefuture.org.

Chapter 3

Minorities and Drugs

Overview

The U.S. Census Bureau estimated the population of the United States at 281,421,906 as of April 2, 2001. The majority of Americans were white (75.1%), followed by black/African Americans (12.3%); Asian (3.6%); American Indian/Alaska Natives (0.9%); Native Hawaiian/ other Pacific Islanders (0.1%); and 12.5% of the population were of Hispanic origin (can be of any race).[1]

Extent of Use

The 2002 National Survey on Drug Use and Health by the Substance Abuse and Mental Health Services Administration (SAMHSA) showed that the highest rate of lifetime illicit drug use was among American Indians/Alaskan Natives (58.4%), followed by persons with multiple races (54%), whites (48.5%), and black/African Americans (43.8%). The lowest rate of lifetime illicit drug use was among Hispanics (38.9%) and Asians (25.6%).[2]

The rates of current illicit drug use for major racial/ethnic groups were 9.7% for blacks/African Americans, 8.5% for whites, and 7.2% for Hispanics. The rate was highest among multiple races (11.4%), followed by American Indian/Alaska Native population (10.1%) and was lowest among Asians (3.5%).[3]

Office of National Drug Control Policy (ONDCP), February 2004.

The Youth Risk Behavior Surveillance System (YRBSS) study by the Centers for Disease Control and Prevention (CDC) surveyed high school students on risk factors including drug and alcohol abuse. The 2001 report showed that 24.6% of Hispanic, 24.4% of white, and 21.8% of black high school students were current marijuana users.[4]

The Monitoring the Future Study (MTF) sponsored by the National Institute on Drug Abuse (NIDA) found similar findings to the YRBSS. According to the 2002 findings, drug use was the lowest among African American youth for most types of drugs. Of 12th graders, whites tended to have the highest rates of use for a number of drugs, including inhalants, hallucinogens, LSD, ecstasy, heroin without a needle, amphetamines, sedatives (barbiturates), tranquilizers, and narcotics other than heroin. Hispanic seniors had the highest rate of usage for a number of the most dangerous drugs, including heroin with a needle, crack, and crystal methamphetamine (ice).[5]

Health Effects

According to the Drug Abuse Warning Network emergency department (ED) data, there were a total of 670,307 drug-related ED episodes during 2002. The majority of the episodes involved whites (372,727), followed by African Americans (142,974) and Hispanics (79,098).[6]

Table 3.1. Reported Drug Use by High School Students, by Race/Ethnicity, 2001.

	White	Black	Hispanic
Lifetime marijuana use	42.8%	40.2%	44.7%
Current marijuana use	24.4	21.8	24.6
Lifetime cocaine use	9.9	2.1	14.9
Current cocaine use	4.2	1.3	7.1
Lifetime inhalant use	16.3	5.8	15.2
Current inhalant use	4.9	2.6	5.5
Lifetime heroin use	3.3	1.7	3.1
Lifetime methamphetamine use	11.4	2.1	9.1
Lifetime illegal steroid use	5.3	3.2	4.2
Lifetime injecting illegal drug use	2.4	1.6	2.5
Tried marijuana before age 13 years	9.5	11.4	12.9

Table 3.2. Definitions

Drug Episode: A drug-related ED episode is an ED visit that was induced by or related to the use of drug(s).

Drug Mention: A drug mention refers to a substance that was recorded during an ED episode. Because up to four drugs can be reported for each drug abuse episode, there are more mentions than episodes.

Treatment

According to the Treatment Episode Data Set (TEDS) during 2000, 59.7% of those admitted to treatment were white. The remaining treatment admissions were black (23.6%), Hispanic (11.7%), American Indian (2.1%), other (1.7%), Asian/Pacific (0.9%), and Alaska Native (0.3%).[7]

Arrests and Sentencing

During 2002, there were a total of 1,103,017 state and local arrests for drug abuse violations in the United Sates. Of the 1,101,547 drug abuse violations with race information available, 66.2% of those arrested were white, 32.5% were black, 0.7% were Asian or Pacific Islanders, and 0.6% were American Indians or Alaskan Natives.[8]

In FY 2001, there were a total of 24,255 federal defendants charged with a drug offense. More than a quarter of the defendants were white (26%), nearly one third were black (30.5%), and the majority were Hispanic (43.1%). The most common drug type for Hispanic defendants was heroin and marijuana; for black defendants it was crack cocaine; and for white defendants it was methamphetamine and other.[9]

Of the drug offenders convicted in state courts during 1998, 42% were black and 29% were white.[10]

During 2001, there were a total of 1,208,700 sentenced state prison inmates, 246,100 of whom were incarcerated for drug offenses. The majority of drug offenders held in state prisons were black (139,700), followed by whites (57,300), and Hispanics (47,000).[11]

A 1997 Bureau of Justice Statistics (BJS) survey of prison inmates showed that prior drug use among state prison inmates varied little by race. Approximately 84% of both white and black inmates and 81% of Hispanic inmates had used drugs in the past. The percentage of inmates that used drugs at the time of their offense was also similar for all races. Approximately one third of Hispanic (33.0%), black (31.9%), and white (33.9%) state prison inmates had used drugs at the time of their offense.[12]

During 1995 there were a total of 2,065,896 state and local probationers; of that total, 20% (414,832) were on probation for a drug offense. White probationers (73%) had the highest rate of prior drug use, followed by black probationers (68%) and Hispanics (56%). Drug use at the time of the offense was similar for white (14%) and black (15%) probationers, and lowest for Hispanics (11%).[13]

The Arrestee Drug Abuse Monitoring (ADAM) program reports on drug use among adult and juvenile arrestees in over 30 sites around the U.S., and provides data on arrestee drug use by race. For example, during 1999 in Los Angeles, California, 80.6% of black male arrestees and 71.4% of black females tested positive for drug use at the time of their arrest. Drug use among white females (74%) was higher than black and Hispanic (35%) females or white males (65%). Hispanic male (52%) and female (35%) arrestees' drug use rates were lower than rates for both black and white arrestees. Over half (58.3%) of black male juvenile arrestees in Los Angeles tested positive for drugs at the time of their arrest, followed by Hispanic juveniles (53%) and white juveniles (47%).[14]

Notes

1. U.S. Census Bureau, *Percent of Population by Race and Hispanic or Latino Origin, for the United States, Regions, Divisions, and States, and for Puerto Rico: 2000* (PDF), April 2001.

2. Substance Abuse and Mental Health Services Administration, *Results from the 2002 National Survey on Drug Use and Health: National Findings*, September 2003.

3. Ibid.

4. Centers for Disease Control and Prevention, *Youth Risk Behavior Surveillance System (YRBSS)*, 2001, June 2002.

5. National Institute on Drug Abuse and University of Michigan, *Monitoring the Future National Survey Results on Drug Use, 1975–2002, Volume II: College Students & Adults Ages 19–40* (PDF), 2003.

6. Substance Abuse and Mental Health Services Administration, *Emergency Department Trends from the Drug Abuse Warning Network, Final Estimates 1995–2002*, July 2003.

7. Substance Abuse and Mental Health Services Administration, *Treatment Episode Data Set (TEDS): 1992–2001*, December 2003.

8. Federal Bureau of Investigation, *Crime in the United States, 2002*, October 2003.

9. U.S. Sentencing Commission, *2001 Sourcebook of Federal Sentencing Statistics*, 2002.

10. Bureau of Justice Statistics, *State Court Sentencing of Convicted Felons, 1998* (PDF), December 2001.

11. Bureau of Justice Statistics, *Prisoners in 2002*, July 2003.

12. Bureau of Justice Statistics, *Substance Abuse and Treatment of State and Federal Prisoners, 1997*, December 1998.

13. Bureau of Justice Statistics, *Substance Abuse and Treatment of Adults on Probation, 1995*, March 1998.

14. National Institute of Justice, *1999 Annual Report on Drug Use Among Adult and Juvenile Arrestees* (PDF), June 2000. *Adult Findings* (PDF) and *Juvenile Findings* (PDF).

Chapter 4

Women, Pregnancy, and Drug Use Trends

Women and Drugs—An Overview

A three-year study on women and young girls (ages eight to 22) from the National Center on Addiction and Substance Abuse (CASA) at Columbia University revealed that girls and young women use substances for reasons different than boys and young men. The study also found that the signals and situations of higher risk are different and that girls and young women are more vulnerable to abuse and addiction: they get hooked faster and suffer the consequences sooner than boys and young men.[1]

In 2002, lifetime, past year, and past month drug use rates were lower for women than for men.[2] Women accounted for 30% of the nationwide admissions to treatment during 2000.[3]

Extent of Use

According to the 2002 National Survey on Drug Use and Health, approximately 50.7 million women ages 12 and older reported using an illicit drug at some point in their lives, representing 41.7% of the females ages 12 and older. Approximately 12.5% of females ages 12 and older reported past month use of an illicit drug and 6.4% reported past month use of an illicit drug.[4]

This chapter contains "Women and Drugs," Office of National Drug Control Policy (ONDCP), February 2004; and "Pregnancy and Drug Use Trends," National Institute on Drug Abuse (NIDA), June 2003.

Approximately 3.3% of pregnant women between the ages of 15 and 44 reported using an illicit drug in the month before being interviewed in 2002. This was significantly lower than the rate among non-pregnant women in the same age group (10.3%). The drug with the highest prevalence of use among pregnant women ages 15–44 was marijuana, with 2.9% reporting past month marijuana use.[5]

According to the Centers for Disease Control and Prevention (CDC), in 2001, nearly 40% of female high school students surveyed nationwide used marijuana during their lifetime.[6]

The 2002 National Survey on Drug Use and Health asked respondents how easy it was to obtain illegal drugs. Females ages 12–17 were more likely than males ages 12–17 to report that marijuana, cocaine, crack, heroin, and LSD were fairly or very easy to obtain.[7]

According to preliminary data from the Arrestee Drug Abuse Monitoring (ADAM) Program, a median of 67.1% of adult female arrestees tested positive for either cocaine, marijuana, methamphetamine, opiates, or PCP. Approximately 21% of female arrestees were positive for more than one of these drugs. This data was compiled by testing female arrestees in 23 U.S. sites.[8]

Table 4.1. Percent of Females Reporting Illicit Drug Use, 2002.

Drug Type	Lifetime	Past Year	Past Month
Any illicit drug	41.7%	12.5%	6.4%
Marijuana/hashish	36.0	8.4	4.4
Cocaine	11.2	1.6	0.
Crack	2.5	0.4	0.1
Heroin	0.9	0.1	0.0
Hallucinogens	11.7	1.6	0.4
LSD	8.0	0.3	0.0
PCP	2.2	0.1	0.0
MDMA/Ecstasy	3.6	1.1	0.2
Inhalants	6.5	0.6	0.2
Methamphetamine	4.1	0.6	0.2

Table 4.2. Percent of High School Students Reporting Drug Use, 2001.

Drug Type	Female	Male	Total
Lifetime marijuana use	38.4%	46.5%	42.4%
Current marijuana use	20.0	27.9	23.9
Lifetime cocaine use	8.4	10.3	9.4
Current cocaine use	3.7	4.7	4.2
Lifetime inhalant use	14.9	14.7	14.7
Current inhalant use	4.2	5.1	4.7
Lifetime heroin use	2.5	3.8	3.1
Lifetime methamphetamine use	9.2	10.5	9.8

Table 4.3. Definitions.

Drug Episode: A drug-related ED episode is an ED visit that was induced by or related to the use of drug(s).

Drug Mention: A drug mention refers to a substance that was recorded during an ED episode. Because up to four drugs can be reported for each drug abuse episode, there are more mentions than episodes.

Table 4.4. Percent of Female Arrestees Testing Positive for Drugs, 2002.

Drug Category	Percent
Cocaine	30.7%
Opiates	6.2
Marijuana	28.4
Methamphetamine	12.0
Any drug	67.1
Multiple drugs	20.6

Health Effects

A National Vital Statistics Report found that 21,683 persons died of drug-induced causes in 2001. Of the drug-induced deaths, 7,439 (34%) were females. Drug-induced deaths include deaths from dependent and nondependent use of drugs (legal and illegal use) and poisoning from medically prescribed and other drugs. It excludes accidents, homicides, and other causes indirectly related to drug use. Also excluded are newborn deaths due to mother's drug use.[9]

The Drug Abuse Warning Network (DAWN) collects data on drug-related visits to emergency departments (ED) nationwide. In 2002, there were 670,307 ED episodes. Of these episodes, 308,098 involved females, a 22% increase from the 252,128 female ED episodes in 1995. In 2002, there were 1,209,938 ED drug mentions reported to DAWN, 553,874 of which involved females.[10]

Table 4.5. Number of Female ED Drug Mentions, 2000–2002.

Drug Type	2000	2001	2002
Alcohol in combination	80,948	85,328	79,957
Cocaine	59,314	65,713	69,852
Heroin	30,146	30,023	31,173
Marijuana	33,334	37,781	41,707
Methamphetamine	4,841	6,680	6,565
MDMA (ecstasy)	2,011	2,331	1,987
LSD	948	820	112
PCP	1,720	1,683	2,738
Total mentions	513,271	538,166	553,874

Treatment

According to the Treatment Episode Data Set (TEDS), 484,475 females were admitted to treatment facilities in the United States during 2000, representing 30.4% of the total treatment admissions. Admissions in which smoked cocaine was the primary substance of abuse represented 13.9% of the female admissions.[11]

Additional TEDS data indicate that more than half of the treatment admissions for tranquilizers and sedatives in 2000 involved women.[12]

Table 4.6. Percent of Female Admissions to Treatment, 2000.

Drug Category	Percent
Alcohol only	20.2%
Alcohol with secondary drug	17.4
Heroin	16.6
Other opiates	2.6
Smoked cocaine	13.9
Cocaine by other route	4.3
Marijuana/hashish	11.8
Methamphetamine/amphetamines	7.9

Table 4.7. Admissions to Treatment, by Sex, 2000.

	Male	Female
Alcohol	76.3	23.7
Heroin	66.9	33.1
Other opiates	51.5	48.5
Cocaine-smoked	57.4	42.6
Cocaine-other route	64.9	35.1
Marijuana	75.9	24.1
Methamphetamine/amphetamine	52.9	47.1
Other stimulants	60.3	39.7
Tranquilizers	41.5	58.5
Sedatives	45.1	54.9
Hallucinogens	73.7	26.3
PCP	63.7	36.3
Inhalants	72.4	27.6
Other	62.4	37.6
All admissions	69.6	30.4

A SAMHSA report on females admitted to treatment with a dual diagnosis of a substance abuse problem and a psychiatric disorder found that almost half (46%) had alcohol as a primary substance of abuse. The report also found that dually diagnosed female admissions were more likely to have had prior treatments than non-dually diagnosed female admissions (72% vs. 60%).[13]

Arrests and Sentencing

According to the Federal Bureau of Investigation, there were 199,361 state and local female arrests in 2002 for drug abuse violations.[14]

In FY 2001, the U.S. Marshals Service arrested and booked 17,249 female suspects for federal offenses, representing 14.3% of the total arrests made by the U.S. Marshals Service. Of the U.S. Marshals Service arrestees booked on drug offense charges, 15.3% were female. Also in FY 2001, the Drug Enforcement Administration (DEA) arrested 5,452 females, representing 16.6% of the DEA arrests. Approximately 28% (1,528) of the female DEA arrests in FY 2001 involved methamphetamine.[15]

From October 1, 2000 to September 30, 2001, there were 8,898 female offenders convicted of a federal offense. Approximately 82% of the female offenders convicted of felony drug offenses in FY 2001 were sentenced to incarceration. On September 30, 2001, there were 9,604 female offenders in federal prison. Females accounted for 8.2% of the federal prisoners serving time for drug offenses.[16]

In 2001, there were 76,200 sentenced female prisoners under state jurisdiction. Approximately 23,000 of these females were incarcerated for drug offenses. From 1995 to 2001, drug offenses accounted for 12.8% of the total prison growth among female inmates.[17]

Table 4.8. Females Arrested by the DEA, by Type of Drug, FY 2001.

Drug Category	Total Arrested
Powered cocaine	948
Crack cocaine	714
Marijuana	973
Methamphetamine	1,528
Opiates	561
Other or non-drug	728

A Bureau of Justice Statistics (BJS) report found that about half of women offenders confined in state prisons had been using alcohol, drugs, or both at the time of the offense for which they had been incarcerated. About 6 in 10 women in state prison described themselves as using drugs in the month before the offense and 5 in 10 described themselves as a daily user of drugs. Nearly 1 in 3 women serving time in state prisons said they had committed the offense that brought them to prison in order to obtain money to support their need for drugs.[18]

A report from the Office of Juvenile Justice and Delinquency Prevention (OJJDP) that summarized research on female gangs states that drug offenses are among the most common offenses committed by female gang members. In Los Angeles County, an analysis of lifetime arrest records of female gang members revealed that drug offenses were the most frequent cause for arrest. A special tabulation from Chicago showed that between 1993 and 1996, either drug offenses or violent offenses were the most common cause for arrest of female gang members.[19]

Pregnancy and Drug Use Trends—An Overview

Drug abuse can occur at any stage in a woman's life. Of women who use illicit drugs, however, about half are in the childbearing age group of 15 to 44. In 1992/1993, NIDA conducted a nationwide hospital survey to determine the extent of drug abuse among pregnant women in the United States. This National Pregnancy and Health Survey still provides the most recent national data available.

The survey found that of the 4 million women who gave birth during the period, 757,000 women drank alcohol products and 820,000 women smoked cigarettes during their pregnancies. There was a strong link among cigarette, alcohol, and illegal drug use. Thirty-two percent of those who reported use of one drug also smoked cigarettes and drank alcohol.

Survey results showed that 221,000 women used illegal drugs during their pregnancies that year, with marijuana and cocaine being the most prevalent: 119,000 women reported use of marijuana and 45,000 reported use of cocaine. The survey estimated that the number of babies born to these women was 222,000, a close parallel to the number of mothers. Generally, rates of any illegal drug use were higher in women who were not married, had less than 16 years of formal education, were not working, and relied on some public source of funding to pay for their hospital stay.

Despite a generally decreasing trend in the use of drugs from three months before pregnancy and through the pregnancy, women did not discontinue drug use. However, findings from other NIDA research on women in treatment, for example, indicate that once women are successfully detoxified and enrolled in a treatment program, their motivator to stay drug free is their children.

The survey also pointed to issues of prevalence differences among ethnic groups. While the rates of illegal substance abuse were higher for African Americans, the estimated number of white women using drugs during pregnancy was larger at 113,000 than the number of African-American women at 75,000, or Hispanic women at 28,000.

As for the legal drugs, estimates of alcohol use were also highest among white women at about 588,000, compared to 105,000 among African-American women, and 54,000 among Hispanic women. Whites had the highest rates of cigarette use as well: 632,000 compared with 132,000 for African Americans and 36,000 for Hispanics.

Rates of marijuana use were highest among those under 25 and rates of cocaine use were higher among those 25 and older.

Notes

1. National Center on Addiction and Substance Abuse at Columbia University, *The Formative Years: Pathways to Substance Abuse Among Girls and Young Women Ages 8–22* (PDF), February 2003.

2. Substance Abuse and Mental Health Services Administration, *Results from the 2002 National Survey on Drug Use and Health: National Findings*, September 2003.

3. Substance Abuse and Mental Health Services Administration, *Treatment Episode Data Set (TEDS) 1992–2000: National Admissions to Substance Abuse Treatment Services*, December 2002.

4. Substance Abuse and Mental Health Services Administration, *Results from the 2002 National Survey on Drug Use and Health: National Findings*, September 2003.

5. Ibid.

6. Centers for Disease Control and Prevention, *Youth Risk Behavior Surveillance System (YRBSS), 2001*, June 2002.

7. Substance Abuse and Mental Health Services Administration, *Results from the 2002 National Survey on Drug Use and Health: National Findings, Detailed Tables* (PDF), September 2003.

8. National Institute of Justice, *Preliminary Data on Drug Use & Related Matters Among Adult Arrestees & Juvenile Detainees, 2002* (PDF), 2003.

9. Centers for Disease Control and Prevention, *Deaths: Final Data for 2001* (PDF), September 2003.

10. Substance Abuse and Mental Health Services Administration, *Emergency Department Trends from the Drug Abuse Warning Network, Final Estimates 1995–2002*, July 2003.

11. Substance Abuse and Mental Health Services Administration, *Treatment Episode Data Set (TEDS): 1992–2001*, December 2003.

12. Ibid.

13. Substance Abuse and Mental Health Services Administration, *Dually Diagnosed Female Substance Abuse Treatment Admissions: 1999*, October 2002.

14. Federal Bureau of Investigation, *Crime in the United States, 2002*, October 2003.

15. Bureau of Justice Statistics, *Compendium of Federal Justice Statistics, 2001*, November 2003.

16. Bureau of Justice Statistics, *Compendium of Federal Justice Statistics, 2001*, November 2003.

17. Bureau of Justice Statistics, *Prisoners in 2002*, July 2003.

18. Bureau of Justice Statistics, *Women Offenders*, December 1999.

19. Office of Juvenile Justice and Delinquency Prevention, *Female Gangs: A Focus on Research*, March 2001.

Chapter 5

Drug Use and Crime

At the Time of the Offense

Drug-Related Crime

In 1998 an estimated 61,000 convicted jail inmates said they had committed their offense to get money for drugs.[1]

Of convicted property and drug offenders, about 1 in 4 had committed their crimes to get money for drugs. A higher percentage of drug offenders in 1996 (24%) than in 1989 (14%) were in jail for a crime committed to raise money for drugs.

Table 5.1. Percent of Jail Inmates Who Committed Offense to Get Money for Drugs.

Offense	1996	1989
Total	15.8%	13.3%
Violent	8.8	11.5
Property	25.6	24.4
Drugs	23.5	14.0
Public-order	4.2	3.3

Source: BJS, *Profile of Jail Inmates, 1996*, NCJ 164620, April 1998.

Bureau of Justice Statistics, December 2003.

In 1997, 19% of state prisoners and 16% of federal inmates said they committed their current offense to obtain money for drugs. These percentages represent a slight increase from 1991, when 17% of state and 10% of federal prisoners identified drug money as a motive for their current offense.[2]

The Uniform Crime Reporting Program (UCR) of the Federal Bureau of Investigation (FBI) reported that in 2002, 4.7% of the 14,054 homicides in which circumstances were known were narcotics related. Murders that occurred specifically during a narcotics felony, such as drug trafficking or manufacturing, are considered drug related.

Table 5.2. Drug-Related Homicides.

Year	Number of homicides	Percent drug related
1987	17,963	4.9%
1988	17,971	5.6
1989	18,954	7.4
1990	20,273	6.7
1991	21,676	6.2
1992	22,716	5.7
1993	23,180	5.5
1994	22,084	5.6
1995	20,232	5.1
1996	16,967	5.0
1997	15,837	5.1
1998	14,276	4.8
1999	13,011	4.5
2000	13,230	4.5
2001	14,061	4.1
2002	14,054	4.7

Note: The percentages are based on data from the Supplementary Homicide Reports (SHR) while the totals are from the Uniform Crime Reports (UCR). Not all homicides in the UCR result in reports in the SHR.

Source: Table constructed by ONDCP Drug Policy Information Clearinghouse staff from FBI, Uniform Crime Reports, *Crime in the United States*, annually.

Offenders under the Influence at the Time of the Offense

Victim's Perception

According to the National Crime Victimization Survey (NCVS), in 2002, there were 5.3 million violent victimizations of residents age 12 or older. Victims of violence were asked to describe whether they perceived the offender to have been drinking or using drugs.

- About 29% of the victims of violence reported that the offender was using drugs, alone or in combination with alcohol.

- Based on victim perceptions, about 1.0 million violent crimes occurred each year in which victims were certain that the offender had been drinking. For about 1 in 5 of these violent victimizations involving alcohol use by the offender, victims believed the offender was also using drugs at the time of the offense.

Table 5.3. Victim's Perception of the Use of Alcohol and Drugs by the Violent Offender, 2002.

	Percent of victims of violent crime
Alcohol only	17.0
Alcohol and drugs	4.6
Alcohol or drugs	1.5
Drugs only	5.6
No drugs or alcohol	27.7
Don't know	43.3

Source: Table constructed by staff from the U.S. Census Bureau for the *National Crime Victimization Survey*, March 2003.

Victims of workplace violence.[3] Of workplace victims of violence:

- 35% believed the offender was drinking or using drugs at the time of the incident

- 36% did not know if the offender had been drinking or using drugs

- 27% of all workplace offenders had not been drinking or using drugs

Victims of workplace violence varied in their perception of whether the offender used alcohol or drugs by occupation:

- 47% in law enforcement perceived the offender to be using alcohol or drugs
- 35% in the medical field
- 31% in retail sales

American Indian victims. Alcohol and drug use was a factor in more than half of violent crimes against American Indians.

Substantial differences can be found by race in the reports of victims of violence of their perceptions of drug and alcohol use by offenders. Among those who could describe alcohol or drug use by offenders, American Indian victims of violence were the most likely to report such perceived use by the offender.

Overall, in 55% of American Indian violent victimizations, the victim said the offender was under the influence of alcohol, drugs, or both. The offender's use of alcohol and/or drugs was somewhat less likely in violent crimes committed against whites (44%) or blacks (35%).

Table 5.4. Violent Crime, by the Perceived Drug or Alcohol Use of the Offender and by Race of Victim, 1992–96.

	Perceived drug or alcohol use by offender				
Race of victim	Total	Alcohol	Drugs	Both	Neither
Total	100%	28%	8%	7%	57%
American Indian	100	38	9	8	45
White	100	29	8	7	56
Black	100	21	7	7	65
Asian	100	20	3	2	75

Note: Table excludes those respondents who were unable to report whether or not they perceived the offender to have been using drugs or alcohol.

Source: BJS, *American Indians and Crime*, NCJ 173386, February 1999.

Perspectives of Probationers, Prisoners, and Jail Inmates

Probationers. The first national survey of adults on probation, conducted in 1995, reported that 14% of probationers were on drugs when they committed their offense.[4]

Among probationers, 49% of the mentally ill and 46% of others reported alcohol or drug use at the time of the offense.[5]

Prisoners. In the 1997 Survey of Inmates in State and Federal Correctional Facilities, 33% of state prisoners and 22% of federal prisoners said they had committed their current offense while under the influence of drugs. Drug offenders (42%) and property offenders (37%) reported the highest incidence of drug use at the time of the offense.[6]

About 60% of mentally ill and 51% of other inmates in state prison were under the influence of alcohol or drugs at the time of their current offense.[7]

Abused state inmates were more likely than those reporting no abuse to have been using illegal drugs at the time of their offense. This pattern occurred especially among female inmates. Forty-six percent of the abused women committed their current offense under the influence of illegal drugs. Among women who were not abused, 32% committed their offense while on drugs.[8]

According to the 1997 Survey of Inmates in State and Federal Correctional Facilities, veterans in state prisons (26%) were less likely than nonveterans (34%) to have been under the influence of drugs while committing their offense. In federal prisons, about the same percentages of veterans (21%) and nonveterans (34%) reported drug use at the time of their offense.[9]

A third of the parents in state prison reported committing their current offense while under the influence of drugs. Parents were most likely to report the influence of cocaine-based drugs (16%) and marijuana (15%) while committing their crime. About equal percentages of parents in state prison reported the use of opiates (6%) and stimulates (5%) at the time of their offense, while 2% used depressants or hallucinogens.

Thirty-two percent of mothers in state prison reported committing their crime to get drugs or money for drugs, compared to 19% of fathers.[10]

Jail inmates. In 1998 an estimated 138,000 convicted jail inmates (36%) were under the influence of drugs at the time of the offense.[11]

In 1996, those jail inmates convicted of drug trafficking (60%), drug possession (57%), fraud (45%), or robbery (44%) were most likely to have reported to be using drugs at the time of the offense.[12]

According to the *Survey of Inmates in Local Jails, 1996,* more than half of prison of the jail inmates with an intimate victim had been drinking or using drugs when they committed the violent crime.[13]

Sixty-five percent of mentally ill jail inmates and 57% of other jail inmates were under the influence of both alcohol and drug use at the time of the offense. These percentages were the highest compared to state inmates and probationers.[14]

Based on data from the 1996 *Survey of Inmates in Local Jails*, 29% of veterans and 32% of nonveterans in local jails were under the influence of drugs at the time of offense.[15]

Drug Use at Arrest

The Arrestee Drug Abuse Monitoring (ADAM) program collects data from adult arrestees in 38 sites across the country. In most sites, a half or more of the adult arrestees tested positive for at least one drug.

In 2000 the ADAM program reported that adult male arrestees tested positive for at least one drug almost as often as adult female arrestees. In 35 of the 38 ADAM sites, 64% of male arrestees tested positive; compared to 63% of female arrestees in 29 of the sites.

Marijuana. In 2000 men were generally more likely than women to test positive for marijuana.

For adult arrestees testing positive for marijuana use ranged from:

- 57% in Oklahoma City to 29% in Laredo for males.
- 45% in Oklahoma City to 17% in Laredo for females.

A comparison between 1999 and 2000 results indicated that marijuana-positive percentages relatively remained the same in most of the sites.

Cocaine. In 2000 women were more likely than men to test positive for cocaine.

For adult arrestees testing positive for cocaine use ranged from:

- 49% in Atlanta and New York to 11% in Des Moines for males.
- 59% in Chicago to 8% in San Jose for females.

A comparison between 1999 and 2000 results indicated that cocaine-positive percentages increased in most of the sites.

Methamphetamine. In 2000 methamphetamine use was more likely in the Western region, and more prevalent for women than men.

For adult arrestees testing positive for methamphetamine use ranged from:

- 36% in Honolulu to 11% in Oklahoma City and Omaha for males.
- 47% in Honolulu to 21% in Las Vegas for females.

In comparison between 1999 and 2000 results indicated that methamphetamine-positive percentages increased some in most of the sites.

Juvenile detainees. Data were collected from more than 2,000 juvenile male arrestees in 9 sites, and more than 400 juvenile female arrestees in 8 sites. In most sites, half or more of juvenile arrestees tested positive for at least one drug. Juvenile arrestees interviewed by ADAM ranged from ages 12 to 18. In 2000, the largest proportion was between ages 15 and 17. Among those who tested positive for use of any drug, the largest group was age 17. In half the sites, 70% of more of the juvenile detainees said they were still in school, with the range 55% in Phoenix to 93% in San Antonio.

- Marijuana was the leading drug use among juveniles.
- Cocaine came in a distant second; the percentages testing positive for methamphetamine were also low.[16]

Prior Drug Use by Offenders

Probationers

In 1995 the first national survey of adults on probation reported:

- nearly 70% of probationers reported past drug use
- 32% said they were using illegal drugs in the month before their offense.

Marijuana (10%) was the most commonly used drug among probationers at the time of the offense.

In 1995 adults age 44 years old or younger on probation (87% of all probationers) reported similar levels of prior drug abuse, and their incidence of drug use was consistently higher than that of older probationers. Over 70% of probationers under age 45 reported some prior drug use, compared to 37% of those age 45 or older. Thirty-five percent of probationers under age 45—but 9% of older probationers—reported drug use in the month before their offense.[17]

Two-thirds of Driving While Intoxicated (DWI) offenders on probation reported using drugs in the past. Among DWI probationers, marijuana (65%) and stimulants (29%) were the most commonly used drugs. Seventeen percent of those on probation reported drug use in the month prior to arrest.

Among DWI offenders, the most commonly reported experience associated with drug use was domestic disputes:

- 19% of probationers said they had arguments with their family, friends, spouse, or boyfriend/girlfriend while under the influence of drugs.

- About 1 in 10 of those on probation for DWI had been arrested or held in a police station as a result of their drug use.

- 3% of those on probation had lost a job because of their drug use.

- 8% of those on probation said they had been in a physical fight while under the influence of drugs.[18]

Table 5.5. Prior Drug Use of Adults on Probation at the Time of Offense, by Type of Drugs, 1995.

Type of drug	Percent of adults on probation who were under the influence of drugs at the time of offense
Any drug	14%
Marijuana/hashish	10
Cocaine/crack	4
Heroin and other opiates	1
Barbiturates	1
Stimulants	2
Hallucinogens	1

Note: Excludes 11,712 probationers for whom information on drug use was not provided.

Source: BJS, *Substance Abuse and Treatment of Adults on Probation, 1995*, NCJ 166611, March 1998.

Nearly 40% of mentally ill probationers and 30% of other probationers reported using drugs in the month before their offense.[19]

Jail Inmates

Of those inmates held in local jails, only convicted offenders were asked if they had used drugs in the time leading up to their current offense. In 1996, 55% of convicted jail inmates reported they had used illegal drugs during the month before their offense, up from 44% in 1989. Use of marijuana in the month before the offense increased from 28% to 37% and of stimulants from 5% to 10%. Reported cocaine or crack use was stable at about 24%.

Half of inmates in both 1989 and 1996 reported trying cocaine. Overall, 82% of all jail inmates in 1996 said they had ever used an

Table 5.6. Prior Drug Use Reported by Probationers.

| | Percent of probationers | |
Level of prior drug use	DWI offenders	Other offenders
Ever used drugs/a	67.9%	69.9%
Marijuana/hashish	64.6	67.2
Cocaine/crack	28.1	31.7
Heroin/opiates	5.7	8.8
Depressants/b	14.6	15.6
Stimulants/c	28.5	24.4
Hallucinogens/d	19.9	19.6
Ever used drugs regularly/e	55.6%	64.2%
Used drugs in month before arrest	16.6%	35.7%
Used drugs at time of arrest	3.3%	16.1%

a/Other unspecified drugs are included in the totals
b/Includes barbiturates, tranquilizers, and Quaaludes
c/Includes amphetamines and methamphetamines
d/Includes LSD and PCP
e/Used drugs at least once a week for at least a month

Source: BJS, *DWI Offenders under Correctional Supervision*, NCJ 172212, June 1999.

Table 5.7. Prior Drug Use of Jail Inmates, by Type of Drug, 1996 and 1989.

Type of drug	Ever used drugs		Ever used drugs regularly/a		Used drugs in the month before the offense		Used drugs at the time of the offense	
	1996	1989	1996	1989	1996	1989	1996	1989
Any drug	82.4%	77.7%	64.2%	58.0%	55.0%	43.8%	35.6%	27.0%
Marijuana	78.2	70.7	54.9	47.8	36.8	28.0	18.5	9.0
Cocaine or crack	50.4	50.4	31.0	30.7	24.1	23.5	15.2	13.7
Heroin or opiates	23.9	18.6	11.8	11.8	8.8	7.2	5.6	4.9
Depressants/c	29.9	21.1	10.4	9.0	5.9	3.9	2.4	1.2
Stimulants/d	33.6	22.1	16.5	12.1	10.4	5.4	6.1	2.2
Hallucinogens/e	32.2	23.7	10.5	9.4	4.6	3.2	1.6	1.6
Inhalants	16.8	—	4.8	—	1.0	—	0.3	—

Note: Detail add to more than total because inmates may have used more than one drug.

—Not reported

a/Used drugs at least once week for a month

b/Other unspecified drugs are included in the totals

c/Includes barbiturates, tranquilizers, and Quaaludes

d/Includes amphetamines and methamphetamines

e/Includes LSD and PCP

Source: BJS, *Profile of Jail Inmates, 1996*, NCJ 164620, April 1998.

illegal drug, up from 78% in 1989. A higher percentage of jail inmates in 1996 than in 1989 reported ever using for every other type of drug:

- marijuana rose from 71% to 78%;

- stimulants (amphetamine and methamphetamine) from 22% to 34%;

- hallucinogens, including LSD and PCP, from 24% to 32%;

- depressants, including Quaalude, barbiturates, and tranquilizers without a doctor's prescription, from 21% to 30%; and

- heroin or other opiates from 19% to 24%.[20]

Over three-quarters of DWI offenders in jail reported using drugs in the past. Among jail inmates held for DWI, marijuana (73%) and cocaine-based drugs including crack (41%) were the most commonly used drugs. Thirty percent of those in jail reported drug use in the month prior to arrest.

Domestic disputes were also one of the most commonly reported experiences associated with drug use:

- 25% of jail inmates said they had arguments with their family, friends, spouse, or boyfriend/girlfriend while under the influence of drugs.

- Nearly 1 in 5 of those in jail for DWI had been arrested or held in a police station as a result of their drug use.

- About 10% of DWI offenders in jail had lost a job because of their drug use.

- About 15% of jail inmates said they had been in a physical fight while under the influence of drugs.[21]

Fifty-eight percent of mentally ill jail inmates and 47% of other jail inmates were using drugs in the month before the offense.[22]

In local jails, veterans (81%) reported levels of prior drug use similar to nonveterans (83%), but lower levels (44%) of drug use in the month prior to the offense than nonveterans (50%) in 1997.[23]

State and Federal Prison Inmates

In the 1997 Survey of Inmates in State and Federal Correctional Facilities, over 570,000 of the nation's prisoners (51%) reported the use of alcohol or drugs while committing their offense.

61

In 1991, 60% of federal prisoners reported prior drug use, compared to 79% of state prisoners. In 1997 this gap in prior drug use was narrowed, as the percentage of federal inmates reporting past drug use rose to 73%, compared to 83% of state inmates. This increase was mostly due to a rise in the percentage of federal prisoners reporting prior use of marijuana (from 53% in 1991 to 65% in 1997) and cocaine-based drugs (from 37% in 1991 to 45% in 1997).

Most other drug types showed modest increases over this period. A fifth of federal prisoners had used stimulants and hallucinogens, followed by depressants and opiates, including heroin (both 16%). About 1 in 12 federal prisoners reported the prior use of inhalants.

Although the proportion of federal prisoners held for drug offenses rose from 58% in 1991 to 63% in 1997, the percentage of all federal inmates who reported using drugs in the month before the offense rose more dramatically from 32% to 45%.

The proportion of state prison inmates reporting the past use of cocaine or crack remained stable between 1991 and 1997:

- Marijuana (77%) use had increased slightly since 1991 (74%), and remained the most commonly used drug.

- Past use of cocaine-based drugs remained unchanged at 49% since 1991.

Table 5.8. Drug Use by State Prisoners, 1997 and 1991.

Percent of inmates who had ever used drugs

Type of drug	1997	1991
Any drug	83%	79%
Marijuana	77	74
Cocaine/crack	49	49
Heroin/opiates	24	25
Depressants	24	24
Stimulants	28	30
Hallucinogens	29	27

Source: BJS, *Substance Abuse and Treatment, State and Federal Prisoners, 1997*, NCJ 172871, January 1999.

- Twenty percent of all inmates reported the past use of intravenous drugs, down from 25% in 1991.

Nineteen percent of state inmates told interviewers that they had been physically or sexually abused before their current offense. For state prisoners reporting prior abuse, 89% had ever used illegal drugs: 76% of the men and 80% of the women had used them regularly. Of those not reporting prior abuse, 82% had used illegal drugs: 68% of the men and 65% of the women had used them regularly.

Illegal drug use was more common among abused state prison inmates than among those who said they were not abused. An estimated 76% of abused men and 80% of abused women had used illegal drugs regularly, compared to 68% of men and 65% of women who had not been abused.

Table 5.9. Current and Past Violent Offenses and Past Drug Use, by Whether Abused before Admission to State Prison, 1997.

Percent of State Prison Inmates

Offense history and drug use	Reported being abused			Reported being not abused		
	Total	Males	Females	Total	Males	Females
Current or past violent offense	70.4%	76.5%	45.0%	60.2%	61.2%	29.1%
Used an illegal drug						
Ever	88.6%	88.5%	88.9%	81.8%	81.9%	77.4%
Ever regularly	76.3	75.5	79.7	67.9	67.9	65.0
In month before offense	61.4	59.7	68.6	55.3	55.3	54.0
At time of offense	39.6	38.0	46.2	30.7	30.7	32.0

Source: BJS, *Prior Abuse Reported by Inmates and Probationers*, NCJ 172879, April 1999.

About 60% of mentally ill state prisoners and 56% of other inmates were using drugs in the month before their offense.[24]

In 1997 a majority of parents in state prison reported some type of prior drug use:

- 85% reported any past drug use
- 58% reported use in the month before the current offense.

Nonparents in state prison reported slightly lower levels of prior drug use:

- 80% reported any past drug use
- 55% reported use in the month before the current offense.

In 1997 mothers in state prison were more likely than fathers to report drug use in the month before their offense: 65% for mothers and 58% for fathers. Cocaine/crack was the most common drug used: 45% for mothers and 26% for fathers.

Table 5.10. Percent of Parents in State Prison Who Used Drugs in the Month Before the Current Offense, 1997.

Marijuana	39%
Cocaine/crack	27
Heroin/opiates	10
Stimulates	9
Depressants	5
Hallucinogens	3
Inhalants	1

Table 5.11. Prior Drug Use of Veterans in State Prison, 1997.

	Percent of veterans who reported prior drug use	
Drug use	Combat	Noncombat
Any prior drug use	69%	82%
In the month before	30	49
Prior use of intravenous drugs	23	25

Nearly half of parents in federal prison reported using drugs in the month before their offense and 3 in 4 had ever used drugs. Nearly a quarter of parents in federal prison were under the influence of drugs when committing their offense. Aside from marijuana use (higher among fathers), mothers and fathers in federal prison reported similar drug use histories.[25]

Seventy-nine percent of veterans in state prison reported prior drug use during their military service.

Vietnam-era veterans varied little from other veterans in state prison concerning prior drug abuse:

- 77% of Vietnam-era veterans compared to 80% of other veterans reported ever using drugs.

- 41% of Vietnam-era veterans compared to 47% of other veterans used drugs in the month before the offense.[26]

Notes

1. BJS, *Drug Use, Testing, and Treatment in Jails*, 1998, NCJ 179999, May 2000.

2. BJS, *Substance Abuse and Treatment, State and Federal Prisoners*, 1997, NCJ 172871, January 1999.

3. BJS, *Violence in the Workplace*, 1993–99, NCJ 190076, December 2001.

4. BJS, *Substance Abuse and Treatment of Adults on Probation*, 1995, NCJ 166611, March 1998.

5. BJS, *Mental Health and Treatment and Inmates and Probationers*, NCJ 174463, July 1999.

6. BJS, *Substance Abuse and Treatment, State and Federal Prisoners*, 1997, NCJ 172871, January 1999.

7. BJS, *Mental Health and Treatment and Inmates and Probationers*, NCJ 174463, July 1999.

8. BJS, *Prior Abuse Reported by Inmates and Probationers*, NCJ 172879, April 1999.

9. BJS, *Veterans in Prison or Jail*, NCJ 178888, January 2000.

10. BJS, *Incarcerated Parents and Their Children*, NCJ 182335, August 2000.

11. BJS, *Drug Use, Testing, and Treatment in Jails*, NCJ 179999, May 2000.

12. BJS, *Profile of Jail Inmates*, 1996, NCJ 164620, April 1998.

13. BJS, *Violence by Intimates*, NCJ 167237, March 1998.

14. BJS, *Mental Health and Treatment of Inmates and Probationers*, NCJ 174463, July 1999.

15. BJS, *Veterans in Prison or Jail*, NCJ 178888, January 2000.

16. *2000 Annual Report on Drug Use Among Adult and Juvenile Arrestees, Arrestees Drug Abuse Monitoring Program (ADAM)*, National Institute of Justice, NCJ 193013, April 2003.

17. BJS, *Substance Abuse and Treatment of Adults on Probation*, 1995, NCJ 166611, March 1998.

18. BJS, *DWI Offenders under Correctional Supervision*, NCJ 172212, June 1999.

19. BJS, *Mental Health and Treatment and Inmates and Probationers*, NCJ 174463, July 1999.

20. BJS, *Profile of Jail Inmates*, 1996, NCJ 164620, April 1998.

21. BJS, *DWI Offenders under Correctional Supervision*, NCJ 172212, June 1999.

22. BJS, *Mental Health and Treatment and Inmates and Probationers*, NCJ 174463, July 1999.

23. BJS, *Veterans in Prison or Jail*, NCJ 178888, January 2000.

24. BJS, *Mental Health and Treatment and Inmates and Probationers*, NCJ 174463, July 1999.

25. BJS, *Incarcerated Parents and Their Children*, NCJ 182335, August 2000.

26. BJS, *Veterans in Prison or Jail*, NCJ 178888, January 2000.

Chapter 6

The Controlled Substances Act

The Controlled Substances Act (CSA), Title II of the Comprehensive Drug Abuse Prevention and Control Act of 1970, is the legal foundation of the government's fight against abuse of drugs and other substances. This law is a consolidation of numerous laws regulating the manufacture and distribution of narcotics, stimulants, depressants, hallucinogens, anabolic steroids, and chemicals used in the illicit production of controlled substances.

Controlling Drugs or Other Substances

Formal Scheduling

The CSA places all substances which were in some manner regulated under existing Federal law into one of five schedules. This placement is based upon the substance's medical use, potential for abuse, and safety or dependence liability. The Act also provides a mechanism for substances to be controlled, or added to a schedule; decontrolled, or removed from control; and rescheduled or transferred from one schedule to another. The procedure for these actions is found in Section 201 of the Act (21 U.S.C. 811).

Proceedings to add, delete, or change the schedule of a drug or other substance may be initiated by the Drug Enforcement Administration

Excerpted from *Drugs of Abuse*, U.S. Department of Justice, Drug Enforcement Administration (DEA), 1997. According to DEA, this information is still current as of 2004.

(DEA), the Department of Health and Human Services (HHS), or by petition from any interested party: the manufacturer of a drug, a medical society or association, a pharmacy association, a public interest group concerned with drug abuse, a state or local government agency, or an individual citizen. When a petition is received by DEA, the agency begins its own investigation of the drug.

The agency also may begin an investigation of a drug at any time based upon information received from law enforcement laboratories, state and local law enforcement and regulatory agencies, or other sources of information.

Once DEA has collected the necessary data, the Administrator of DEA, by authority of the Attorney General, requests from HHS a scientific and medical evaluation and recommendation as to whether the drug or other substance should be controlled or removed from control. This request is sent to the Assistant Secretary of Health of HHS. HHS solicits information from the Commissioner of the Food and Drug Administration (FDA), evaluations and recommendations from the National Institute on Drug Abuse, and on occasion from the scientific and medical community at large. The Assistant Secretary, by authority of the Secretary, compiles the information and transmits back to DEA a medical and scientific evaluation regarding the drug or other substance, a recommendation as to whether the drug should be controlled, and in what schedule it should be placed.

The medical and scientific evaluations are binding on DEA with respect to scientific and medical matters. The recommendation on scheduling is binding only to the extent that if HHS recommends that the substance not be controlled, DEA may not control the substance.

Once DEA has received the scientific and medical evaluation from HHS, the Administrator will evaluate all available data and make a final decision whether to propose that a drug or other substance should be controlled and into which schedule it should be placed.

The threshold issue is whether the drug or other substance has potential for abuse. If a drug does not have a potential for abuse, it cannot be controlled. Although the term "potential for abuse" is not defined in the CSA, there is much discussion of the term in the legislative history of the Act. The following items are indicators that a drug or other substance has a potential for abuse:

1. There is evidence that individuals are taking the drug or other substance in amounts sufficient to create a hazard to their health or to the safety of other individuals or to the community; or

2. There is significant diversion of the drug or other substance from legitimate drug channels; or

3. Individuals are taking the drug or other substance on their own initiative rather than on the basis of medical advice from a practitioner licensed by law to administer such drugs; or

4. The drug is a new drug so related in its action to a drug or other substance already listed as having a potential for abuse to make it likely that the drug will have the same potential for abuse as such drugs, thus making it reasonable to assume that there may be significant diversions from legitimate channels, significant use contrary to or without medical advice, or that it has a substantial capability of creating hazards to the health of the user or to the safety of the community. Of course, evidence of actual abuse of a substance is indicative that a drug has a potential for abuse.

In determining into which schedule a drug or other substance should be placed, or whether a substance should be decontrolled or rescheduled, certain factors are required to be considered. Specific findings are not required for each factor. These factors are listed in Section 201 (c), [21 U.S.C. 811 (c)], of the CSA and are as follows:

1. The drug's actual or relative potential for abuse.

2. Scientific evidence of the drug's pharmacological effects. The state of knowledge with respect to the effects of a specific drug is, of course, a major consideration. For example, it is vital to know whether or not a drug has a hallucinogenic effect if it is to be controlled because of that. The best available knowledge of the pharmacological properties of a drug should be considered.

3. The state of current scientific knowledge regarding the substance. Criteria (2) and (3) are closely related. However, (2) is primarily concerned with pharmacological effects and (3) deals with all scientific knowledge with respect to the substance.

4. Its history and current pattern of abuse. To determine whether or not a drug should be controlled, it is important to know the pattern of abuse of that substance, including the socioeconomic characteristics of the segments of the population involved in such abuse.

5. The scope, duration, and significance of abuse. In evaluating existing abuse, the Administrator must know not only the pattern of abuse but whether the abuse is widespread. In reaching his decision, the Administrator should consider the economics of regulation and enforcement attendant to such a decision. In addition, he should be aware of the social significance and impact of such a decision upon those people, especially the young, that would be affected by it.

6. What, if any, risk there is to the public health. If a drug creates dangers to the public health, in addition to or because of its abuse potential, then these dangers must also be considered by the Administrator.

7. The drug's psychic or physiological dependence liability. There must be an assessment of the extent to which a drug is physically addictive or psychologically habit-forming, if such information is known.

8. Whether the substance is an immediate precursor of a substance already controlled. The CSA allows inclusion of immediate precursors on this basis alone into the appropriate schedule and thus safeguards against possibilities of clandestine manufacture.

After considering the above listed factors, the Administrator must make specific findings concerning the drug or other substance. This will determine into which schedule the drug or other substance will be placed. These schedules are established by the CSA. They are as follows:

Schedule I

- The drug or other substance has a high potential for abuse.

- The drug or other substance has no currently accepted medical use in treatment in the United States.

- There is a lack of accepted safety for use of the drug or other substance under medical supervision.

- Some Schedule I substances are heroin, LSD, marijuana, and methaqualone.

Schedule II

- The drug or other substance has a high potential for abuse.

- The drug or other substance has a currently accepted medical use in treatment in the United States or a currently accepted medical use with severe restrictions.

- Abuse of the drug or other substance may lead to severe psychological or physical dependence.

- Schedule II substances include morphine, PCP, cocaine, methadone, and methamphetamine.

Schedule III

- The drug or other substance has a potential for abuse less than the drugs or other substances in Schedules I and II.

- The drug or other substance has a currently accepted medical use in treatment in the United States.

- Abuse of the drug or other substance may lead to moderate or low physical dependence or high psychological dependence.

- Anabolic steroids, codeine, and hydrocodone with aspirin or Tylenol®, and some barbiturates are Schedule III substances.

Schedule IV

- The drug or other substance has a low potential for abuse relative to the drugs or other substances in Schedule III.

- The drug or other substance has a currently accepted medical use in treatment in the United States.

- Abuse of the drug or other substance may lead to limited physical dependence or psychological dependence relative to the drugs or other substances in Schedule III.

- Included in Schedule IV are Darvon®, Talwin®, Equanil®, Valium® and Xanax®.

Schedule V

- The drug or other substance has a low potential for abuse relative to the drugs or other substances in Schedule IV.

- The drug or other substance has a currently accepted medical use in treatment in the United States.

71

- Abuse of the drug or other substances may lead to limited physical dependence or psychological dependence relative to the drugs or other substances in Schedule IV.

- Over-the-counter cough medicines with codeine are classified in Schedule V.

When the Administrator of DEA has determined that a drug or other substance should be controlled, decontrolled, or rescheduled, a proposal to take action is published in the *Federal Register*. The proposal invites all interested persons to file comments with DEA. Affected parties may also request a hearing with DEA. If no hearing is requested, DEA will evaluate all comments received and publish a final order in the *Federal Register*, controlling the drug as proposed or with modifications based upon the written comments filed. This order will set the effective dates for imposing the various requirements imposed under the CSA.

If a hearing is requested, DEA will enter into discussions with the party or parties requesting a hearing in an attempt to narrow the issue for litigation. If necessary, a hearing will then be held before an Administrative Law Judge. The judge will take evidence on factual issues and hear arguments on legal questions regarding the control of the drug. Depending on the scope and complexity of the issues, the hearing may be brief or quite extensive. The Administrative Law Judge, at the close of the hearing, prepares findings of fact and conclusions of law and a recommended decision which is submitted to the Administrator of DEA. The Administrator will review these documents, as well as the underlying material, and prepare his/her own findings of fact and conclusions of law (which may or may not be the same as those drafted by the Administrative Law Judge). The Administrator then publishes a final order in the *Federal Register* either scheduling the drug or other substance or declining to do so.

Once the final order is published in the Federal Register, interested parties have 30 days to appeal to a U.S. Court of Appeals to challenge the order. Findings of fact by the Administrator are deemed conclusive if supported by "substantial evidence." The order imposing controls is not stayed during the appeal, however, unless so ordered by the Court.

Emergency or Temporary Scheduling

The CSA was amended by the Comprehensive Crime Control Act of 1984. This Act included a provision which allows the Administrator of DEA to place a substance, on a temporary basis, into Schedule I when necessary to avoid an imminent hazard to the public safety.

This emergency scheduling authority permits the scheduling of a substance which is not currently controlled, is being abused, and is a risk to the public health while the formal rule making procedures described in the CSA are being conducted. This emergency scheduling applies only to substances with no accepted medical use. A temporary scheduling order may be issued for one year with a possible extension of up to six months if formal scheduling procedures have been initiated. The proposal and order are published in the *Federal Register* as are the proposals and orders for formal scheduling. [21 U.S.C. 811 (1)]

Controlled Substance Analogues

A new class of substances was created by the Anti-Drug Abuse Act of 1986. Controlled substance analogues are substances which are not controlled substances, but may be found in the illicit traffic. They are structurally or pharmacologically similar to Schedule I or II controlled substances and have no legitimate medical use. A substance which meets the definition of a controlled substance analogue and is intended for human consumption is treated under the CSA as if it were a controlled substance in Schedule I.

International Treaty Obligations

U. S. treaty obligations may require that a drug or other substance be controlled under the CSA, or rescheduled if existing controls are less stringent than those required by a treaty. The procedures for these scheduling actions are found in Section 201 (d) of the Act. [21 U.S.C. 811 (d)]

The United States is a party to the Single Convention on Narcotic Drugs of 1961, designed to establish effective control over international and domestic traffic in narcotics, coca leaf, cocaine, and cannabis. A second treaty, the Convention on Psychotropic Substances of 1971, which entered into force in 1976, is designed to establish comparable control over stimulants, depressants, and hallucinogens. Congress ratified this treaty in 1980.

Regulation

The CSA creates a closed system of distribution for those authorized to handle controlled substances. The cornerstone of this system is the registration of all those authorized by DEA to handle controlled substances. All individuals and firms that are registered are required to maintain complete and accurate inventories and records of all transactions involving controlled substances, as well as security for the storage of controlled substances.

Registration

Any person who handles or intends to handle controlled substances must obtain a registration issued by DEA. A unique number is assigned to each legitimate handler of controlled drugs: importer, exporter, manufacturer, distributor, hospital, pharmacy, practitioner, and researcher. This number must be made available to the supplier by the customer prior to the purchase of a controlled substance. Thus, the opportunity for unauthorized transactions is greatly diminished.

Recordkeeping

The CSA requires that complete and accurate records be kept of all quantities of controlled substances manufactured, purchased, and sold. Each substance must be inventoried every two years. Some limited exceptions to the recordkeeping requirements may apply to certain categories of registrants.

From these records it is possible to trace the flow of any drug from the time it is first imported or manufactured through the distribution level, to the pharmacy or hospital that dispensed it, and then to the actual patient who received the drug. The mere existence of this requirement is sufficient to discourage many forms of diversion. It actually serves large drug corporations as an internal check to uncover diversion, such as pilferage by employees.

There is one distinction between scheduled items for recordkeeping requirements. Records for Schedule I and II drugs must be kept separate from all other records of the handler; records for Schedule III, IV, and V substances must be kept in a "readily retrievable" form. The former method allows for more expeditious investigations involving the highly abusable substances in Schedules I and II.

Distribution

The keeping of records is required for distribution of a controlled substance from one manufacturer to another, from manufacturer to distributor, and from distributor to dispenser. In the case of Schedule I and II drugs, the supplier must have a special order form from the customer. This order form (DEA Form 222) is issued by DEA only to persons who are properly registered to handle Schedules I and II. The form is preprinted with the name and address of the customer. The drugs must be shipped to this name and address. The use of this device is a special reinforcement of the registration requirement; it makes doubly certain that only authorized individuals may obtain Schedule I and II drugs. Another benefit of the form is the special monitoring it permits. The form is issued in triplicate: the customer keeps one copy; two copies go to the supplier who, after filling the order, keeps a copy and forwards the third copy to the nearest DEA office.

For drugs in Schedules III, IV, and V, no order form is necessary. The supplier in each case, however, is under an obligation to verify the authenticity of the customer. The supplier is held fully accountable for any drugs which are shipped to a purchaser who does not have a valid registration.

Manufacturers must submit periodic reports of the Schedule I and II controlled substances they produce in bulk and dosage forms. They also report the manufactured quantity and form of each narcotic substance listed in Schedules III, IV, and V, as well as the quantity of synthesized psychotropic substances listed in Schedules I, II, III, and IV. Distributors of controlled substances must report the quantity and form of all their transactions of controlled drugs listed in Schedules I and II and narcotics listed in Schedule III. Both manufacturers and distributors are required to provide reports of their annual inventories of these controlled substances. This data is entered into a system called the Automated Reports and Consolidated Orders System (ARCOS). It enables DEA to monitor the distribution of controlled substances throughout the country, and to identify retail level registrants that receive unusual quantities of controlled substances.

Dispensing to Patients

The dispensing of a controlled substance is the delivery of the controlled substance to the ultimate user, who may be a patient or research subject. Special control mechanisms operate here as well. Schedule I drugs are those which have no currently accepted medical use in the United States; they may, therefore, be used in the United States only in research situations. They generally are supplied by only a limited number of firms to properly registered and qualified researchers. Controlled substances may be dispensed by a practitioner by direct administration, by prescription, or by dispensing from office supplies. Records must be maintained by the practitioner of all dispensing of controlled substances from office supplies and of certain administrations. The CSA does not require the practitioner to maintain copies of prescriptions, but certain states require the use of multiple copy prescriptions for Schedule II and other specified controlled substances.

The determination to place drugs on prescription is within the jurisdiction of the FDA. Unlike other prescription drugs, however, controlled substances are subject to additional restrictions. Schedule II prescription orders must be written and signed by the practitioner; they may not be telephoned into the pharmacy except in an emergency. In addition, a prescription for a Schedule II drug may not be refilled; the patient must see the practitioner again in order to obtain more drugs. For Schedule III and IV drugs, the prescription order may be either written or oral (that is, by telephone to the pharmacy). In addition, the patient may (if authorized by the practitioner) have the prescription refilled up to five times and at anytime within six months from the date of the initial dispensing.

Schedule V includes some prescription drugs and many over-the-counter narcotic preparations, including antitussives and antidiarrheals. Even here, however, the law imposes restrictions beyond those normally required for the over-the-counter sales; for example, the patient must be at least 18 years of age, must offer some form of identification, and have his or her name entered into a special log maintained by the pharmacist as part of a special record.

Quotas

DEA limits the quantity of Schedule I and II controlled substances which may be produced in the United States in any given calendar year. By utilizing available data on sales and inventories of these controlled substances, and taking into account estimates of drug usage provided by the FDA, DEA establishes annual aggregate production quotas for Schedule I and II controlled substances. The aggregate production quota is allocated among the various manufacturers who are registered to manufacture the specific drug. DEA also allocates the amount of bulk drug which may be procured by those companies which prepare the drug into dosage units.

Security

DEA registrants are required by regulation to maintain certain security for the storage and distribution of controlled substances. Manufacturers and distributors of Schedule I and II substances must store controlled substances in specially constructed vaults or highly rated safes, and maintain electronic security for all storage areas. Lesser physical security requirements apply to retail level registrants such as hospitals and pharmacies.

All registrants are required to make every effort to ensure that controlled substances in their possession are not diverted into the illicit market. This requires operational as well as physical security. For example, registrants are responsible for ensuring that controlled substances are distributed only to other registrants that are authorized to receive them, or to legitimate patients and consumers.

Penalties

The CSA provides penalties for unlawful manufacturing, distribution, and dispensing of controlled substances. The penalties are basically determined by the schedule of the drug or other substance, and sometimes are specified by drug name, as in the case of marijuana. As the statute has been amended since its initial passage in 1970, the penalties have been altered by Congress.

User Accountability/Personal Use Penalties

On November 19, 1988, Congress passed the Anti-Drug Abuse Act of 1988, P. L. 100690. Two sections of this Act represent the Federal Government's attempt to reduce drug abuse by dealing not just with the person who sells the illegal drug, but also with the person who buys it. The first new section is titled "User Accountability" and is codified at 21 U.S.C. § 862 and various sections of Title 42, U.S.C. The second involves "personal use amounts" of illegal drugs, and is codified at 21 U.S.C. § 844a.

User Accountability

The purpose of User Accountability is to not only make the public aware of the Federal Government's position on drug abuse, but to describe new programs intended to decrease drug abuse by holding drug abusers personally responsible for their illegal activities, and imposing civil penalties on those who violate drug laws.

It is important to remember that these penalties are in addition to the criminal penalties drug abusers are already given, and do not replace those criminal penalties.

The new User Accountability programs call for more instruction in schools, kindergarten through senior high, to educate children on the dangers of drug abuse. These programs will include participation by students, parents, teachers, local businesses and the local, state and Federal Government.

User Accountability also targets businesses interested in doing business with the Federal Government. This program requires those businesses to maintain a drug-free workplace, principally through educating employees on the dangers of drug abuse, and by informing employees of the penalties they face if they engage in illegal drug activity on company property.

There is also a provision in the law that makes public housing projects drug-free by evicting those residents who allow their units to be used for illegal drug activity, and denies Federal benefits, such as housing assistance and student loans, to individuals convicted of illegal drug activity. Depending on the offense, an individual may be prohibited from ever receiving any benefit provided by the Federal Government.

Personal Use Amounts

This section of the 1988 Act allows the government to punish minor drug offenders without giving the offender a criminal record if the offender is in possession of only a small amount of drugs. This law is designed to impact the "user" of illicit drugs, while simultaneously saving the government the costs of a full-blown criminal investigation. Under this section, the government has the option of imposing only a civil fine on individuals possessing only a small quantity of an illegal drug. Possession of this small quantity, identified as a "personal use amount" carries a civil fine of up to $10,000.

In determining the amount of the fine in a particular case, the drug offender's income and assets will be considered. This is accomplished through an administrative proceeding rather than a criminal trial, thus reducing the exposure of the offender to the entire criminal justice system, and reducing the costs to the offender and the government.

The value of this section is that it allows the government to punish a minor drug offender without saddling the offender with a criminal record. This section also gives the drug offender the opportunity to fully redeem himself or herself, and have all public record of the proceeding destroyed. If this was the drug offender's first offense, and the offender has paid all fines, can pass a drug test, and has not been convicted of a crime after three years, the offender can request that all proceedings be dismissed.

If the proceeding is dismissed, the drug offender can lawfully say he or she had never been prosecuted, either criminally or civilly, for a drug offense.

Congress has imposed two limitations on this section's use. It may not be used if (1) the drug offender has been previously convicted of a Federal or state drug offense; or (2) the offender has already been fined twice under this section.

Chapter 7

Speaking Out against Drug Legalization

Fact 1: We have made significant progress in fighting drug use and drug trafficking in America. Now is not the time to abandon our efforts.

Demand Reduction

- Legalization advocates claim that the fight against drugs has not been won and is, in fact, unconquerable. They frequently state that people still take drugs, drugs are widely available, and that efforts to change this are futile. They contend that legalization is the only workable alternative.

- The facts are to the contrary to such pessimism. On the demand side, the United States has reduced casual use, chronic use and addiction, and prevented others from even starting using drugs. Overall drug use in the United States is down by more than a third since the late 1970s. That's 9.5 million people fewer using illegal drugs. We've reduced cocaine use by an astounding 70% during the last 15 years. That's 4.1 million fewer people using cocaine.

- Almost two-thirds of teens say their schools are drug-free, according to a new survey of teen drug use conducted by The National Center on Addiction and Substance Abuse (CASA) at

U.S. Department of Justice, Drug Enforcement Administration (DEA), March 2003.

Columbia University. This is the first time in the seven-year history of the study that a majority of public school students report drug-free schools.

• The good news continues. According to the 2001–2002 PRIDE survey, student drug use has reached the lowest level in nine years. According to the author of the study, "following 9/11, Americans seemed to refocus on family, community, spirituality, and nation." These statistics show that U.S. efforts to educate kids about the dangers of drugs is making an impact. Like smoking cigarettes, drug use is gaining a stigma which is the best cure for this problem, as it was in the 1980s, when government, business, the media and other national institutions came together to do something about the growing problem of drugs and drug-related violence. This is a trend we should encourage—not send the opposite message of greater acceptance of drug use.

• The crack cocaine epidemic of the 1980s and early 1990s has diminished greatly in scope. And we've reduced the number of chronic heroin users over the last decade. In addition, the number of new marijuana users and cocaine users continues to steadily decrease.

• The number of new heroin users dropped from 156,000 in 1976 to 104,000 in 1999, a reduction of 33%.

• Of course, drug policy also has an impact on general crime. In a 2001 study, the British Home Office found violent crime and property crime increased in the late 1990s in every wealthy country except the United States. Our murder rate is too high, and we have much to learn from those with greater success—but this reduction is due in part to a reduction in drug use.

• There is still much progress to make. There are still far too many people using cocaine, heroin and other illegal drugs. In addition, there are emerging drug threats like ecstasy and methamphetamine. But the fact is that our current policies balancing prevention, enforcement, and treatment have kept drug usage outside the scope of acceptable behavior in the United States.

• To put things in perspective, less than 5% of the population uses illegal drugs of any kind. Think about that: More than 95% of Americans do not use drugs. How could anyone but the most hardened pessimist call this a losing struggle?

Supply Reduction

- There have been many successes on the supply side of the drug fight, as well. For example, Customs officials have made major seizures along the U.S.-Mexico border during a six-month period after September 11th, seizing almost twice as much as the same period in 2001. At one port in Texas, seizures of methamphetamine are up 425% and heroin by 172%. Enforcement makes a difference—traffickers' costs go up with these kinds of seizures.

- Purity levels of Colombian cocaine are declining too, according to an analysis of samples seized from traffickers and bought from street dealers in the United States. The purity has declined by 9%, from 86% in 1998, to 78% in 2001. There are a number of possible reasons for this decline in purity, including DEA supply reduction efforts in South America.

- One DEA program, Operation Purple, involves 28 countries and targets the illegal diversion of chemicals used in processing cocaine and other illicit drugs. DEA's labs have discovered that the oxidation levels for cocaine have been greatly reduced, suggesting that Operation Purple is having a detrimental impact on the production of cocaine.

- Another likely cause is that traffickers are diluting their cocaine to offset the higher costs associated with payoffs to insurgent and paramilitary groups in Colombia. The third possible cause is that cocaine traffickers simply don't have the product to simultaneously satisfy their market in the United States and their rapidly growing market in Europe. As a result, they are cutting the product to try to satisfy both.

- Whatever the final reasons for the decline in drug purity, it is good news for the American public. It means less potent and deadly drugs are hitting the streets, and dealers are making less profit—that is, unless they raise their own prices, which helps price more and more Americans out of the market.

- Purity levels have also been reduced on methamphetamine by controls on chemicals necessary for its manufacture. The average purity of seized methamphetamine samples dropped from 72% in 1994 to 40% in 2001.

- The trafficking organizations that sell drugs are finding that their profession has become a lot more costly. In the mid-1990s, the DEA helped dismantle Burma's Shan United Army, at the time the world's largest heroin trafficking organization, which in two years helped reduce the amount of Southeast Asian heroin in the United States from 63% of the market to 17% of the market. In the mid-1990s, the DEA helped disrupt the Cali cartel, which had been responsible for much of the world's cocaine.

- Progress does not come overnight. America has had a long, dark struggle with drugs. It's not a war we've been fighting for 20 years. We've been fighting it for 120 years. In 1880, many drugs, including opium and cocaine, were legal. We didn't know their harms, but we soon learned. We saw the highest level of drug use ever in our nation, per capita. There were over 400,000 opium addicts in our nation. That's twice as many per capita as there are today. And like today, we saw rising crime with that drug abuse. But we fought those problems by passing and enforcing tough laws and by educating the public about the dangers of these drugs. And this vigilance worked—by World War II, drug use was reduced to the very margins of society. And that's just where we want to keep it. With a 95% success rate—bolstered by an effective, three-pronged strategy combining education/prevention, enforcement, and treatment—we shouldn't give up now.

Fact 2: A balanced approach of prevention, enforcement, and treatment is the key in the fight against drugs.

- Over the years, some people have advocated a policy that focuses narrowly on controlling the supply of drugs. Others have said that society should rely on treatment alone. Still others say that prevention is the only viable solution. As the 2002 National Drug Strategy observes, "What the nation needs is an honest effort to integrate these strategies."

- Drug treatment courts are a good example of this new balanced approach to fighting drug abuse and addiction in this country. These courts are given a special responsibility to handle cases involving drug-addicted offenders through an extensive supervision and treatment program. Drug court programs use the varied experience and skills of a wide variety of law enforcement and treatment professionals: judges, prosecutors, defense counsels, substance abuse treatment specialists, probation officers, law enforcement and correctional personnel, educational and vocational experts, community leaders and others—all focused on one goal: to help cure addicts of their addiction, and to keep them cured.

- Drug treatment courts are working. Researchers estimate that more than 50% of defendants convicted of drug possession will return to criminal behavior within two to three years.

  Those who graduate from drug treatment courts have far lower rates of recidivism, ranging from 2% to 20%. That's very impressive when you consider that; for addicts who enter a treatment program voluntarily, 80% to 90% leave by the end of the first year. Among such dropouts, relapse within a year is generally the rule.

- What makes drug treatment courts so different? Graduates are held accountable for sticking with the program. Unlike other, purely voluntary treatment programs, the addict—who has a physical need for drugs—can't simply quit treatment whenever he or she feels like it.

- Law enforcement plays an important role in the drug treatment court program. It is especially important in the beginning of the process because it often triggers treatment for people who need it. Most people do not volunteer for drug treatment. It is more often an outside motivator, like an arrest, that gets—and keeps—people in treatment. And it is important for judges to keep people in incarceration if treatment fails.

- There are already more than 123,000 people who use heroin at least once a month, and 1.7 million who use cocaine at least once a month. For them, treatment is the answer. But for most Americans, particularly the young, the solution lies in prevention, which in turn is largely a matter of education and enforcement, which aims at keeping drug pushers away from children and teenagers.

- The role of strong drug enforcement has been analyzed by R. E. Peterson. He has broken down the past four decades into two periods. The first period, from 1960 to 1980, was an era of permissive drug laws. During this era, drug incarceration rates fell almost 80%. Drug use among teens, meanwhile, climbed by more than 500%. The second period, from 1980 to 1995, was an era of stronger drug laws. During this era, drug use by teens dropped by more than a third.

- Enforcement of our laws creates risks that discourage drug use. Charles Van Deventer, a young writer in Los Angeles, wrote about this phenomenon in an article in *Newsweek*. He said that from his experience as a casual user—and he believes his experience with illegal drugs is "by far the most common"—drugs aren't nearly as easy to buy as some critics would like people to believe.

  Being illegal, they are too expensive, their quality is too unpredictable, and their purchase entails too many risks. "The more barriers there are," he said, "be they the cops or the hassle or the fear of dying, the less likely you are to get addicted.... The road to addiction was just bumpy enough," he concluded, "that I chose not to go down it. In this sense, we are winning the war on drugs just by fighting them."

- The element of risk, created by strong drug enforcement policies, raises the price of drugs, and therefore lowers the demand. A research paper, *Marijuana and Youth*, funded by the Robert Wood Johnson Foundation, concludes that changes in the price of marijuana "contributed significantly to the trends in youth marijuana use between 1982 and 1998, particularly during the contraction in use from 1982 to 1992." That contraction was a product of many factors, including a concerted effort among federal agencies to disrupt domestic production and distribution; these factors contributed to a doubling of the street price of marijuana in the space of a year.

- The 2002 National Drug Control Strategy states that drug control policy has just two elements: modifying individual behavior to discourage and reduce drug use and addiction, and disrupting the market for illegal drugs. Those two elements call for a balanced approach to drug control, one that uses prevention, enforcement, and treatment in a coordinated policy. This is a simple strategy and an effective one. The enforcement side of the fight against drugs, then, is an integrated part of the overall strategy.

Fact 3: Illegal drugs are illegal because they are harmful.

- There is a growing misconception that some illegal drugs can be taken safely—with many advocates of legalization going so far as to suggest it can serve as medicine to heal anything from headaches to bipolar diseases. Today's drug dealers are savvy businessmen. They know how to market to kids. They imprint ecstasy pills with cartoon characters and designer logos. They promote parties as safe and alcohol-free. Meanwhile, the drugs can flow easier than water. Many young people believe the new "club drugs," such as ecstasy, are safe, and tablet testing at raves has only fueled this misconception.

- Because of the new marketing tactics of drug promoters, and because of a major decline in drug use in the 1990s, there is a growing perception among young people today that drugs are harmless. A decade ago, for example, 79% of 12th graders thought regular marijuana use was harmful; only 58% do so today. Because peer pressure is so important in inducing kids to experiment with drugs, the way kids perceive the risks of drug use is critical. There always have been, and there continues to be, real health risks in using illicit drugs.

- Drug use can be deadly, far more deadly than alcohol. Although alcohol is used by seven times as many people as drugs, the numbers of deaths induced by those substances are not far apart. According to the Centers for Disease Control and Prevention (CDC), during 2000, there were 15,852 drug-induced deaths; only slightly less than the 18,539 alcohol-induced deaths.

Ecstasy

- Ecstasy has rapidly become a favorite drug among young party goers in the United States and Europe, and it is now being used within the mainstream as well. According to the 2001 *National Household Survey on Drug Abuse*, ecstasy use tripled among Americans between 1998 and 2001. Many people believe, incorrectly, that this synthetic drug is safer than cocaine and heroin. In fact, the drug is addictive and can be deadly. The drug often results in severe dehydration and heat stroke in the user, since it has the effect of "short-circuiting" the body's temperature signals to the brain. Ecstasy can heat your body up to temperatures as high as 117 degrees. Ecstasy can cause hypothermia, muscle breakdown, seizures, stroke, kidney and cardiovascular system failure, as well as permanent brain damage during repetitive use, and sometimes death. The psychological effects of ecstasy include confusion, depression, anxiety, sleeplessness, drug craving, and paranoia.

- The misconception about the safety of club drugs, like ecstasy, is often fueled by some governments' attempts to reduce the harm

85

of mixing drugs. Some foreign governments and private organizations in the United States have established ecstasy testing at rave parties. Once the drug is tested, it is returned to the partygoers. This process leads partygoers to believe that the government has declared their pill safe to consume. But the danger of ecstasy is the drug itself—not simply its purity level.

Cocaine

- Cocaine is a powerfully addictive drug. Compulsive cocaine use seems to develop more rapidly when the substance is smoked rather than snorted. A tolerance to the cocaine high may be developed, and many addicts report that they fail to achieve as much pleasure as they did from their first cocaine exposure.

- Physical effects of cocaine use include constricted blood vessels and increased temperature, heart rate, and blood pressure. Users may also experience feelings of restlessness, irritability, and anxiety. Cocaine-related deaths are often the result of cardiac arrest or seizures followed by respiratory arrest. Cocaine continues to be the most frequently mentioned illicit substance in U.S. emergency departments, present in 30% of the emergency department drug episodes during 2001.

Marijuana

- Drug legalization advocates in the United States single out marijuana as a different kind of drug, unlike cocaine, heroin, and methamphetamine. They say it's less dangerous. Several European countries have lowered the classification of marijuana. However, as many people are realizing, marijuana is not as harmless as some would have them believe. Marijuana is far more powerful than it used to be. In 2000, there were six times as many emergency room mentions of marijuana use as there were in 1990, despite the fact that the number of people using marijuana is roughly the same. In 1999, a record 225,000 Americans entered substance abuse treatment primarily for marijuana dependence, second only to heroin—and not by much.

- At a time of great public pressure to curtail tobacco because of its effects on health, advocates of legalization are promoting the use of marijuana. Yet, according to the National Institute on Drug Abuse, "Studies show that someone who smokes five joints per week may be taking in as many cancer-causing chemicals as someone who smokes a full pack of cigarettes every day." Marijuana contains more than 400 chemicals, including the most harmful substances found in tobacco smoke. For example, smoking one marijuana cigarette deposits about four times more tar into the lungs than a filtered tobacco cigarette.

- Those are the long-term effects of marijuana. The short-term effects are also harmful. They include: memory loss, distorted perception, trouble with thinking and problem solving, loss of motor skills, decrease in muscle strength, increased heart rate, and anxiety. Marijuana impacts young people's mental development, their ability to concentrate in school, and their motivation and initiative to reach goals. And marijuana affects people of all ages: Harvard University researchers report that the risk of a heart attack is five times higher than usual in the hour after smoking marijuana.

Fact 4. Smoked marijuana is not scientifically approved medicine. Marinol, the legal version of medical marijuana, is approved by science.

- Medical marijuana already exists. It's called Marinol.

- A pharmaceutical product, Marinol, is widely available through prescription. It comes in the form of a pill and is also being studied by researchers for suitability via other delivery methods, such as an inhaler or patch. The active ingredient of Marinol is synthetic THC, which has been found to relieve the nausea and vomiting associated with chemotherapy for cancer patients and to assist with loss of appetite with AIDS patients.

- Unlike smoked marijuana—which contains more than 400 different chemicals, including most of the hazardous chemicals found in tobacco smoke—Marinol has been studied and approved by the medical community and the Food and Drug Administration (FDA), the nation's watchdog over unsafe and harmful food and drug products. Since the passage of the 1906 Pure Food and Drug Act, any drug that is marketed in the United States must undergo rigorous scientific testing. The approval process mandated by this act ensures that claims of safety and therapeutic value are supported by clinical evidence and keeps unsafe, ineffective, and dangerous drugs off the market.

- There are no FDA-approved medications that are smoked. For one thing, smoking is generally a poor way to deliver medicine. It is difficult to administer safe, regulated dosages of medicines in smoked form. Secondly, the harmful chemicals and carcinogens that are byproducts of smoking create entirely new health problems. There are four times the level of tar in a marijuana cigarette, for example, than in a tobacco cigarette.

- Morphine, for example, has proven to be a medically valuable drug, but the FDA does not endorse the smoking of opium or heroin. Instead, scientists have extracted active ingredients from opium, which are sold as pharmaceutical products like morphine, codeine, hydrocodone or oxycodone. In a similar vein, the FDA has not approved smoking marijuana for medicinal purposes, but has approved the active ingredient—THC—in the form of scientifically regulated Marinol.

- The DEA helped facilitate the research on Marinol. The National Cancer Institute approached the DEA in the early 1980s regarding their study of THC's in relieving nausea and vomiting. As a result, the DEA facilitated the registration and provided regulatory support and guidance for the study. California, researchers are studying the potential use of marijuana and its ingredients on conditions such as multiple sclerosis and pain. At this time, however, neither the medical community nor the scientific community has found sufficient data to conclude that smoked marijuana is the best approach to dealing with these important medical issues.

- The most comprehensive, scientifically rigorous review of studies of smoked marijuana was conducted by the Institute of Medicine, an organization chartered by the National Academy of Sciences. In a report released in 1999, the Institute did not recommend the use of smoked marijuana, but did conclude that active ingredients in marijuana could be isolated and developed into a variety of pharmaceuticals, such as Marinol.

- In the meantime, the DEA is working with pain management groups, such as Last Acts, to make sure that those who need access to safe, effective pain medication can get the best medication available.

Fact 5: Drug control spending is a minor portion of the U.S. budget. Compared to the social costs of drug abuse and addiction, government spending on drug control is minimal.

- Legalization advocates claim that the United States has spent billions of dollars to control drug production, trafficking, and use, with few, if any, positive results. As shown in previous chapters, the results of the American drug strategy have been positive indeed—with a 95% rate of Americans who do not use drugs. If the number of drug abusers doubled or tripled, the social costs would be enormous.

Social Costs

- In the year 2000, drug abuse cost American society an estimated $160 billion. More important were the concrete losses that are imperfectly symbolized by those billions of dollars—the destruction of lives, the damage of addiction, fatalities from car accidents, illness, and lost opportunities and dreams.

- Legalization would result in skyrocketing costs that would be paid by American taxpayers and consumers. Legalization would significantly increase drug use and addiction—and all the social costs that go with it. With the removal of the social and legal sanctions against drugs, many experts estimate the user population would at least double. For example, a 1994 article in the *New England Journal of Medicine* stated that it was probable, that if cocaine were legalized, the number of cocaine addicts in America would increase from 2 million to at least 20 million.

- Drug abuse drives some of America's most costly social problems—including domestic violence, child abuse, chronic mental illness, the spread of AIDS, and homelessness. Drug treatment costs, hospitalization for long-term drug-related disease, and treatment of the consequences of family violence burden our already strapped health care system. In 2000, there were more than 600,000 hospital emergency department drug episodes in the United States. Health care costs for drug abuse alone were about $15 billion.

- Drug abuse among the homeless has been conservatively estimated at better than 50%. Chronic mental illness is inextricably linked with drug abuse. In Philadelphia, nearly half of the VA's mental patients abused drugs. The Centers for Disease Control and Prevention has estimated that 36% of new HIV cases are directly or indirectly linked to injecting drug users.

- In 1998, Americans spent $67 billion for illegal drugs, a sum of money greater than the amount spent that year to finance public higher education in the United States. If the money spent on illegal drugs were devoted instead to public higher education, for example, public colleges would have the financial ability to accommodate twice as many students as they already do.

- In addition, legalization—and the increased addiction it would spawn—would result in lost workforce productivity—and the unpredictable damage that it would cause to the American economy. The latest drug use surveys show that about 75% of adults who reported current illicit drug use—which means they've used drugs once in the past month—are employed, either full or part-time. In 2000, productivity losses due to drug abuse cost the economy $110 billion. Drug use by workers leads not only to more unexcused absences and higher turnover, but also presents an enormous safety problem in the workplace. Studies have confirmed what common sense dictates: Employees who abuse drugs are five times more likely than other workers to injure themselves or coworkers and they cause 40% of all industrial fatalities. They were more likely to have worked for three or more employers and to have voluntarily left an employer in the past year.

- Legalization would also result in a huge increase in the number of traffic accidents and fatalities. Drugs are already responsible for a significant number of accidents. Marijuana, for example, impairs the ability of drivers to maintain concentration and show good judgment. A study by the National Institute on Drug Abuse surveyed 6,000 teenage drivers. It studied those who drove more than six times a month after using marijuana. The study found that they were about two-and-a-half times more likely to be involved in a traffic accident than those who didn't smoke before driving.

- Legalizers fail to mention the hidden consequences of legalization.

- Will the right to use drugs imply a right to the access to drugs? One of the arguments for legalization is that it will end the need for drug trafficking cartels. If so, who will distribute drugs? Government employees? The local supermarket? The college bookstore? In view of the huge settlement agreed to by the tobacco companies, what marketer would want the potential liability for selling a product as harmful as cocaine or heroin— or even marijuana?

- Advocates also argue that legalization will lower prices. But that raises a dilemma: If the price of drugs is low, many more people will be able to afford them and the demand for drugs will explode. For example, the cost of cocaine production is now as low as $3 per gram. At a market price of, say, $10 a gram, cocaine could retail for as little as ten cents a hit. That means a young person could buy six hits of cocaine for the price of a candy bar. On the other hand, if legal drugs are priced too high, through excise taxes, for example, illegal traffickers will be able to undercut it.

- Advocates of legalization also argue that the legal market could be limited to those above a certain age level, as it is for alcohol and cigarettes. Those under the age limits would not be permitted to buy drugs at authorized outlets. But teenagers today have found many ways to circumvent the age restrictions, whether by using false identification or by buying liquor and cigarettes from older friends. According to the 2001 *National Household Survey on Drug Abuse*, approximately 10.1 million young people aged 12–20 reported past month alcohol use (28.5% of this age group). Of these, nearly 6.8 million (19%) were binge drinkers. With drugs, teenagers would have an additional outlet: the highly organized illegal trafficking networks that exist today and that would undoubtedly concentrate their marketing efforts on young people to make up for the business they lost to legal outlets.

Costs to the Taxpayer

- The claim that money allegedly saved from giving up on the drug problem could be better spent on education and social problems is readily disputed. When compared to the amount of funding that is spent on other national priorities, federal drug control spending is minimal. For example, in 2002, the amount of money spent by the federal government on drug control was less than $19 billion in its entirety. And unlike critics of American drug policy would have you believe, all of those funds did not go to enforcement policy only. Those funds were used for treatment, education and prevention, as well as enforcement. Within that budget, the amount of money Congress appropriated for the Drug Enforcement Administration was roughly $1.6 billion, a sum that the Defense Department runs through about every day-and-a-half or two days.

- In FY 2002, the federal drug budget is $18.8 billion. One-third of that budget is invested in demand reduction: prevention and treatment efforts. This fiscal year, we have budgeted more than $3 billion for drug abuse treatment, a 27% increase over 1999.

- By contrast, our country spent about $650 billion, in total, in 2000 on our nation's educational system. And most of us would agree that it was money well spent, even if our educational system isn't perfect. Education is a long-term social concern, with new problems that arise with every new generation. The same can be said of drug abuse and addiction. Yet nobody suggests that we should give up on our children's education. Why, then, would we give up on helping to keep them off drugs and out of addiction?

- Even if drug abuse had not dropped as much as it has in the last 20 years—by more than a third—the alternative to spending money on controlling drugs would be disastrous. If the relatively modest outlays of federal dollars were not made, drug abuse and the attendant social costs ($160 billion in 2000) would be far greater.

- On the surface, advocates of legalization present an appealing, but simplistic, argument that by legalizing drugs we can move vast sums of money from enforcing drug laws to solving society's ills. But as in education and drug addiction, vast societal problems can't be solved overnight. It takes time, focus, persistence—and resources.

- Legalization advocates fail to note the skyrocketing social and welfare costs, not to mention the misery and addiction, that would accompany outright legalization of drugs.

- Legalizers also fail to mention that, unless drugs are made available to children, law enforcement will still be needed to deal with the sale of drugs to minors. In other words, a vast black market will still exist. Since young people are often the primary target of pushers, many of the criminal organizations that now profit from illegal drugs would continue to do so.

- Furthermore, it is reasonable to assume that the health and societal costs of drug legalization would also increase exponentially. Drug treatment costs, hospitalization for long-term drug-related diseases, and treatment of family violence would also place additional demands on our already overburdened health system. More taxes would have to be raised to pay for an American health care system already bursting at the seams.

- Criminal justice costs would likely increase if drugs were legalized. It is quite likely that violent crime would significantly increase with greater accessibility to dangerous drugs—whether the drugs themselves are legal or not. According to a 1991 Justice Department study, six times as many homicides are committed by people under the influence of drugs as by those who are looking for money to buy drugs. More taxes would have to be raised to pay for additional personnel in law enforcement, which is already overburdened by crimes and traffic fatalities associated with alcohol. Law enforcement is already challenged by significant alcohol-related crimes. More users would probably result in the commission of additional crimes, causing incarceration costs to increase as well.

Fact 6: Legalization of drugs will lead to increased use and increased levels of addiction. Legalization has been tried before, and failed miserably.

- Legalization proponents claim, absurdly, that making illegal drugs legal would not cause more of these substances to be consumed, nor would addiction increase. They claim that many people can use drugs in moderation and that many would choose not to use drugs, just as many abstain from alcohol and tobacco now. Yet how much misery can already be attributed to alcoholism and smoking? Is the answer to just add more misery and addiction?

- It's clear from history that periods of lax controls are accompanied by more drug abuse and that periods of tight controls are accompanied by less drug abuse.

- During the 19th century, morphine was legally refined from opium and hailed as a miracle drug. Many soldiers on both sides

93

of the Civil War who were given morphine for their wounds became addicted to it, and this increased level of addiction continued throughout the 19th century and into the 20th. In 1880, many drugs, including opium and cocaine, were legal—and, like some drugs today, seen as benign medicine not requiring a doctor's care and oversight.

Addiction skyrocketed. There were over 400,000 opium addicts in the United States. That is twice as many per capita as there are today.

- By 1900, about one American in 200 was either a cocaine or opium addict. Among the reforms of this era was the Federal Pure Food and Drug Act of 1906, which required manufacturers of patent medicines to reveal the contents of the drugs they sold. In this way, Americans learned which of their medicines contained heavy doses of cocaine and opiates—drugs they had now learned to avoid.

- Specific federal drug legislation and oversight began with the 1914 Harrison Act, the first broad anti-drug law in the United States. Enforcement of this law contributed to a significant decline in narcotic addiction in the United States. Addiction in the United States eventually fell to its lowest level during World War II, when the number of addicts is estimated to have been somewhere between 20,000 and 40,000. Many addicts, faced with disappearing supplies, were forced to give up their drug habits.

- What was virtually a drug-free society in the war years remained much the same way in the years that followed. In the mid-1950s, the Federal Bureau of Narcotics estimated the total number of addicts nationwide at somewhere between 50,000 to 60,000. The former chief medical examiner of New York City, Dr. Milton Halpern, said in 1970 that the number of New Yorkers who died from drug addiction in 1950 was 17. By comparison, in 1999, the New York City medical examiner reported 729 deaths involving drug abuse.

- The consequences of legalization became evident when the Alaska Supreme Court ruled in 1975 that the state could not interfere with an adult's possession of marijuana for personal consumption in the home. The court's ruling became a green light for marijuana use. Although the ruling was limited to persons 19 and over, teens were among those increasingly using marijuana.

According to a 1988 University of Alaska study, the state's 12- to 17-year-olds used marijuana at more than twice the national average for their age group. Alaska's residents voted in 1990 to recriminalize possession of marijuana, demonstrating their belief that increased use was too high a price to pay.

- By 1979, after 11 states decriminalized marijuana and the Carter administration had considered federal decriminalization, marijuana use shot up among teenagers. That year, almost 51% of 12th graders reported they used marijuana in the last 12 months. By 1992, with tougher laws and increased attention to the risks of drug abuse, that figure had been reduced to 22%, a 57% decline.

- Other countries have also had this experience. The Netherlands has had its own troubles with increased use of cannabis products. From 1984 to 1996, the Dutch liberalized the use of cannabis. Surveys reveal that lifetime prevalence of cannabis in Holland increased consistently and sharply. For the age group 18–20, the increase is from 15% in 1984 to 44% in 1996.

- The Netherlands is not alone. Switzerland, with some of the most liberal drug policies in Europe, experimented with what became known as Needle Park. Needle Park became the Mecca for drug addicts throughout Europe, an area where addicts could come to openly purchase drugs and inject heroin without police intervention or control. The rapid decline in the neighborhood surrounding Needle Park, with increased crime and violence, led authorities to finally close Needle Park in 1992.

- The British have also had their own failed experiments with liberalizing drug laws. England's experience shows that use and addiction increase with "harm reduction" policy. Great Britain allowed doctors to prescribe heroin to addicts, resulting in an explosion of heroin use, and by the mid-1980s, known addiction rates were increasing by about 30% a year.

- The relationship between legalization and increased use becomes evident by considering two current "legal drugs," tobacco and alcohol. The number of users of these "legal drugs" is far greater than the number of users of illegal drugs. The numbers were explored by the 2001 *National Household Survey on Drug Abuse*. Roughly 109 million Americans used alcohol at least once a month. About 66 million Americans used tobacco at the same rate. But less than 16 million Americans used illegal drugs at least once a month.

- It's clear that there is a relationship between legalization and increasing drug use, and that legalization would result in an unacceptably high number of drug-addicted Americans.

- When legalizers suggest that easy access to drugs won't contribute to greater levels of addiction, they aren't being candid. The question isn't whether legalization will increase addiction levels— it will—it's whether we care or not. The compassionate response is to do everything possible to prevent the destruction of addiction, not make it easier.

Fact 7: Crime, violence, and drug use go hand-in-hand.

- Proponents of legalization have many theories regarding the connection between drugs and violence. Some dispute the connection between drugs and violence, claiming that drug use is a victimless crime and users are putting only themselves in harm's way and therefore have the right to use drugs. Other proponents of legalization contend that if drugs were legalized, crime and violence would decrease, believing that it is the illegal nature of drug production, trafficking, and use that fuels crime and violence, rather than the violent and irrational behavior that drugs themselves prompt.

- Yet, under a legalization scenario, a black market for drugs would still exist. And it would be a vast black market. If drugs were legal for those over 18 or 21, there would be a market for everyone under that age. People under the age of 21 consume the majority of illegal drugs, and so an illegal market and organized crime to supply it would remain—along with the organized crime that profits from it. After Prohibition ended, did the organized crime in our country go down? No. It continues today in a variety of other criminal enterprises. Legalization would not put the cartels out of business; cartels would simply look to other illegal endeavors.

- If only marijuana were legalized, drug traffickers would continue to traffic in heroin and cocaine. In either case, traffic-related violence would not be ended by legalization.

- If only marijuana, cocaine, and heroin were legalized, there would still be a market for PCP and methamphetamine. Where do legalizers want to draw the line? Or do they support legalizing all drugs, no matter how addictive and dangerous?

- In addition, any government agency assigned to distribute drugs under a legalization scenario would, for safety purposes, most likely not distribute the most potent drug. The drugs may also be more expensive because of bureaucratic costs of operating such a distribution system. Therefore, until 100% pure drugs are given away to anyone, at any age, a black market will remain.

- The greatest weakness in the logic of legalizers is that the violence associated with drugs is simply a product of drug trafficking. That is, if drugs were legal, then most drug crime would end. But most violent crime is committed not because people want to buy drugs, but because people are on drugs. Drug use changes behavior and exacerbates criminal activity, and there is ample scientific evidence that demonstrates the links between drugs, violence, and crime. Drugs often cause people to do things they wouldn't do if they were rational and free of the influence of drugs.

- Six times as many homicides are committed by people under the influence of drugs as by those who are looking for money to buy drugs.

- According to the 1999 Arrestee Drug Abuse Monitoring (ADAM) study, more than half of arrestees for violent crimes test positive for drugs at the time of their arrest.

- For experts in the field of crime, violence, and drug abuse, there is no doubt that there is a connection between drug use and violence. As Joseph A. Califano, Jr., of the National Center on Addiction and Substance Abuse at Columbia University stated, "Drugs like marijuana, heroin and cocaine are not dangerous because they are illegal; they are illegal because they are dangerous."

- There are numerous statistics, from a wide variety of sources, illustrating the connection between drugs and violence. The propensity for violence against law enforcement officers, coworkers, family members, or simply people encountered on the street by drug abusers is a matter of record.

97

- A 1997 FBI study of violence against law enforcement officers found that 24% of the assailants were under the influence of drugs at the time they attacked the officers and that 72% of the assailants had a history of drug law violations.

- Many scientific studies also support the connection between drug use and crime. One study investigated state prisoners who had five or more convictions. These are hardened criminals. It found that four out of every five of them used drugs regularly.

- Numerous episodes of workplace violence have also been attributed to illegal drugs. A two-year independent postal commission study looked into 29 incidents resulting in 34 deaths of postal employees from 1986 to 1999. "Most perpetrators (20 of 34) either had a known history of substance abuse or were known to be under the influence of alcohol or illicit drugs at the time of the homicide. The number is likely higher because investigations in most other cases were inconclusive."

- According to the 1998 *National Household Survey on Drug Abuse*, teenage drug users are five times far more likely to attack someone than those who don't use drugs. About 20% of the 12- to 17-year-olds reporting use of an illegal drug in the past year attacked someone with the intent to seriously hurt them, compared to 4.3% of the non-drug users.

- As we see in most cases, the violence associated with drug use escalates and, in many instances, results in increased homicide rates. A 1994 Journal of the American Medical Association article reported that cocaine use was linked to high rates of homicide in New York City.

- As these studies, and others, prove—violence is the hallmark of drug abuse. Drug users are not only harming themselves, but as we can see, they are harming anyone who may have the misfortune of crossing their path. Dr. Mitchell Rosenthal, head of Phoenix House, a major drug treatment center, has pointed out that, "there are a substantial number of abusers who cross the line from permissible self-destruction to become 'driven' people who are 'out of control' and put others in danger of their risk-taking, violence, abuse, or HIV infection."

- It is impossible to claim drug use is victimless crime or deny the relationship between drugs and violence, especially when looking at an Office of National Drug Control Policy (ONDCP) estimate for 1995, which estimates there were almost 53,000 drug-related deaths in that year alone, compared to 58,000 American lives lost in eight and a half years in the Vietnam War. The assertions dismissing the connection between drugs and violence by legalization proponents are simply not true. Drug use, legal or not, is not a victimless crime; it is a crime that destroys communities, families, and lives. Six times as many homicides are committed by people under the influence of drugs as by those who are looking for money to buy drugs.

Fact 8: Alcohol has caused significant health, social, and crime problems in this country, and legalized drugs would only make the situation worse.

- If private companies were to handle distribution—as is done with alcohol—the American consumer can expect a blizzard of profit-driven advertising encouraging drug use, just as we now face with alcohol advertising. If the government were to distribute drugs, either the taxpayer would have to pay for its production and distribution, or the government would be forced to market the drugs to earn the funds necessary to stay in business. Furthermore, the very act of official government distribution of drugs would send a message that drug use is safe. After all, it's the U.S. government that's handing it out, right?

- Drugs are far more addictive than alcohol. According to Dr. Mitchell Rosenthal, director of Phoenix House, only 10% of drinkers become alcoholics, while up to 75% of regular illicit drug users become addicted.

- Even accepting, for the sake of argument, the analogy of the legalizers, alcohol use in the U.S. has taken a tremendous physical and social toll on Americans. Legalization proponents would have the problems multiplied by greatly adding to the class of drug-addicted Americans. To put it in perspective, less than 5% of the population uses illegal drugs of any kind. That's less than 16 million regular users of all illegal drugs compared to 66 million tobacco users and over 100 million alcohol users.

- According to the Centers for Disease Control and Prevention (CDC), during 2000, there were 15,852 drug-induced deaths; only slightly less than the 18,539 alcohol-induced deaths. Yet

99

the personal costs of drug use are far higher. According to a 1995 article by Dr. Robert L. DuPont, an expert on drug abuse, the health-related costs per person is more than twice as high for drugs as it is for alcohol: $1,742 for users of illegal drugs and $798 for users of alcohol. Legalization of drugs would compound the problems in the already overburdened health care, social service, and criminal justice systems. And it would demand a staggering new tax burden on the public to pay for the costs. The cost to families affected by addiction is incalculable.

- Alcohol, a "legal drug," is already abused by people in almost every age and socio-economic group. According to the 2001 *National Household Survey on Drug Abuse*, approximately 10.1 million young people aged 12–20 reported past month alcohol use (28.5% of this age group). Of these, nearly 6.8 million (19%) were binge drinkers. American society can expect even more destructive statistics if drug use were to be made legal and acceptable.

- If drugs were widely available under legalization, they would no doubt be easily obtained by young people, despite age restrictions. According to the 2001 *National Household Survey on Drug Abuse*, almost half (109 million) of Americans aged 12 or older were current drinkers, while an estimated 15.9 million or 7.1% were current illicit drug users.

- The cost of drug and alcohol abuse is not all monetary. In 2001 more than 17,000 people were killed and approximately 275,000 people were injured in alcohol-related crashes. According to the National Highway Transportation Safety Administration, approximately three out of every ten Americans will be involved in an alcohol-related crash at some time in their lives.

Fact 9: Europe's more liberal drug policies are not the right model for America.

- Over the past decade, European drug policy has gone through some dramatic changes toward greater liberalization. The Netherlands, considered to have led the way in the liberalization of drug policy, is only one of a number of West European countries to relax penalties for marijuana possession. Now several European nations are looking to relax penalties on all drugs—including cocaine and heroin—as Portugal did in July 2001, when minor possession of all drugs was decriminalized.

- There is no uniform drug policy in Europe. Some countries have liberalized their laws, while others have instituted strict drug control policies. Which means that the so-called "European Model" is a misnomer. Like America, the various countries of Europe are looking for new ways to combat the worldwide problem of drug abuse.

- The Netherlands has led Europe in the liberalization of drug policy. "Coffee shops" began to emerge throughout the Netherlands in 1976, offering marijuana products for sale. Possession and sale of marijuana are not legal, but coffee shops are permitted to operate and sell marijuana under certain restrictions, including a limit of no more than 5 grams sold to a person at any one time, no alcohol or hard drugs, no minors, and no advertising. In the Netherlands, it is illegal to sell or possess marijuana products. So coffee shop operators must purchase their marijuana products from illegal drug trafficking organizations.

- Apparently, there has been some public dissatisfaction with the government's policy. Recently the Dutch government began considering scaling back the quantity of marijuana available in coffee shops from 5 to 3 grams.

- Furthermore, drug abuse has increased in the Netherlands. From 1984 to 1996, marijuana use among 18- to 25-year-olds in Holland increased twofold. Since legalization of marijuana, heroin addiction levels in Holland have tripled and perhaps even quadrupled by some estimates.

- The increasing use of marijuana is responsible for more than increased crime. It has widespread social implications as well. The head of Holland's best-known drug abuse rehabilitation center has described what the new drug culture has created: The strong form of marijuana that most of the young people smoke, he says, produces "a chronically passive individual— someone who is lazy, who doesn't want to take initiatives, doesn't want to be active—the kid who'd prefer to lie in bed with a joint in the morning rather than getting up and doing something."

- Marijuana is not the only illegal drug to find a home in the Netherlands. The club drug commonly referred to as ecstasy (3, 4-methylenedioxy-methamphetamine or MDMA) also has strong roots in the Netherlands. The majority of the world's ecstasy is produced in clandestine laboratories in the Netherlands and, to a lesser extent, Belgium.

• The growing ecstasy problem in Europe, and the Netherlands' pivotal role in ecstasy production, has led the Dutch government to look once again to law enforcement. In May 2001, the government announced a "Five Year Offensive against the Production, Trade, and Consumption of Synthetic Drugs." The offensive focuses on more cooperation among the enforcement agencies with the Unit Synthetic Drugs playing a pivotal role.

• Recognizing that the government needs to take firm action to deal with the increasing levels of addiction, in April 2001, the Dutch government established the Penal Care Facility for Addicts. Like American Drug Treatment Courts, this facility is designed to detain and treat addicts (of any drug) who repeatedly commit crimes and have failed voluntary treatment facilities. Offenders may be held in this facility for up to two years, during which time they will go through a three-phase program. The first phase focuses on detoxification, while the second and third phases focus on training for social reintegration.

• The United Kingdom has also experimented with the relaxation of drug laws. Until the mid-1960s, British physicians were allowed to prescribe heroin to certain classes of addicts. According to political scientist James Q. Wilson, "a youthful drug culture emerged with a demand for drugs far different from that of the older addicts." Many addicts chose to boycott the program and continued to get their heroin from illicit drug distributors. The British Government's experiment with controlled heroin distribution, says Wilson, resulted in, at a minimum, a 30-fold increase in the number of addicts in ten years.

• Switzerland has some of the most liberal drug policies in Europe. In late 1980s, Zurich experimented with what became known as Needle Park, where addicts could openly purchase drugs and inject heroin without police intervention. Zurich became the hub for drug addicts across Europe, until the experiment was ended, and "Needle Park" was shut down.

• Many proponents of drug legalization or decriminalization claim that drug use will be reduced if drugs were legalized. However, history has not shown this assertion to be true. According to an October 2000 CNN report, marijuana, the illegal drug most often decriminalized, is "continuing to spread in the European Union, with one in five people across the 15-state bloc having tried it at least once."

- It's not just marijuana use that is increasing in Europe. According to the 2001 Annual Report on the State of the Drugs Problem in the European Union, there is a Europe-wide increase in cocaine use. The report also cites a new trend of mixing "base/crack" cocaine with tobacco in a joint at nightspots. With the increase in use, Europe is also seeing an increase in the number of drug users seeking treatment for cocaine use.

- Drug policy also has an impact on general crime. In a 2001 study, the British Home Office found violent crime and property crime increased in the late 1990s in every wealthy country except the United States.

- Not all of Europe has been swept up in the trend to liberalize drug laws. Sweden, Finland, and Greece have the strictest policies against drugs in Europe. Sweden's zero-tolerance policy is widely supported within the country and among the various political parties. Drug use is relatively low in the Scandinavian countries.

- In April 1994, a number of European cities signed a resolution titled "European Cities Against Drugs," commonly known as the Stockholm resolution. It states: "The demands to legalize illicit drugs should be seen against the background of current problems, which have led to a feeling of helplessness. For many, the only way to cope is to try to administer the current situation. But the answer does not lie in making harmful drugs more accessible, cheaper, and socially acceptable. Attempts to do this have not proved successful. By making them legal, society will signal that it has resigned to the acceptance of drug abuse. The signatories to this resolution therefore want to make their position clear by rejecting the proposals to legalize illicit drugs."

Fact 10: Most non-violent drug users get treatment, not just jail time.

- There is a myth in this country that U.S. prisons are filled with drug users. This assertion is simply not true. Actually, only 5%

of inmates in federal prison on drug charges are incarcerated for drug possession. In our state prisons, it's somewhat higher—about 27% of drug offenders. In New York, which has received criticism from some because of its tough Rockefeller drug laws, it is estimated that 97% of drug felons sentenced to prison were charged with sale or intent to sell, not simply possession. In fact, first time drug offenders, even sellers, typically do not go to prison.

- Most cases of simple drug possession are simply not prosecuted, unless people have been arrested repeatedly for using drugs. In 1999, for example, only 2.5% of the federal cases argued in District Courts involved simple drug possession. Even the small number of possession charges is likely to give an inflated impression of the numbers. It is likely that a significant percentage of those in prison on possession charges were people who were originally arrested for trafficking or another more serious drug crime but plea-bargained down to a simple possession charge.

- The Michigan Department of Corrections just finished a study of their inmate population. They discovered that out of 47,000 inmates, only 15 people were incarcerated on first-time drug possession charges. (500 are incarcerated on drug possession charges, but 485 are there on multiple charges or pled down.)

- In Wisconsin the numbers are even lower, with only 10 persons incarcerated on drug possession charges. (769 are incarcerated on drug possession charges, but 512 of those entered prison through some type of revocation, leaving 247 entering prison on a "new sentence." Eliminating those who had also been sentenced on trafficking and/or non-drug related charges; the total of new drug possession sentences came to 10.)

Policy Shift to Treatment

- There has been a shift in the U.S. criminal justice system to provide treatment for non-violent drug users with addiction problems, rather than incarceration. The criminal justice system actually serves as the largest referral source for drug treatment programs.

- Any successful treatment program must also require accountability from its participants. Drug treatment courts are a good example of combining treatment with such accountability. These courts are given a special responsibility to handle cases involving drug-addicted offenders through an extensive supervision and treatment program. Drug treatment court programs use the varied experience and skills of a wide variety of law enforcement and treatment professionals: judges, prosecutors, defense counsels, substance abuse treatment specialists, probation officers, law enforcement and correctional personnel, educational and vocational experts, community leaders and others—all focused on one goal: to help cure addicts of their addiction, and to keep them cured.

- Drug treatment courts are working. Researchers estimate that more than 50% of defendants convicted of drug possession will return to criminal behavior within two to three years. Those who graduate from drug treatment courts have far lower rates of recidivism, ranging from 2 to 20%.

- What makes drug treatment courts so different? Graduates are held accountable to the program. Unlike purely voluntary treatment programs, the addict—who has a physical need for drugs—can't simply quit treatment whenever he or she feels like it.

- Many state governments are also taking the opportunity to divert non-violent drug offenders from prison in the hopes of offering treatment and rehabilitation outside the penal facility. In New York, prosecutors currently divert over 7,000 convicted drug felons from prison each year. Many enter treatment programs.

- States throughout the Midwest are also establishing programs to divert drug offenders from prison and aid in their recovery. In Indiana, 64 of the 92 counties offer community corrections programs to rehabilitate and keep first time non-violent offenders, including nonviolent drug offenders, out of prison. Nonviolent drug offenders participating in the community corrections program are required to attend a treatment program as part of their rehabilitation.

- In July of 2002, the Ohio Judicial Conference conducted a survey of a select group of judges. The results from the survey demonstrated that judges "offer treatment to virtually 100% of

first-time drug offenders and over 95% of second-time drug offenders." According to the survey, these percentages are accurate throughout the state, no matter the jurisdiction or county
size. The Ohio Judicial Conference went a step further, reviewing pre-sentence investigations and records, which demonstrated that "99% of offenders sentenced to prison had one or
more prior felony convictions or multiple charges."

• The assertion that U.S. prisons are filled with drug users is simply untrue. As this evidence shows, more and more minor drug
offenders are referred to treatment centers in an effort to reduce the possibility of recidivism and help drug users get help
for their substance abuse problems. The drug treatment court
program and several other programs set up throughout the
United States have been reducing the number of minor drug offenses that actually end up in the penal system. The reality is
that you have to work pretty darn hard to end up in jail on drug
possession charges.

Chapter 8

Arguing against Marijuana Prohibition

- Very few Americans had even heard about marijuana when it was first federally prohibited in 1937. Today, between 95 and 100 million Americans admit to having tried it.[1,2]

- According to government-funded researchers, high school seniors consistently report that marijuana is easily available, despite decades of a nationwide drug war. With little variation, every year about 85% consider marijuana "fairly easy" or "very easy" to obtain.[3] In an August 2002 Columbia University survey, teens reported that marijuana, which is completely unregulated, was easier to obtain than either beer or cigarettes, which are legally regulated.[4]

- There have been nearly 6.5 million marijuana arrests in the United States since 1993, including 697,082 arrests in 2002. About 88% of all marijuana arrests are for possession—not manufacture or distribution.[5]

- Every comprehensive, objective government commission that has examined the marijuana phenomenon throughout the past 100 years has recommended that adults should not be criminalized for using marijuana.[6]

"Marijuana Prohibition Facts" is reprinted with permission from the Marijuana Policy Project, Washington, DC © 2004 Marijuana Policy Project. All rights reserved. For additional information, visit the Marijuana Policy Project website at http://www.mpp.org.

- Cultivation of even one marijuana plant is a federal felony.

- Lengthy mandatory minimum sentences apply to myriad offenses. For example, a person must serve a five-year mandatory minimum sentence if federally convicted of cultivating 100 marijuana plants—including seedlings or bug-infested, sickly plants. This is longer than the average sentences for auto theft and manslaughter![7]

- A one-year minimum prison sentence is mandated for "distributing" or "manufacturing" controlled substances within 1,000 feet of any school, university, or playground. Most areas in a city fall within these "drug-free zones." An adult who lives three blocks from the edge of a university is subject to a one-year mandatory minimum sentence for selling an ounce of marijuana to another adult—or even growing one marijuana plant in his or her basement.[8]

- Approximately 77,000 marijuana offenders are in prison or jail right now.[9]

- According to the organization Stop Prisoner Rape, "290,000 males were victimized in jail every year, 192,000 of them penetrated. ... Victims are more likely to be young, small, nonviolent, first offenders, middle-class. ..."[10]

- Civil forfeiture laws allow police to seize the money and property of suspected marijuana offenders—charges need not even be filed. The claim is against the property, not the defendant. The owner must then prove that the property is "innocent." Enforcement abuses stemming from forfeiture laws abound.[11]

- MPP estimates that the war on marijuana consumers costs taxpayers nearly $12 billion annually.[12]

- Many patients and their doctors find marijuana a useful medicine as part of the treatment for AIDS, cancer, glaucoma, multiple sclerosis, and other ailments. Yet the federal government allows only seven patients in the United States to use marijuana as a medicine, through a program now closed to all new applicants. Federal laws treat all other patients currently using medical marijuana as criminals. Doctors are presently allowed to prescribe cocaine and morphine—but not marijuana.[13,14]

- Organizations that have endorsed medical access to marijuana include: the AIDS Action Council, American Academy of Family Physicians, American Public Health Association, California Medical Association, California Society of Addiction Medicine, Lymphoma Foundation of America, National Association of People With AIDS, National Nurses Society on Addictions, the *New England Journal of Medicine*, and others.

- A few of the many editorial boards that have endorsed medical access to marijuana include: *Boston Globe, Chicago Tribune, Miami Herald, New York Times, Orange County Register, USA Today, Baltimore's Sun*, and *The Los Angeles Times*.

- Since 1996, a majority of voters in Alaska, Arizona, California, Colorado, the District of Columbia, Maine, Nevada, Oregon, and Washington state have voted in favor of ballot initiatives to remove criminal penalties for seriously ill people who grow or possess medical marijuana.

- Seventy-two percent of Americans believe that marijuana users should not be jailed. Eighty percent support legal access to medical marijuana for seriously ill adults.[2]

- "Decriminalization" involves the removal of criminal penalties for possession of marijuana for personal use. Small fines may be issued (somewhat similarly to traffic tickets), but there is typically no arrest, incarceration, or criminal record. Marijuana is presently decriminalized in 11 states—California, Colorado, Maine, Minnesota, Mississippi, Nebraska, Nevada, New York, North Carolina, Ohio, and Oregon. In these states, cultivation and distribution remain criminal offenses.

- Decriminalization saves a tremendous amount in enforcement costs. California saves $100 million per year.[15]

- In 2001, a National Research Council study sponsored by the U.S. government concluded, "existing research seems to indicate there is little apparent relationship between the severity of sanctions prescribed for drug use and prevalence or frequency of use, and that perceived legal risk explains very little in the variance of individual drug use." The primary evidence cited came from comparisons between states that have decriminalized marijuana and states that have not.[16]

- In the Netherlands, where adult possession and purchase of small amounts of marijuana is allowed under a regulated system, the rate of marijuana use by teenagers is far lower than in the United States.[17,18] Under a regulated system, licensed merchants have an incentive to check ID and avoid selling to minors. Such a system also has the advantage of separating marijuana from the trade in hard drugs such as cocaine and heroin.

- "Zero tolerance" policies against "drugged driving" can result in "DUI" convictions of drivers who are not intoxicated at all. Trace amounts of THC metabolites—detected by commonly used tests—can linger in blood and urine for weeks after any psychoactive effects have worn off. This is the equivalent of convicting someone of "drunk driving" three weeks after he or she drank one beer.[19]

- The arbitrary criminalization of tens of millions of Americans who consume marijuana results in a large-scale lack of respect for the law and the entire criminal justice system.

- Marijuana prohibition subjects users to added health hazards:

  - *Adulterants, contaminants, and impurities*—Marijuana purchased through criminal markets is not subject to the same quality control standards as are legal consumer goods. Illicit marijuana may be adulterated with much more damaging substances; contaminated with pesticides, herbicides, or fertilizers; and/or infected with molds, fungi, or bacteria.

  - *Inhalation of hot smoke*—One of the more well-established hazards of marijuana consumption is the fact that smoke from burning plant material is bad for the respiratory system. Laws that prohibit the sale or possession of paraphernalia make it difficult to obtain and use devices such as vaporizers, which can reduce these risks.[20]

- Because vigorous enforcement of the marijuana laws forces the toughest, most dangerous criminals to take over marijuana trafficking, prohibition links marijuana sales to violence, predatory crime, and terrorism.

- Prohibition invites corruption within the criminal justice system by giving officials easy, tempting opportunities to accept bribes, steal and sell marijuana, and plant evidence on innocent people.

- Because marijuana is typically used in private, trampling the Bill of Rights is a routine part of marijuana law enforcement— e.g., use of drug dogs, urine tests, phone taps, government informants, curbside garbage searches, military helicopters, and infrared heat detectors.

Notes

1. *National Survey on Drug Use and Health*, 2002, Substance Abuse and Mental Health Administration, U.S. Department of Health and Human Services, Table 1.31A.

2. Time/CNN poll of adults, *Time*, Nov. 4, 2002 issue. Forty-seven percent said they had tried marijuana at least once.

3. Johnston, Lloyd D., O'Malley, Patrick M., & Bachman, Jerald G., *Monitoring the Future, National Results on Adolescent Drug Abuse: Overview of Key Findings*, 2002, National Institute on Drug Abuse, U.S. Department of Health and Human Services, 2003.

4. *National Survey of American Attitudes on Substance Abuse VII: Teens, Parents and Siblings*, National Center on Addiction and Substance Abuse, Columbia University, August 20, 2002.

5. Federal Bureau of Investigation, Uniform Crime Reports, *Crime in the United States*, annually.

6. For example, *Report of the Indian Hemp Drugs Commission*, 1894; *The Panama Canal Zone Military Investigations*, 1925; *The Marihuana Problem in the City of New York* (LaGuardia Committee Report), 1944; *Marihuana: A Signal of Misunderstanding* (Nixon–Shafer Report), 1972; *An Analysis of Marijuana Policy* (National Academy of Sciences), 1982; *Cannabis, Our Position for a Canadian Public Policy* (Report of the Senate Special Committee on Illegal Drugs), 2002, and others.

7. 21USC841(b)(1)(B); *1996 Sourcebook of Federal Sentencing Guidelines*, U.S. Sentencing Commission, 1997; p. 24.

8. 21USC860(a); report from Congressional Research Service, June 22, 1995.

9. Estimated by MPP, based on *Prisoners in 2001*, Bureau of Justice Statistics, U.S. Department of Justice; *Prison and Jail*

Inmates at Midyear 2001, Bureau of Justice Statistics, U.S. Department of Justice; *Profile of Jail Inmates*, 1996, Bureau of Justice Statistics, U.S. Department of Justice; *Substance Abuse and Treatment, State and Federal Prisoners, 1997*, Bureau of Justice Statistics.

10. *Rape of Incarcerated Americans: A Preliminary Statistical Look*, Stephen Donaldson; New York, NY: Stop Prisoner Rape, 1995.

11. *Forfeiting Our Property Rights: Is Your Property Safe From Seizure?*, U.S. Rep. Henry Hyde (R-IL); Washington, D.C.: Cato Institute, 1995.

12. In 2002, the federal government spent $18.8 billion on the "drug war." Approximately 53% ($9.964 billion) was spent on enforcement, court, and prison expenses, with the rest used for treatment and education (*National Drug Control Strategy*, Office of National Drug Control Policy; Washington, D.C., 2002). In 1991—the most recent year for which data are available—state and local governments spent a total of nearly $16 billion, of which about 80% was used for enforcement, court, and prison costs (*National Drug Control Strategy*, Office of National Drug Control Policy; Washington, D.C., 1994). State and local spending is estimated to have increased to $20 billion annually in 2002 ("Drug War Retreat? The Pentagon's Double-Edged Plan to Scale Back," *Daytona Beach News-Journal*, Nov. 9, 2002). Hence, the total annual criminal justice system expenditure for federal, state, and local governments is $25.964 billion ($9.964 billion + $16 billion [$20 billion × 80%]). While this total annual expenditure is not broken down by specific drugs, marijuana crimes account for 45.6% of all drug arrests (Federal Bureau of Investigation, *Crime in the United States: 2001*). Assuming that expense and arrest percentages roughly match, the war on marijuana consumers costs taxpayers $11.84 billion annually.

13. "Marihuana as Medicine: A Plea for Reconsideration," *Journal of the American Medical Association*, June 21, 1995.

14. "Medical Marijuana Briefing Paper"; Washington, D.C., Marijuana Policy Project, 2004.

15. "Savings in California Marijuana Law Enforcement Costs Attributable to the Moscone Act of 1976—A Summary," Michael

Aldrich, Ph.D., and Tod Mikuriya, M.D.; *Journal of Psychoactive Drugs*, Vol. 20(1), Jan.–March 1988; Pp. 75–81.

16. *Informing America's Policy on Illegal Drugs: What We Don't Know Keeps Hurting Us*, National Research Council, National Academy Press, 2001; Pp. 192–93.

17. Abraham, Manja D., Hendrien L. Kaal, & Peter D.A. Cohen (2002), *Licit and illicit drug use in the Netherlands 2001.* Amsterdam: CEDRO/Mets en Schilt.

18. Johnston, Lloyd D., O'Malley, Patrick M., & Bachman, Jerald G., *Monitoring the Future, National Results on Adolescent Drug Abuse: Overview of Key Findings, 2002*, National Institute on Drug Abuse, U.S. Department of Health and Human Services, 2003.

19. "The Real Risk of Being Killed When Driving Whilst Impaired by Cannabis," P. Swann, *Australian Studies of Cannabis and Accident Risk, 2000.*

20. Mirken, Bruce, "Vaporizers for Medical Marijuana," *AIDS Treatment News*, Issue #327, September 17, 1999.

Chapter 9

Medical Marijuana: A Controversy

Exposing the Myth of Medical Marijuana

Does marijuana pose health risks to users?

- Marijuana is an addictive drug[1] with significant health consequences to its users and others. Many harmful short-term and long-term problems have been documented with its use.

- The short term effects of marijuana use include: memory loss, distorted perception, trouble with thinking and problem solving, loss of motor skills, decrease in muscle strength, increased heart rate, and anxiety.[2]

- In recent years there has been a dramatic increase in the number of emergency room mentions of marijuana use. From 1993–2000, the number of emergency room marijuana mentions more than tripled.

- There are also many long-term health consequences of marijuana use. According to the National Institutes of Health, studies show that someone who smokes five joints per week may be taking in as many cancer-causing chemicals as someone who smokes a full pack of cigarettes every day.

This chapter includes "Exposing the Myth of Medical Marijuana," U.S. Department of Justice, Drug Enforcement Administration (DEA), 2003; and excerpts from "Frequently Asked Questions," © 2004 National Organization for the Reform of Marijuana Laws (NORML). All rights reserved. For more information, visit http://www.norml.org.

- Marijuana contains more than 400 chemicals, including most of the harmful substances found in tobacco smoke. Smoking one marijuana cigarette deposits about four times more tar into the lungs than a filtered tobacco cigarette.

- Harvard University researchers report that the risk of a heart attack is five times higher than usual in the hour after smoking marijuana.[3]

- Smoking marijuana also weakens the immune system[4] and raises the risk of lung infections.[5] A Columbia University study found that a control group smoking a single marijuana cigarette every other day for a year had a white-blood-cell count that was 39% lower than normal, thus damaging the immune system and making the user far more susceptible to infection and sickness.[6]

- Users can become dependent on marijuana to the point they must seek treatment to stop abusing it. In 1999, more than 200,000 Americans entered substance abuse treatment primarily for marijuana abuse and dependence.

- More teens are in treatment for marijuana use than for any other drug or for alcohol. Adolescent admissions to substance abuse facilities for marijuana grew from 43% of all adolescent admissions in 1994 to 60% in 1999.

- Marijuana is much stronger now than it was decades ago. According to data from the Potency Monitoring Project at the University of Mississippi, the tetrahydrocannabinol (THC) content of commercial-grade marijuana rose from an average of 3.71% in 1985 to an average of 5.57% in 1998. The average THC content of U.S. produced sinsemilla increased from 3.2% in 1977 to 12.8% in 1997.[7]

Does marijuana have any medical value?

- Any determination of a drug's valid medical use must be based on the best available science undertaken by medical professionals. The Institute of Medicine conducted a comprehensive study in 1999 to assess the potential health benefits of marijuana and its constituent cannabinoids. The study concluded that smoking marijuana is not recommended for the treatment of any disease condition. In addition, there are more effective medications currently available. For those reasons, the Institute of Medicine concluded that there is little future in smoked marijuana as a medically approved medication.[8]

- Advocates have promoted the use of marijuana to treat medical conditions such as glaucoma. However, this is a good example of more effective medicines already available. According to the Institute of Medicine, there are six classes of drugs and multiple surgical techniques that are available to treat glaucoma that effectively slow the progression of this disease by reducing high intraocular pressure.

- In other studies, smoked marijuana has been shown to cause a variety of health problems, including cancer, respiratory problems, increased heart rate, loss of motor skills, and increased heart rate. Furthermore, marijuana can affect the immune system by impairing the ability of T-cells to fight off infections, demonstrating that marijuana can do more harm than good in people with already compromised immune systems.[9]

- In addition, in a recent study by the Mayo Clinic, THC was shown to be less effective than standard treatments in helping cancer patients regain lost appetites.[10]

- The American Medical Association recommends that marijuana remain a Schedule I controlled substance.

- The DEA supports research into the safety and efficacy of THC (the major psychoactive component of marijuana), and such studies are ongoing, supported by grants from the National Institute on Drug Abuse.

- As a result of such research, a synthetic THC drug, Marinol, has been available to the public since 1985. The Food and Drug Administration has determined that Marinol is safe, effective, and has therapeutic benefits for use as a treatment for nausea and vomiting associated with cancer chemotherapy, and as a treatment of weight loss in patients with AIDS. However, it does not produce the harmful health effects associated with smoking marijuana.

- Furthermore, the DEA recently approved the University of California San Diego to undertake rigorous scientific studies to assess the safety and efficacy of cannabis compounds for treating certain debilitating medical conditions.

- It's also important to realize that the campaign to allow marijuana to be used as medicine is a tactical maneuver in an overall strategy to completely legalize all drugs. Pro-legalization groups have transformed the debate from decriminalizing drug

117

use to one of compassion and care for people with serious diseases. The New York Times interviewed Ethan Nadelman, Director of the Lindesmith Center, in January 2000. Responding to criticism from former Drug Czar Barry McCaffrey that the medical marijuana issue is a stalking-horse for drug legalization, Mr. Nadelman did not contradict General McCaffrey. "Will it help lead toward marijuana legalization?" Mr. Nadelman said: "I hope so."

Does marijuana harm anyone besides the individual who smokes it?

- Consider the public safety of others when confronted with intoxicated drug users:

- Marijuana affects many skills required for safe driving: alertness, the ability to concentrate, coordination, and reaction time. These effects can last up to 24 hours after smoking marijuana. Marijuana use can make it difficult to judge distances and react to signals and signs on the road.[11]

- In a 1990 report, the National Transportation Safety Board studied 182 fatal truck accidents. It found that just as many of the accidents were caused by drivers using marijuana as were caused by alcohol—12.5% in each case.

- Consider also that drug use, including marijuana, contributes to crime. A large percentage of those arrested for crimes test positive for marijuana. Nationwide, 40% of adult males tested positive for marijuana at the time of their arrest.

Is marijuana a gateway drug?

- Yes. Among marijuana's most harmful consequences is its role in leading to the use of other illegal drugs like heroin and cocaine. Long-term studies of students who use drugs show that very few young people use other illegal drugs without first trying marijuana. While not all people who use marijuana go on to use other drugs, using marijuana sometimes lowers inhibitions about drug use and exposes users to a culture that encourages use of other drugs.

- The risk of using cocaine has been estimated to be more than 104 times greater for those who have tried marijuana than for those who have never tried it.[12]

Notes

1. Herbert Kleber, Mitchell Rosenthal, "Drug Myths from Abroad: Leniency is Dangerous, not Compassionate" Foreign Affairs Magazine, September/October 1998. Drug Watch International "NIDA Director cites Studies that Marijuana is Addictive." "Research Finds Marijuana is Addictive," *Washington Times*, July 24, 1995.

2. National Institute of Drug Abuse, *Journal of the American Medical Association*, *Journal of Clinical Pharmacology*, *International Journal of Clinical Pharmacology and Therapeutics*, *Pharmacology Review*.

3. "Marijuana and Heart Attacks" *Washington Post*, March 3, 2000.

4. I. B. Adams and BR Martin, "Cannabis: Pharmacology and Toxicology in Animals and Humans" *Addiction* 91: 1585–1614. 1996.

5. National Institute of Drug Abuse, "Smoking Any Substance Raises Risk of Lung Infections" NIDA Notes, Volume 12, Number 1, January/February 1997.

6. Dr. James Dobson, "Marijuana Can Cause Great Harm" *Washington Times*, February 23, 1999.

7. *2000 National Drug Control Strategy Annual Report*, page 13.

8. "Marijuana and Medicine: Assessing the Science Base," Institute of Medicine, 1999.

9. See footnotes in response to question 4 regarding marijuana's short and long term health effects.

10. "Marijuana Appetite Boost Lacking in Cancer Study" *The New York Times*, May 13, 2001.

11. *Marijuana: Facts Parents Need to Know*, National Institute on Drug Abuse, National Institutes of Health.

12. *Marijuana: Facts Parents Need to Know*, National Institute on Drug Abuse, National Institutes of Health.

National Organization for the Reform of Marijuana Laws (NORML) Answers Frequently Asked Questions

Critics of the medical use of marijuana say (1) there are traditional medications to help patients and marijuana is not needed; and, (2) permitting the medical use of marijuana sends the wrong message to kids. How do you respond to these concerns?

For many patients, traditional medications do work and they do not require or desire medical marijuana. However, for a significant number of serious ill patients, including patients suffering from AIDS, cancer, multiple sclerosis and chronic pain among others, traditional medications do not provide symptomatic relief as effectively as medicinal cannabis. These patients must not be branded as criminals or forced to suffer needlessly in pain.

Dronabinol (trade name Marinol) is a legal, synthetic THC alternative to cannabis. Nevertheless, many patients claim they find minimal relief from it, particularly when compared to inhaled marijuana. The active ingredient in Marinol, delta-9-tetrahydrocannabinol, is only one of the compounds isolated in marijuana that appears to be medically beneficial to patients. Other compounds such as cannabidiol (CBD), an anticonvulsant, and cannabichromene (CBC), an anti-inflammatory, are unavailable in Marinol, and patients only have access to their therapeutic properties by using cannabis.

Patients prescribed Marinol frequently complain of its high psychoactivity. This is because patients consume the drug orally. Once swallowed, Marinol passes through the liver, where a significant proportion is converted into other chemicals. One of these, the 11-hydroxy metabolite, is four to five times more potent than THC and greatly increases the likelihood of a patient experiencing an adverse psychological reaction. In contrast, inhaled marijuana doesn't cause significant levels of the 11-hydroxy metabolite to appear in the blood.

Marinol's oral administration also delays the drug from taking peak effect until two to four hours after dosing. A 1999 report by the U.S. Institute of Medicine (IOM) concluded: "It is well recognized that Marinol's oral route of administration hampers its effectiveness because of slow absorption and patients' desire for more control over dosing. ... In contrast, inhaled marijuana is rapidly absorbed." In a series of U.S. state studies in the 1980s, cancer patients given a choice between using inhaled marijuana and oral THC overwhelmingly chose cannabis.

As to the message we are sending to kids, NORML hopes the message we are sending is that we would not deny any effective medication to the seriously ill and dying. We routinely permit cancer patients to self-administer morphine in cancer wards all across the country; we allow physicians to prescribe amphetamines for weight loss and to use cocaine in nose and throat operations. Each of these drugs can be abused on the street, yet no one is suggesting we are sending the wrong message to kids by permitting their medical use.

Part Two

The Nature of
Drug Addiction

Chapter 10

Why People Take Drugs

Why Do People, Smart People, Try Drugs?

One reason often heard from people using drugs is that they do them to feel good. For real, it does feel good because most drugs act directly on the "pleasure center"—the limbic system—in the brain. At this point, it can be considered recreational use. Some might light up a cigarette at a party. They might not consider themselves a "smoker," but they do it to feel good or to "look cool." Someone might smoke pot at their friend's house because they think it could be fun. The problem? Drugs don't care what the reason is. The same effects can occur whether you're drinking to have fun or drinking to forget a problem, whether you're doing drugs to see how they feel or doing them to be one of the crowd.

People do drugs to change the way they feel. Often they want to change their situation. If they're depressed, they want to become happy. If they are stressed or nervous, they want to relax, and so on. By taking drugs, people often think they can be the person they want to be. The problem? It isn't real. You haven't changed the situation, you've only distorted it for a little while. Following are some of the reasons people say they do drugs to feel good or change the situation:

National Youth Anti-Drug Media Campaign, a program of the White House Office on National Drug Control Policy (ONDCP), 2004. For more information, visit www.freevibe.com.

1. **Because they want to fit in.** No one wants to be the only one not participating. No one wants to be left out. So sometimes they make bad decisions, like taking drugs, to cover up their insecurities. They don't think about how drugs can isolate you from your friends and family. They forget to look past that one party to see how things could turn out. Or maybe they just don't see the people around them who aren't using drugs.

2. **Because they want to escape or relax.** You'll hear a lot of people saying things like "I'm so stressed, I need to get messed up!" or "Drugs help me relax" or whatever. What they're really saying is "Drinking or doing drugs is just easier than dealing with my problems or reaching out for help." The thing is, the problems are still there when they come down—and not only do they still have to deal with it, they have to deal with it when they're not 100% and feeling guilty or even worse when they're not thinking straight.

3. **Because they're bored.** Lots of people turn to drugs for a little excitement because they say there's nothing else to do but watch the same *Simpsons*' rerun for the 10th time or hang out at the Burger King. But people who make these kinds of decisions usually find out that drugs are ultimately really a waste and painful. Drugs don't change the situation, and they just might make it worse.

4. **Because the media says it's cool.** Even though there's an antidrug ad on every minutes and more rock stars and ball players than you can shake a stick at tell you to stay away from drugs, the truth is the entertainment world still manages to make drugs appear very attractive. Kind of like how they encourage people to be really skinny even when they say anorexia is bad. Or when they say you should be super muscular but steroids are bad. But if you're wise, you'll understand that the entertainment world is not the real world, and basing your life on these messages is superficial.

5. **Because they think it makes them seem grown-up.** This is one of the weirdest reasons. Think about it...Why would an adult want to use drugs? Probably for many of the same reasons you would consider. The reality is that the most grown-up people out there aren't users. They're too busy living their lives to bother with stuff, like drugs, that will interfere.

6. **Because they want to rebel.** Sometimes people turn to drugs not so much for themselves, but to make a statement against someone else, such as their families or society in general. Somehow taking drugs makes them outlaws or more individual. The problem is taking drugs, ultimately, robs these people of their ability to be independent, because it makes them dependent—on drugs and their drug connections.

7. **Because they want to experiment.** It's human nature to want to experiment. Trying things out helps you decide if they're right for you. But it's also human nature to avoid things that are obviously bad for you. You wouldn't experiment with jumping off the Brooklyn Bridge. The point is, there are a zillion better things to experiment with: sports, music, dying your hair, seeing bad movies, eating spicy food...

Are Drugs Always Bad?

Illegal drugs are always bad. There's no good use for sniffing glue or snorting heroin.

But many drugs were developed as medications by doctors to help treat patients with very specific medical conditions. And for those people, drugs make sense. Unfortunately, many of these drugs are used by people who don't need them. Which, if you think about it, is kind of like going for chemotherapy when you don't have cancer. In other words, really dumb.

Physical Effects

What Do Drugs Feel Like?

Depending on the drug, many people report feelings like happiness, confidence, serenity, or even euphoria when they take drugs. But even when they're feeling these things, there's a sense that it's not real, that the happiness is going to disappear any moment. Kind of like when you cover up a big zit on your face. You can't see it, but it's still there.

Unfortunately, in most cases these feelings are followed by even more powerful ones like depression, anxiety, nausea, guilt, embarrassment, loneliness, and wanting more drugs.

What Do Drugs Do to Your Body in the Short Term?

Every drug is different, but the general idea is, they interfere with your nervous system's basic functions. Sometimes they alter your muscles and how they function too. That's why people feel different—their brains and nerves and muscles have been juggled around, making them have sensations they aren't used to.

Besides making you feel different and playing around with your nerves and brain synapses, almost all drugs can make it tougher to sleep. Some cause major weight gain, some cause unhealthy weight loss. Your eyes get all glassy and bloodshot, your heart races, sometimes you get diarrhea. Some drugs like glue or butane can cause immediate death. Cocaine, ecstasy, and meth can give even healthy people a heart attack on the spot.

On a more cosmetic note, most any drug out there will make your hair and skin much less healthy, and many will make you break out—not just on your face, but on your body. Smoking pot can make your teeth yellow, kind of like cigarettes. Oh, and we've never been able to figure out where the myth that drugs make your sex life better came from...While they might make you believe you're on top of the game, in fact, they generally interfere with, ahem, performance.

What Do Drugs Do to Your Body in the Long Term?

It all depends on the drug. Using drugs over and over for a long period of time can cause lots of medical problems, from lung cancer (pot) to liver problems (alcohol) to big time brain damage (ecstasy, alcohol).

In other words, every drug is different, but all the long term effects aren't good. Besides the physical drawbacks, drugs cause major long term brain issues. Depression is a serious problem for many addicts. Also, they can really hurt people—telling lies, stealing money for drugs, sometimes even getting violent with people they love. Their biggest ambition becomes getting high, instead of setting high goals. And so on, and so on.

Why Do People Keep Taking Drugs?

Many people don't become addicted to drugs, but may continue to do drugs for the same reasons they started: because they want to fit in, because they want to escape, because they're bored, whatever. These are people who have issues with insecurity, and are scared or unwilling to deal with problems in a straight-up, intelligent way—like talking to friends, counselors, even parents!

For other people, once they've started taking drugs, they become physically or mentally addicted. They want more—in fact, they feel like they need more. Eventually, trying to get drugs becomes the most important thing in their lives, using up all their time, money, and energy, and really hurting people they're close to.

Can You Get Addicted Even Though You Only Do It Once in a While?

No one wakes up and says today I'm going to be an addict. Addiction is a process—not an event. Everyone starts using drugs once in a while. The problem is some drugs can make you feel so good that you're always searching for that initial feeling—that big high; that rush. The truth is you never quite get the feeling you want, so some folks keep searching and taking more or different drugs. Meanwhile things are happening in your brain—permanent changes are happening—you are beginning to get addicted. That once in a while use of drugs quickly changes to frequently doing drugs to often doing drugs. You get the picture. No one knows when the "chemical switch" goes off in your brain or who will get addicted. It's a lot like playing Russian Roulette—you just never know. The only thing we do know is that the more you do drugs, the closer you get to an addiction.

Chapter 11

How Casual Drug Use Leads to Addiction

It is an all-too-common scenario: A person experiments with an addictive drug like cocaine. Perhaps he intends to try it just once, for "the experience" of it. It turns out, though, that he enjoys the drug's euphoric effect so much that in ensuing weeks and months he uses it again—and again. But in due time, he decides he really should quit. He knows that despite the incomparable short-term high he gets from using cocaine, the long-term consequences of its use are perilous. So he vows to stop using it.

His brain, however, has a different agenda. It now demands cocaine. While his rational mind knows full well that he shouldn't use it again, his brain overrides such warnings. Unbeknown to him, repeated use of cocaine has brought about dramatic changes in both the structure and function of his brain. In fact, if he'd known the danger signs for which to be on the lookout, he would have realized that the euphoric effect derived from cocaine use is itself a sure sign that the drug is inducing a change in the brain—just as he would have known that as time passes, and the drug is used with increasing regularity, this change becomes more pronounced, and indelible, until finally his brain has become addicted to the drug.

And so, despite his heartfelt vow never again to use cocaine, he continues using it. Again and again.

"Oops: How Casual Drug Use Leads to Addiction," by Alan I. Leshner, PhD, Director of National Institute of Drug Abuse (NIDA), National Institutes of Health (NIH), May 2003.

His drug use is now beyond his control. It is compulsive. He is addicted.

While this turn of events is a shock to the drug user, it is no surprise at all to researchers who study the effects of addictive drugs. To them, it is a predictable outcome.

To be sure, no one ever starts out using drugs intending to become a drug addict. All drug users are just trying it, once or a few times. Every drug user starts out as an occasional user, and that initial use is a voluntary and controllable decision. But as time passes and drug use continues, a person goes from being a voluntary to a compulsive drug user. This change occurs because over time, use of addictive drugs changes the brain—at times in big dramatic toxic ways, at others in more subtle ways, but always in destructive ways that can result in compulsive and even uncontrollable drug use.

The fact is, drug addiction is a brain disease. While every type of drug of abuse has its own individual "trigger" for affecting or transforming the brain, many of the results of the transformation are strikingly similar regardless of the addictive drug that is used—and of course in each instance the result is compulsive use. The brain changes range from fundamental and long-lasting changes in the biochemical makeup of the brain, to mood changes, to changes in memory processes and motor skills. And these changes have a tremendous impact on all aspects of a person's behavior. In fact, in addiction the drug becomes the single most powerful motivator in the life of the drug user. He will do virtually anything for the drug.

This unexpected consequence of drug use is what I have come to call the oops phenomenon. Why oops? Because the harmful outcome is in no way intentional. Just as no one starts out to have lung cancer when they smoke, or no one starts out to have clogged arteries when they eat fried foods that in turn usually cause heart attacks, no one starts out to become a drug addict when they use drugs. But in each case, though no one meant to behave in a way that would lead to tragic health consequences, that is what happened just the same, because of the inexorable, and undetected, destructive biochemical processes at work.

While we haven't yet pinpointed precisely all the triggers for the changes in the brain's structure and function that culminate in the "oops" phenomenon, a vast body of hard evidence shows that it is virtually inevitable that prolonged drug use will lead to addiction. From this we can soundly conclude that drug addiction is indeed a brain disease.

I realize that this flies in the face of the notion that drug addiction boils down to a serious character flaw—that those addicted to drugs are just too weak-willed to quit drug use on their own. But the moral weakness notion itself flies in the face of all scientific evidence, and so it should be discarded.

It should be stressed, however, that to assert that drug addiction is a brain disease is by no means the same thing as saying that those addicted to drugs are not accountable for their actions, or that they are just unwitting, hapless victims of the harmful effects that use of addictive drugs has on their brains, and in every facet of their lives.

Just as their behavior at the outset was pivotal in putting them on a collision course with compulsive drug use, their behavior after becoming addicted is just as critical if they are to be effectively treated and to recover.

At minimum, they have to adhere to their drug treatment regimen. But this can pose an enormous challenge. The changes in their brain that turned them into compulsive users make it a daunting enough task to control their actions and complete treatment. Making it even more difficult is the fact that their craving becomes more heightened and irresistible whenever they are exposed to any situation that triggers a memory of the euphoric experience of drug use. Little wonder, then, that most compulsive drug users can't quit on their own, even if they want to (for instance, at most only 7% of those who try in any one year to quit smoking cigarettes on their own actually succeed). This is why it is essential that they enter a drug treatment program, even if they don't want to at the outset.

Clearly, a host of biological and behavioral factors conspires to trigger the oops phenomenon in drug addiction. So the widely held sentiment that drug addiction has to be explained from either the standpoint of biology or the standpoint of behavior, and never the twain shall meet, is terribly flawed. Biological and behavioral explanations of drug abuse must be given equal weight and integrated with each other if we are to gain an in-depth understanding of the root causes of drug addiction and then develop more effective treatments. Modern science has shown us that we reduce one explanation to the other—the behavioral to the biological, or vice versa—at our own peril. We have to recognize that brain disease stemming from drug use cannot and should not be artificially isolated from its behavioral components, as well as its larger social components. They all are critical pieces of the puzzle that interact with and impact on one another at every turn.

A wealth of scientific evidence, by the way, makes it clear that rarely if ever are any forms of brain disease only biological in nature. To the contrary, such brain diseases as stroke, Alzheimer's, Parkinson's, schizophrenia, and clinical depression all have their behavioral and social dimensions. What is unique about the type of brain disease that results from drug abuse is that it starts out as voluntary behavior. But once continued use of an addictive drug brings about structural and functional changes in the brain that cause compulsive use, the disease-ravaged brain of a drug user closely resembles that of people with other kinds of brain diseases.

It's also important to bear in mind that we now see addiction as a chronic, virtually life-long illness for many people. And relapse is a common phenomenon in all forms of chronic illness—from asthma and diabetes, to hypertension and addiction. The goals of successive treatments, as with other chronic illnesses, are to manage the illness and increase the intervals between relapses, until there are no more.

An increasing body of scientific evidence makes the compelling case that the most effective treatment programs for overcoming drug addiction incorporate an array of approaches—from medications, to behavior therapies, to social services and rehabilitation. The National Institute on Drug Abuse recently published *Principles of Effective Drug Addiction Treatment*, which features many of the most promising drug treatment programs to date. As this booklet explains, the programs with the most successful track records treat the whole individual. Their treatment strategies place just as much emphasis on the unique social and behavioral aspects of drug addiction treatment and recovery as on the biological aspects. By doing so, they better enable those who have abused drugs to surmount the unexpected consequences of drug use and once again lead fruitful lives.

Chapter 12

Early Marijuana Use Is Associated with Later Abuse of Other Drugs

Individuals who used marijuana before age 17 years were more likely to use other drugs, abuse drugs, or become dependent on alcohol or other drugs, according to an article in the January 22/29, 2003, issue of *The Journal of the American Medical Association*.

According to background information in the article, in 1999 there were 220,000 marijuana-related admissions to publicly funded substance abuse treatment programs in the United States. This represented 14% of all such treatment admissions, with admissions occurring primarily among youth: approximately one-third of all marijuana-related admissions were for youths aged 12 to 17 years old. The idea that early marijuana use may increase the risk of an individual later using other drugs has been a major cause for concern. This idea, known as the gateway hypothesis, states that there is an order in the progression of drug use, with marijuana use preceding the use of "harder" drugs like cocaine and heroin.

Michael T. Lynskey, Ph.D., of Washington University School of Medicine, St. Louis, and colleagues studied marijuana use and its effects on later drug use among 311 sets of same-sex twins (average age at the start of the study, 30 years old) where only one twin used marijuana before age 17 years. The study was conducted among a national volunteer sample in Australia between 1996 and 2000.

The researchers found that individuals who used marijuana before age 17 had odds of other drug use, alcohol dependence and drug abuse/dependence that were 2.1 to 5.2 times higher than those of their twins who did not use marijuana before age 17. Adjustments to the data for known risk factors for drug abuse, such as early use of alcohol and tobacco, parental conflicts or separation, childhood sexual abuse, conduct disorder, major depression and social anxiety, had little effect on the results. The associations found between marijuana use and other drug and alcohol use did not differ between monozygotic (identical) twins and dizygotic (fraternal) twins.

The researchers write, "The results of our co-twin analysis indicated that early initiation of cannabis use was associated with significantly increased risks for other drug use and abuse/dependence and were consistent with early cannabis use having a causal role as a risk factor for other drug use and for any drug abuse or dependence."

"Associations between early cannabis [marijuana] use and later drug use and abuse/dependence cannot solely be explained by common predisposing genetic or shared environmental factors. The association may arise from the effects of the peer and social context within which cannabis is used and obtained. In particular, early access to the use of cannabis may reduce perceived barriers against the use of other illegal drugs and provide access to these drugs," the authors write.

Editor's Note [in the original document]: This work was supported by U.S. National Institutes of Health grants as well as grants from the National Health and Medical Research Council of Australia.

Editorial: Does Marijuana Use Cause the Use of Other Drugs?

In an accompanying editorial, Denise B Kandel, Ph.D., of Columbia University and New York State Psychiatric Institute, New York, writes "... Lynskey et al find that early marijuana use by itself, even after control for other covariates, increases significantly the use of other illicit drugs. As the authors emphasize, the strength of the twin design is that twins are assumed to share the same environment and family experiences, and monozygotic [identical] pairs share the same genetic risk."

Dr. Kandel writes, "Whether or not a true causal link exists between the use of marijuana and other drugs, the association between the two has been well established. It is important, however, to appreciate that the progression is not inevitable. Not all those who try marijuana will subsequently use cocaine or become heroin addicts. For policy makers, the gateway hypothesis raises two issues depending on whether the population of interest has or has not yet used marijuana. For a population of nonusers, the issue is: will preventing the use of marijuana prevent the use of other illicit drugs?

Hopefully, it will, for prevention efforts will presumably affect the underlying risk and protective factors related to the onset of marijuana use, whether or not these factors are shared with the onset of the use of other illicit drugs. For youths who have already used marijuana, the issue is: can and should intervention programs be developed to target this group at very high risk for progressing to other substances? It appears so. A marijuana user is at risk for using other illicit drugs, and measures to prevent subsequent use of these drugs are warranted."

Chapter 13

Teen Cigarette Smoking and Marijuana Abuse

In 1994, The National Center on Addiction and Substance Abuse (CASA) at Columbia University issued its report, *Cigarettes, Alcohol, Marijuana: Gateways to Illicit Drug Use*, a statistical analysis which found that teens who smoked cigarettes were 12 times likelier to use marijuana and more than 19 times likelier to use cocaine. Similar analyses have also been conducted by a number of distinguished researchers, including Denise Kandel, PhD (1992). In recent years, scientists have found evidence that sheds light on this statistical relationship: studies at the University of Cagliari in Italy, Cumplutense University in Madrid, and Scripps Research Institute in California reveal that marijuana affects levels of dopamine (the substance that gives pleasure) in the brain in a manner similar to nicotine, heroin and cocaine. Dr. Nora Volkow, Director of the National Institute on Drug Abuse, has stated that "cigarette smoking may also facilitate consumption of other drugs." As a smoked drug, cigarettes initiate teens into the sensation of inhaling a drug and desensitize them to the feeling of smoke entering their lungs.

These findings—and their implications for American teenagers—led us to examine how prevalent marijuana was in the life of teenage smokers. As a result, The National Center on Addiction and Substance

Abuse (CASA) at Columbia University and the American Legacy Foundation included in CASA's 2003 back to school survey of 12- to 17-year-olds—the *CASA National Survey of American Attitudes on Substance Abuse VIII: Teens and Parents*—questions regarding the extent to which marijuana is part of the life of a teenage smoker.

This report on the results of this survey by CASA and the American Legacy Foundation finds that marijuana is pervasive in the life of a teenage cigarette smoker. Teens who smoke nicotine cigarettes are 14 times likelier to try marijuana, six times likelier to be able to buy marijuana in an hour or less and 18 times likelier to report that most of their friends smoke marijuana. Among teens who are repeat marijuana users, 60% tried cigarettes first. The findings indicate that reducing teen smoking can be a singularly effective way to reduce teen marijuana use.

There is a powerful message for the administration and Congress in these findings: the media and public service awareness campaigns to prevent teen drug use—such as the National Youth Anti-Drug Media Campaign of the White House Office of National Drug Control Policy and that of the Partnership for a Drug-Free America—should devote a significant amount of their energy and time to discourage cigarette smoking among teens. President George W. Bush last year committed to reduce illegal drug use by 10% over two years and 25% over five years. He can only achieve such dramatic declines by sharp reductions in marijuana use. This report suggests one powerful way to help the administration attain its stated goal. We urge the administration to take advantage of this opportunity and educate the nation on the dangers of tobacco use.

There is also a powerful message for parents in these findings: To the extent that biological activation and desensitization play a role, preventing teen initiation of cigarette use can significantly reduce teen involvement with other drugs—especially drugs that are typically smoked, such as marijuana. This underscores—for parents, teachers, policymakers and anyone else concerned with the welfare of American children—the importance of intervening to end teen cigarette smoking in order to prevent other drug use.

Introduction and Key Findings

For eight years, CASA has been engaged in the unprecedented undertaking of surveying attitudes of teens and those who most influence them—parents, teachers and school principals. While other surveys seek to measure the extent of substance abuse in the population, the *CASA*

National Survey of American Attitudes on Substance Abuse VIII: Teens and Parents probes substance-abuse risk and identifies factors that increase or diminish the likelihood that teens will abuse tobacco, alcohol or illegal drugs. We regard this effort as a work in progress and strive to refine it each year.

This year, for the first time, working with the American Legacy Foundation, CASA asked a series of questions to examine statistical associations between teen cigarette smoking and teen marijuana use.

The troubling findings:

- Teens who smoke cigarettes are 14 times likelier than those who do not to try marijuana.

- Among teens who admit to having tried marijuana, those who do not smoke cigarettes are likelier to have tried marijuana only once.

- Teens who have tried marijuana and are current cigarette smokers are 60% likelier to be repeat (as opposed to one-time) marijuana users.

- Teens who are current cigarette smokers are six times likelier than those who have never smoked cigarettes to report that they can buy marijuana in an hour or less.

- Fifty-five percent of teens who are current cigarette smokers report more than half their friends use marijuana, compared with only 3% of those who have never smoked cigarettes.

- Among teens who are repeat marijuana users, 60% tried cigarettes first.

- Seventy-seven percent of teens believe that a teen who smokes cigarettes is more likely to use marijuana.

Cigarette Smoking and Marijuana

A teen who is a current smoker (i.e., one who smoked within the past 30 days) is 14 times likelier to try marijuana than a teen who has never smoked cigarettes (84% vs. 6%). A teen who is a current smoker is almost twice as likely to try marijuana than a teen who has tried cigarettes but is not a current smoker (84% vs. 45%).

Of teens who have tried marijuana once, 20% are current cigarette smokers. Of teens who are repeat marijuana users, 43% are current cigarette smokers.

Among teens who have tried marijuana:

- 57% smoked cigarettes first;
- 29% have not smoked cigarettes;
- 13% smoked cigarettes at about the same time or after they tried marijuana.

Thus, a 50% reduction in teen cigarette smoking could effect a substantial reduction in teen marijuana use—as much as 16.5% to 28.5%. The high end of the range assumes that half of the 57% of teens who smoked cigarettes first would not have smoked marijuana if they had not smoked cigarettes. The low end assumes that 42% of the 57% of teens who smoked cigarettes first might use marijuana even if they had not smoked cigarettes first.

Repeat Marijuana Use More Common among Teens Who Smoke Cigarettes

Among teens who have tried marijuana, some have tried marijuana only once and others are repeat marijuana users. Whether a teen is a one-time user or a repeat user of marijuana is associated with the teen's cigarette smoking experience.

Among those teens who have tried marijuana and are current cigarette smokers, 62% are repeat marijuana users and 38% used marijuana only once. The results flip when the teens are not current smokers: Among teens who have tried marijuana and have also tried cigarettes but are not current cigarette smokers, 38% are repeat marijuana users and 60% used marijuana only once. Among teens who have tried marijuana but have never smoked cigarettes, 31% are repeat marijuana users and 67% used marijuana only once.

Teens who are repeat marijuana users are likely to have started by smoking nicotine cigarettes: Among teens who are repeat marijuana users, 60% tried cigarettes first.

Availability of Marijuana

Marijuana is a pervasive presence for those teens who smoke cigarettes. Seventy-six percent of those teens who are current cigarette smokers can buy marijuana in an hour or less. Thirty-six percent of those teens who have tried cigarettes but are not current smokers can buy marijuana in an hour or less. Thirteen percent of teens who have never smoked cigarettes can buy marijuana in an hour or less.

Teen current cigarette smokers are more likely than teen nonsmokers to report that most of their friends use marijuana. Fifty-five percent of teen smokers report that more than half of their friends use marijuana, compared with 15% of those teens who have tried cigarettes but are not current smokers and 3% of those teens who have never smoked.

Teen Perceptions about Cigarette Smoking and Marijuana Use

Teens perceive a connection between cigarette smoking and marijuana use: When asked whether they think that a teen who smokes cigarettes is more likely to use marijuana, 77% respond in the affirmative.

Cigarette Smoking and Drugs in Schools

Drugs Are Likelier to Be Used, Kept, or Sold at Schools where Smoking Occurs

In schools where smoking occurs, 36% are drug free (i.e., schools where drugs are not used, kept or sold) and 62% are not drug free. In schools where smoking cigarettes on school grounds is not tolerated, 73% are drug free and 26% are not.

Chapter 14

Stress and Drug Abuse

Stress—What Is It?

- Stress is a term we all know and use often, but what does it really mean? It is hard to define because it means different things to different people. Stress is a normal reaction to life for people of all ages. It is caused by our body's instinct to protect itself from emotional or physical pressure or, in extreme situations, from danger.

- Stressors differ for each of us. What is stressful for one person may or may not be stressful for another; each of us responds to stress in an entirely different way. How a person copes with stress—by reaching for a beer or cigarette or by heading to the gym—also plays an important role in the impact that stress will have on our bodies.

- By using their own support systems, some people are able to cope effectively with the emotional and physical demands brought on by stressful and traumatic experiences. However, individuals who experience prolonged reactions to stress that disrupt their daily functioning may benefit from consulting with a trained and experienced mental health professional.

"NIDA Community Drug Alert Bulletin: Stress and Substance Abuse," National Institute on Drug Abuse (NIDA), National Institutes of Health (NIH) January 2002.

The Body's Response to Stress

- The stress response is mediated by a highly complex, integrated network that involves the central nervous system, the adrenal system, the immune system, and the cardiovascular system.

- Stress activates adaptive responses. It releases the neurotransmitter norepinephrine, which is involved with memory. This may be why people remember stressful events more clearly than they do nonstressful situations.

- Stress also increases the production of a hormone in the body known as corticotropin releasing factor (CRF). CRF is found throughout the brain and initiates our biological response to stressors. During all negative experiences, certain regions of the brain show increased levels of CRF. Interestingly, almost all drugs of abuse have also been found to increase CRF levels, which suggests a neurobiological connection between stress and drug abuse.

- Mild stress may cause changes that are useful. For example, stress can actually improve our attention and increase our capacity to store and integrate important and life-protecting information. But if stress is prolonged or chronic, those changes can become harmful.

Stress and Drug Abuse

- Stressful events may influence profoundly the use of alcohol or other drugs. Stress is a major contributor to the initiation and continuation of addiction to alcohol or other drugs, as well as to relapse or a return to drug use after periods of abstinence.

- Stress is one of the major factors known to cause relapse to smoking, even after prolonged periods of abstinence.

- Children exposed to severe stress may be more vulnerable to drug use. A number of clinical and epidemiological studies show a strong association between psychosocial stressors early in life (e.g., parental loss, child abuse) and an increased risk for depression, anxiety, impulsive behavior, and substance abuse in adulthood.

144

Stress, Drugs, and Vulnerable Populations

- Stressful experiences increase the vulnerability of an individual to relapse to drugs even after prolonged abstinence.

- Individuals who have achieved abstinence from drugs must continue to sustain their abstinence—avoiding environmental triggers, recognizing their psychosocial and emotional triggers, and developing healthy behaviors to handle life's stresses.

- A number of relapse prevention approaches have been developed to help clinicians address relapse. Treatment techniques that foster coping skills, problem-solving skills, and social support play a role in successful treatment.

- Physicians should be aware of what medications their patients are taking but should not discourage the use of medical prescriptions to help alleviate stress. Some people may need medications for stress-related symptoms or for treatment of depression and anxiety.

What Is PTSD?

- Post-traumatic stress disorder (PTSD) is an anxiety disorder that can develop in some people after exposure to a terrifying event or ordeal in which grave physical harm occurred or was threatened.

- Generally, PTSD has been associated with the violence of modern combat. However, many people other than combat soldiers are susceptible. PTSD can result from many kinds of tragic incidents in which the patient was a witness, victim, or survivor, including violent or personal attacks, natural or human-caused disasters, or accidents.

- Symptoms of PTSD can include re-experience of the trauma; emotional numbness; avoidance of people, places, and thoughts connected to the event; and arousal, which may include trouble sleeping, exaggerated startle response, and hypervigilance.

- PTSD can occur in people of any age, including children and adolescents.

PTSD and Substance Abuse

- An emerging body of research has documented a very strong association between PTSD and substance abuse. In most cases, substance use begins after the exposure to trauma and the development of PTSD, thus making PTSD a risk factor for drug abuse.

- Early intervention to help children and adolescents who have suffered trauma from violence or a disaster is critical. Children who witness or are exposed to a traumatic event and are clinically diagnosed with PTSD have a greater likelihood for developing later drug and/or alcohol use disorders.

- Of individuals with substance use disorders, 30% to 60% meet the criteria for comorbid PTSD.

- Patients with substance abuse disorders tend to suffer from more severe PTSD symptoms than do PTSD patients without substance use disorders.

Helping Those Who Suffer from PTSD and Drug Abuse

- Health care professionals must be alert to the fact that PTSD frequently co-occurs with depression, anxiety disorders, and alcohol or other substance abuse. Patients who are experiencing the symptoms of PTSD need support from physicians and health care providers.

- The likelihood of treatment success increases when these concurrent disorders are appropriately identified and treated as well.

- In some cases, medications such as the antidepressant sertraline (Zoloft™), have been shown to be helpful in treating patients who suffer from PTSD and substance use disorders.

- Some reports suggest that successful detoxification of these comorbid patients will likely require inpatient admission to permit vigorous control of withdrawal and PTSD-related arousal symptoms.

- Although there is no standardized, effective treatment developed for individuals with this disorder, studies show that patients who suffer from PTSD can improve with cognitive behavioral therapy, group therapy, or exposure therapy, in which the patient gradually and repeatedly relives the frightening experience under controlled conditions to help him or her work through the trauma.

- Exposure therapy is thought to be one of the most effective ways to manage PTSD when it is conducted by a trained therapist. It has not yet been widely used with comorbid disorders, but recent studies suggest that some individuals with PTSD and comorbid cocaine addiction can be successfully treated with exposure therapy. Patients in a recent study who suffered from both disorders showed significant reductions in all PTSD symptoms and in overall cocaine use.

- Finally, support from family and friends can play an important role in recovery.

Chapter 15

The Addicted Brain: Why Such Poor Decisions?

One central puzzle haunts any consideration of drug addiction, for research scientists as well as for the rest of the population: Why do men and women who have developed addiction obsessively seek and use drugs, even after the drugs no longer produce pleasure? Why do individuals who are addicted to drugs persist in behavior that damages their health and corrodes the quality of their lives? How can they make such poor decisions?

We are far from having complete answers to these questions, but National Institute on Drug Abuse (NIDA)-sponsored research has begun to provide clues that might lead to answers. We are beginning to understand that drugs exert persistent neurobiological effects that extend beyond the midbrain centers of pleasure and reward to disrupt the function of the brain's frontal cortex—the thinking region of the brain, where risks and benefits are weighed and decisions made.

The exploration of drugs' effects on decision making is a logical extension of NIDA's decades-long scientific inquiry into the neurobiology of drug abuse and addiction, which was the focus of a two-day symposium held in May to honor the accomplishments of the late Dr. Roger Brown, associate director for neuroscience in NIDA's Division of Neuroscience and Behavioral Research. Many of the presentations

By Nora Volkow, M.D., Director of National Institute on Drug Abuse (NIDA), National Institutes of Health (NIH), *NIDA Notes*, Vol. 18, No. 4 (November 2003).

given at that meeting summarized research that has led to our detailed understanding of crucial midbrain dopamine pathways in the ventral tegmental area and nucleus accumbens, where drugs trigger pleasure and establish reinforcement—the desire to repeat the behavior that produces the pleasure.

Other presentations described changes in distribution and density of dopamine receptors in the frontal cortex in animals and humans after drug use. Still other presentations depicted the network of neural circuits that use dopamine and other neurotransmitters to maintain finely tuned two-way communication among brain regions. These networks allow the midbrain regions, where drugs act as reinforcers, to influence and be influenced by the frontal cortical regions, the site of control over motivation, behavior, and inhibition. Taken together, these presentations sketch a rough outline of addiction as an integrated process that may explain how exposure to a drug triggers changes throughout the brain, leading from initial intoxication and reinforcement through craving to compulsive, continued drug use despite destructive consequences.

NIDA-supported research has established that the brain's frontal regions, in particular the orbitofrontal cortex, play a role in all stages of the development of addiction. For example, imaging studies conducted within NIDA's Intramural Research Program (IRP) and at Harvard Medical School show changes in cortical blood flow during initial drug exposure. Research described in this issue shows that drug addiction is associated with altered cortical activity and decision making that appears to overvalue reward, undervalue risk, and fail to learn from repeated errors.

These recent studies illustrate the similarity of addiction to some disorders that are not associated with drugs. For example, compulsive behavior and poor choices are hallmarks of obsessive-compulsive disorder and pathological gambling. These disorders, too, are characterized by disruption of the frontal brain's capacity for reason and control. NIDA and the National Institute of Mental Health are collaborating to investigate such commonalities by developing new chemical "labels" that will allow us to use brain imaging techniques to study in more detail the structure and activity of frontal brain regions in patients suffering addiction or other decision-making disorders.

The emerging picture of addiction as a disease of compulsion and disrupted control (the frontal brain) and not merely pursuit of pleasure (the midbrain) suggests new possibilities for treatment. The neural networks that link brain regions—particularly the interwoven connections between the ventral tegmental area, nucleus accumbens, and prefrontal cortex—may offer targets for pharmacological therapies to modulate signaling that results in compulsive behavior or destructive choice.

Studying the role of frontal brain function also will contribute to development of new behavioral therapies, which help patients recognize conditions that trigger drug craving and alter their behavior to resist the compulsion. Investigators can test these cognitive-behavioral therapies in the same way, and with the same patients, that they have employed to study craving and decision making—through imaging that provides real-time images of the functioning brain.

How do drugs lead to such destructive decisions? Answering this question will not answer all questions about drug abuse and addiction. It will not tell us what role genetics or environment plays in the progression from initial pleasure to crippling compulsion. It will not explain whether a dysfunction in decision making predisposes one person to drug use, while in another person drug use triggers such a dysfunction. But looking for the answer will bring us closer to developing a comprehensive understanding of addiction and, more important, closer to more effective treatment for men and women whose lives are diminished by decisions that bring only harm.

Chapter 16

Exploring Myths about Drug Addiction

Myth: Drug addiction is voluntary behavior.

A person starts out as an occasional drug user, and that is a voluntary decision. But as times passes, something happens, and that person goes from being a voluntary drug user to being a compulsive drug user. Why? Because over time, continued use of addictive drugs changes your brain—at times in dramatic, toxic ways, at others in more subtle ways, but virtually always in ways that result in compulsive and even uncontrollable drug use.

Myth: More than anything else, drug addiction is a character flaw.

Drug addiction is a brain disease. Every type of drug of abuse has its own individual mechanism for changing how the brain functions. But regardless of which drug a person is addicted to, many of the effects it has on the brain are similar: they range from changes in the molecules and cells that make up the brain, to mood changes, to changes in memory processes and in such motor skills as walking and talking. And these changes have a huge influence on all aspects of a person's behavior. The drug becomes the single most powerful motivator in a drug abuser's existence. He or she will do almost anything

"Exploring Myths about Drug Abuse," by Alan I. Leshner, PhD, Director, National Institute on Drug Abuse (NIDA), National Institutes of Health (NIH), January 2001.

for the drug. This comes about because drug use has changed the individual's brain and its functioning in critical ways.

Myth: You have to want drug treatment for it to be effective.

Virtually no one wants drug treatment. Two of the primary reasons people seek drug treatment are because the court ordered them to do so, or because loved ones urged them to seek treatment. Many scientific studies have shown convincingly that those who enter drug treatment programs in which they face "high pressure" to confront and attempt to surmount their addiction do comparatively better in treatment, regardless of the reason they sought treatment in the first place.

Myth: Treatment for drug addiction should be a one-shot deal.

Like many other illnesses, drug addiction typically is a chronic disorder. To be sure, some people can quit drug use "cold turkey," or they can quit after receiving treatment just one time at a rehabilitation facility. But most of those who abuse drugs require longer-term treatment and, in many instances, repeated treatments.

Myth: We should strive to find a "magic bullet" to treat all forms of drug abuse.

There is no "one size fits all" form of drug treatment, much less a magic bullet that suddenly will cure addiction. Different people have different drug abuse-related problems. And they respond very differently to similar forms of treatment, even when they're abusing the same drug. As a result, drug addicts need an array of treatments and services tailored to address their unique needs.

Chapter 17

Eating Disorders and Drug Abuse

For the past three years, The National Center on Addiction and Substance Abuse (CASA) at Columbia University has been examining the link between substance abuse and eating disorders. The result of this intensive study—the most comprehensive ever undertaken on the subject—is this report, *Food for Thought: Substance Abuse and Eating Disorders*. The findings are deeply troubling.

Individuals with eating disorders are up to five times likelier to abuse alcohol or illicit drugs and those who abuse alcohol or illicit drugs are up to 11 times likelier to have eating disorders.

Both problems afflict the very young and quickly spiral out of control. High school girls with eating disorder symptoms are much likelier to smoke cigarettes, drink alcohol or use drugs than those without such symptoms. Girls who smoke, drink or use drugs are much likelier to report past month eating disorder symptoms than those who do not use such substances.

Even middle-school girls—typically age 10 to 14—who have dieted in the previous month and evidence no eating pathology are almost twice as likely to become smokers as nondieters. Girls this age who report dieting more than once a week are nearly four times likelier to become smokers compared to nondieters. The more severely girls and young woman diet, the more likely they are to drink frequently and heavily as well as to use marijuana and other illicit drugs.

People with eating disorders abuse caffeine, tobacco, alcohol, amphetamines, cocaine, heroin, and over-the-counter medications such as diuretics, emetics or laxatives to suppress appetite, increase metabolism, and purge themselves. Substance abuse also occurs in people with eating disorders who are trying to self-medicate the negative feelings and emotions that typically accompany such disorders.

Eating disorders and substance abuse have a number of characteristics in common. Shared risk factors for these disorders include common brain chemistry and common family history; both emerge in times of stress or transition; both are more likely to develop in individuals with low self-esteem, depression, anxiety or a history of physical or sexual abuse; and both may be influenced by unhealthy parental substance use or dieting behaviors, social pressures, and the advertising, marketing, and entertainment industries.

Other shared characteristics of the disorders include an obsessive preoccupation with a substance (food or a drug), intense craving, compulsive behavior, attempts to keep the problem a secret, social isolation, and risk for suicide. The two disorders also have similar effects on the brain and both are linked to other psychiatric disorders such as obsessive-compulsive disorder and mood disorders. Finally, both are chronic, recurring, life-threatening diseases.

In America the message that one can never be too thin broadcasts loud and clear to millions of women and adolescent girls. Many products, including tobacco and weight loss drugs, are marketed to women and girls as passkeys to beauty, joy, success—and slimness.

This report constitutes the most extensive analysis of the current state of knowledge on the link between eating disorders and substance abuse. The findings are based on CASA's analyses of national data sets and on a review of nearly 500 articles, books, and reports from the most current scientific literature available addressing these issues.

Key Findings

Up to 50% of individuals with an eating disorder abuse alcohol or illicit drugs compared to approximately 9% in the general population. Up to 35% of alcohol or illicit drug abusers have an eating disorder compared to up to 3% in the general population.

Although rates of eating disorders are relatively low, disordered weight-related attitudes and behaviors are rampant. Teenage girls are particularly vulnerable. While only 15% of teenage girls and boys can be classified as overweight:

- 62.3% of teenage girls report trying to lose weight (compared to 28.8% of teenage boys), 58.6% are actively dieting (compared to 28.2% of boys) and 68.4% exercise with the goal of losing weight or to avoid gaining weight (compared to 51% of boys).

- 19.1% of teenage girls fast for 24 hours or more (compared to 7.6% of teenage boys), 12.6% use diet pills, powders, or liquids (compared to 5.5% of boys) and 7.8% vomit or take laxatives to lose weight or to avoid gaining weight (compared to 2.9% of boys).

Many individuals who engage in unhealthy weight-control behaviors or have full-blown eating disorders use or abuse substances such as caffeine, tobacco, alcohol, cocaine, heroin, and over-the-counter medications such as appetite suppressants, diuretics, laxatives, and emetics.

- Caffeine is used to alleviate hunger or boost energy. People with eating disorders often consume large amounts of diet sodas, which frequently are high in caffeine content.

- People with eating disorders smoke cigarettes to suppress their appetite and provide themselves with an alternative oral activity to eating. The link between smoking and weight concerns can be seen in girls and women of all ages.

- Alcohol abuse is common in people with eating disorders, particularly bulimia. Bulimic women who are alcohol dependent report a higher rate of suicide attempts, anxiety disorders, personality disorders, conduct disorder, and other substance dependence than bulimic women who are not alcohol dependent.

- Illicit drug use is particularly common among bulimics. Drugs such as heroin and cocaine are used to facilitate weight loss by suppressing appetite, increasing metabolism and purging.

- In addition to appetite suppressants, other over-the-counter medications that are used by people with eating disorders—often inappropriately to facilitate purging—include diuretics, emetics, and laxatives.

Like substance abuse, the adverse effects of eating disorders are well documented and often quite severe, ranging from hair loss, tooth decay, and osteoporosis to heart failure and a destabilization of virtually all body systems. Severe cases may be fatal.

Eating disorders occur in five to 10 million Americans, mostly girls and young women. Although white, upper-middle class girls and young women are the primary victims, the population afflicted by these disorders is becoming more diverse.

- Hispanic girls report some symptoms of eating disorders—such as fasting, vomiting, and taking laxatives to lose weight or to avoid gaining weight—at higher rates than white or black girls.

- Eating disorders appear to be on the rise among middle-aged women and preadolescent girls.

- Approximately one million boys and men suffer from eating disorders and this number is growing; a high proportion of males with eating disorders are gay.

Western culture idealizes thin women and, as a result, many women equate being thin with self-worth. The advertising, marketing and entertainment industries, which inundate adults and children with iconic images of thin beauty, have become a major force in the development of women's body dissatisfaction and disordered eating attitudes and behaviors.

Women's magazines contain 10.5 times more ads and articles related to weight loss than men's magazines—the same sex ratio reported for eating disorders. While the average American woman is 5'4" tall and weighs approximately 140 pounds, the average model is 5'11" tall and weighs 117 pounds.

The commercial world, including the diet, cigarette, and alcohol industries, have not shied away from targeting women's desire to be thin in order to promote their products. In particular, the tobacco companies understood the relationship between smoking and weight control long before the public health experts.

- The 1920s Lucky Strike cigarette advertising campaign encouraged women to "reach for a Lucky instead of a sweet." The Virginia Slims brand tagline was "slimmer, longer, not like those fat cigarettes men smoke." The slogan for Misty cigarettes is "slim n' sassy." Capri cigarette ads claim, "there's no slimmer way to smoke" and call Capri cigarettes "the slimmest slim in town."

Unfortunately, public health professionals, including prevention and treatment specialists are way behind the commercial industries in recognizing the link between substance use and disordered eating. This report demonstrates clearly that it is time for action by health professionals.

What Parents Can Do

To help prevent eating disorders and substance abuse in their children, parents should model and promote healthy, positive and reasonable messages about eating and exercise as well as consistent messages about the dangers of substance use.

What Schools Can Do

Schools should make it a priority to educate parents, teachers, administrators and coaches to recognize the relationship of eating disorders and substance abuse and intervene quickly and effectively.

What Health Professionals Can Do

The public health community, including doctors, dentists, nurses, and prevention and treatment specialists, should educate their patients and the public about nutrition and the negative health effects of eating disorders and substance abuse.

The link between eating disorders and substance abuse is not well understood and often is overlooked by health care professionals. Health care practitioners should routinely screen all patients for both of these disorders so that they can catch them in time and get patients who need it into treatment. Unfortunately, despite their high rates of co-occurrence, few treatment programs exist that address both eating disorders and substance abuse simultaneously and effectively. Prevention programs that target both disorders are rare as well.

What the Advertising, Marketing and Entertainment Industries Can Do

Many commercial industries, including the diet and fashion industries, prey on women's weight concerns to market their products. When this type of marketing approach is used by the tobacco and alcohol industries, it is particularly pernicious given the serious health consequences associated with the abuse of their products. Tobacco and alcohol companies should refrain from linking smoking and drinking to unrealistically thin images of women. The entertainment industry, including television, film and music, also should refrain from making positive associations between thinness and smoking, drinking, and using drugs.

What Policymakers Can Do

Policymakers should increase public awareness about the connection between substance abuse and eating disorders and inform the public about how to recognize the warning signs of these disorders and how best to help combat unhealthy societal messages. Managed care program policies should be modified to cover both mental and physical health treatments for substance use and eating disorders.

What Researchers Can Do

More research is needed on the genetic and biological bases of substance use and eating disorders as well as on co-occurring psychiatric disorders. Research also is needed to develop new and better approaches to preventing, assessing, diagnosing, and treating substance use and eating disorders.

Substance Abuse and Eating Disorders: What Is the Link and Who Is at Risk?

Eating disorders, which include anorexia nervosa, bulimia nervosa and binge eating disorder, affect more than five million Americans. Millions more display some configuration of symptoms, if not the full-blown disorder. Eating disorders can have devastating physical and mental health consequences, not the least of which is the increased potential for substance use and abuse. Between 30% and 50% of individuals with bulimia and between 12% and 18% of those with anorexia abuse or are dependent on alcohol or drugs, compared to approximately 9% in the general population. Up to 35% of individuals who abuse or are dependent on alcohol or drugs also have an eating disorder, compared to up to 3% in the general population. Girls and young women are particularly vulnerable to the development of eating disorders, but the problem is increasing among males and racial/ethnic minorities.

Co-Occurring Eating Disorders and Substance Abuse

When an individual demonstrates distorted or extreme weight-related attitudes or behaviors or when extreme weight control measures occur among those who are not overweight, it may signal a pathological eating disorder.

The substances most frequently abused by individuals with eating disorders or with sub-clinical symptoms of these disorders include: caffeine, tobacco, alcohol, laxatives, emetics, diuretics, appetite suppressants (amphetamines), heroin, and cocaine.

Anorexia Nervosa

Anorexia nervosa is a disorder characterized by the pursuit of thinness and refusal to maintain weight at or above a minimally acceptable standard for age and height. Anorexia typically develops in adolescent girls and is characterized by the denial of illness, an overriding and irrational fear of becoming overweight, and a distorted perception of body image. Although the most common ages of onset of anorexia nervosa are the mid-teens, up to 5% of anorexic patients experience the onset of the disorder in their early 20s, increasing numbers of adults are seeking treatment for it, and more and more preadolescents are exhibiting early signs of the disorder.

Anorexia occurs in about 0.5% to 1% of women in the general population, and 10 to 20 times more often in females than in males. The incidence of anorexia nervosa has increased in the past 30 years both in the United States and Western Europe.

Bulimia Nervosa

Bulimia nervosa, which only was recognized as diagnostically distinct from anorexia nervosa in 1980, is characterized by recurrent episodes of binge eating and vomiting, laxative use, fasting, and/or excessive exercise to counteract the binge eating.

Bulimia nervosa typically is accompanied by feelings of being out of control and unable to voluntarily stop eating. Unlike patients with anorexia nervosa, those with bulimia often maintain a normal body weight, making it more difficult to detect the disease. About one-fourth to one-third of bulimia nervosa patients have had a previous history of anorexia nervosa. The onset of bulimia often occurs later in adolescence than anorexia or in early adulthood. Individuals, ages 12 to 35, are prime candidates for bulimia, with an average age of onset of 18.

161

Bulimia is more prevalent than anorexia nervosa and occurs in approximately 1% to 3% of young women. Like anorexia, bulimia is significantly more common in females than in males. More than one in 10 girls in grades nine through 12 (11.4%) and almost one in every 20 boys of the same age (4.7%) have at least four of the five symptoms of the disorder. In addition to the full-blown disorder, symptoms of bulimia, such as occasional episodes of binge eating and purging, occur in up to 40% of college women.

Other Types of Eating Disorders

Individuals with disordered eating symptoms or behaviors who do not meet the full diagnostic criteria for either anorexia or bulimia are classified as having an "eating disorder not otherwise specified." Some of these individuals have symptoms of both anorexia and bulimia (sometimes referred to as being bulimirexic) but do not meet the full diagnostic criteria for either one; nevertheless, they often suffer greatly from their disorder.

Binge eating disorder, another type of eating disorder, is similar to bulimia in that it involves a pattern of eating excessive amounts of food in one sitting. However, individuals with binge eating disorder are not obsessed with body shape and weight and do not engage in purging, but they do tend to feel anxious about the amount of food consumed.

The majority of persons with binge eating disorder are obese. Obesity is a growing problem in the United States. Approximately 64% of American adults are either overweight or obese and 15% of children, ages six to 19 years, are overweight. Although obese individuals may demonstrate certain addictive qualities (e.g., compulsive behavior, substance-seeking behavior) and brain chemistry (e.g., low dopamine receptor levels) as individuals who are addicted to drugs, they appear to be less likely than individuals without a binge eating disorder to abuse illicit drugs.

Eating Disorders and Caffeine Use

Individuals with eating disorders or eating disorder symptoms may rely on coffee or caffeinated diet beverages to help alleviate hunger and boost energy. An eight-ounce serving of brewed coffee contains 135 milligrams of caffeine, an eight-ounce serving of diet Mountain Dew contains 37 milligrams of caffeine and an eight-ounce serving of Diet Coke contains even more caffeine than regular Coke (31 milligrams compared to 23 milligrams). Regular caffeine use may result in tolerance and withdrawal symptoms—effects that may be exacerbated in low-weight women and men who drink large amounts of diet, caffeinated beverages.

Data from a survey of girls and young women conducted for CASA's report, *The Formative Years: Pathways to Substance Abuse Among Girls and Young Women Ages 8–22*, indicate that girls and young women who drink coffee with caffeine are significantly likelier than those who do not to report that they are trying to lose weight (35.9% vs. 25.1%) or that they take diet pills to help them control their weight (15.7% vs. 6%). The data also indicate that girls and young women who take diet pills to help them control their weight drink coffee more frequently than those who do not take diet pills.

Eating Disorders and Tobacco Use

Dieting and eating disorder symptoms are strongly related to smoking. Weight loss is an important motivational factor for smoking, particularly among girls and young women. Smoking not only suppresses appetite, but also provides an alternative oral activity to eating, which is particularly enticing to individuals with eating disorders who often are obsessed with food. Recent research, however, contradicts the popular belief among girls that smoking enhances weight loss. In one study, teens who initiated smoking actually demonstrated an increase in body mass index (BMI) for up to two years after initiation. Furthermore, no difference was found in average body weight between teens who smoked for three or more years and those who never smoked. Finally, teens who were followed for up to three years after initiating smoking demonstrated no significant reductions in their body weight.

Among adolescent girls with eating disorders, those who smoke have the highest levels of eating disordered thoughts and attitudes. Smoking is common among bulimics—even more so than among anorexics—and it is particularly prevalent in people with bulimia who vomit as a compensatory behavior for caloric intake.

Even nondisordered weight-control behaviors significantly increase the risk of smoking, perhaps because of the perceived weight loss benefits of smoking. Teen girls who smoke report greater body image concerns than nonsmokers. Conversely, adolescent girls who have a poor body image and who engage in disordered weight control behaviors are more than four times likelier to initiate smoking as other girls.

Weight concerns are related to smoking in the long-term as well. Girls who report trying to lose weight at ages 11 or 12 are approximately twice as likely to engage in daily smoking in their late teens. Over the course of one year, 10- to 15-year-old girls and boys with strong weight concerns were approximately twice as likely to begin smoking as those less concerned about their weight. Middle-school girls who are "normal" dieters—dieting once per week or less in the previous month and showing no signs of eating pathology—are almost twice as likely to become smokers as nondieters. Girls this age who report more frequent dieting (i.e., more than once per week) are nearly four times likelier to become smokers compared to nondieters.

Girls and young women who smoke to suppress their appetite are a potential group of new nicotine addicts, making females who are concerned about their weight particularly vulnerable targets for the tobacco industry.

Females who smoke are more than twice as likely as males to cite weight concerns as a reason not to quit. Young women also are far more likely than young men to report weight gain as a cause of smoking relapse. In one study of college students, 39% of female students and 25% of male students stated that smoking was a dieting strategy. Among those in this study who attempted to quit smoking, 20% of females and 7% of males cited weight gain as the reason for relapse.

Eating Disorders and Alcohol Use

Extensive research documents an association between eating disorders and alcohol misuse and abuse. This relationship can be found across the continuum from chronic dieting to full-blown eating disorders. The prevalence of alcohol abuse in females with eating disorders is much higher than in the general female population and, conversely, females with alcohol use disorders report eating-disordered behavior more often than the general population.

The relationship between alcohol use and abuse and eating disorders appears to be strongest for individuals with bulimia nervosa and the combination can be particularly damaging. Bulimic women who also are alcohol dependent report a higher rate of suicide attempts, anxiety disorders, personality disorders (such as borderline and histrionic personality disorders), conduct disorder, and other substance dependence than bulimic women who are not alcohol dependent.

Even nondisordered weight-control behaviors are related to alcohol use and abuse. Preadolescent and early adolescent girls who report being highly concerned about their weight are nearly twice as likely to begin getting drunk as girls who are less concerned about their weight. The reverse pattern is also true. Girls who have a history of getting drunk are at approximately three times the risk of beginning to purge in order to control their weight as girls who have never consumed enough alcohol to get drunk.

Girls who drink more alcohol are significantly likelier to perceive themselves as overweight, to want to lose weight and to engage in unhealthy dieting behaviors, such as fasting, taking diet pills, vomiting or taking laxatives. CASA's report, *The Formative Years: Pathways to Substance Abuse Among Girls and Young Women Ages 8–22*, indicates that girls who engaged in unhealthy dieting behaviors, such as fasting, taking diet pills, or bingeing and purging, reported drinking significantly more alcohol than nondieters.

The more severely a young woman diets, the more likely she is to use alcohol. A study of incoming female college freshmen showed that 72% of at-risk and bulimic dieters reported using alcohol in the past month compared to 44% of those who did not diet. Another study found that chronic dieters may not drink more frequently than other women, but when they do drink they consume significantly greater quantities of alcohol. Although excessive dieting generally is related to restraint from alcohol use because of the high caloric content of alcohol, when a chronic dieter who significantly restricts food intake does consume alcohol, she is at greater risk for binge drinking than a woman who engages in less dietary restraint.

Eating Disorders and the Misuse of Over-the-Counter Medications

Individuals with eating disorders often resort to prescription and over-the-counter (OTC) drugs to reduce water retention rapidly or to induce purging. In 2001, 12.6% of female high school students reported that in the previous month they had taken diet pills, powders, or liquids without a doctor's advice to lose weight or to keep from gaining weight.

Diuretics, which are available both OTC and in prescription form, are used to increase urination and reduce water retention. Diuretics are considered safe when used within the recommended guidelines but when used in large quantities, they can produce nausea, vomiting, and gastrointestinal distress. Tolerance develops with repeated use and withdrawal symptoms may occur when stopped.

Some individuals with eating disorders use emetic agents—substances that induce vomiting—to control their weight. A common drug of this type is syrup of ipecac, a readily available OTC substance. Ipecac produces short-term weight reduction but when used frequently, it can result in muscle weakness, nausea and excessive vomiting or diarrhea. Because it remains in the body for a long time, repeated use can result in toxic buildup that can produce severe and even lethal gastrointestinal, cardiac, and neuromuscular complications.

The use of laxatives—drugs that relieve constipation—also is common among individuals with bulimia (and among anorexics of the binge eating/purging type). Bulimics (and some anorexics) self-administer laxatives to lose weight and reduce feelings of bloating following bingeing. Common complaints of individuals abusing laxatives include diarrhea, weakness, abdominal pain, nausea, and dehydration. Both tolerance and withdrawal occur with repeated laxative use. Though rare, chronic abuse of laxatives can be fatal.

Most OTC diet pills used to contain varying strengths of phenylpropanolamine (PPA), an ingredient that helps suppress appetite and that serves as a nasal and bronchial decongestant. First introduced as a replacement to ephedrine, in November of 2000, the Food and Drug Administration (FDA) issued a public health advisory concerning PPA, which was found to increase the risk of hemorrhagic stroke (bleeding into the brain or into tissue surrounding the brain), and began taking steps to remove PPA from all OTC drug products.

Diet pills containing the ingredient ephedra, which are used by some people trying to control their weight, are currently at the center of a regulatory debate. Ephedra is a naturally occurring substance and is not regulated as a drug; however its principal active ingredient, ephedrine, is regulated as a drug by the FDA if it is chemically synthesized. Dietary supplements containing ephedra (often combined with or "stacked" on top of caffeine, aspirin, or both) often are marketed as weight loss pills that "burn fat" and increase metabolic rates. They also are marketed as athletic performance enhancers.

A recent study by the RAND Corporation found that while there is an association between short-term weight loss and the short-term use of ephedrine/ephedra or ephedrine/ephedra plus caffeine, there are no studies that examine the long-term effects of these substances. The study also found that the use of ephedrine/ephedra or ephedrine/ephedra plus caffeine was associated with two to three times the risk of nausea, vomiting, psychiatric symptoms such as anxiety and mood change, hyperactivity and heart palpitations. Furthermore, from thousands of case reports that were examined, researchers identified five deaths, five heart attacks, 11 strokes, four seizures, and eight psychiatric cases that might reasonably be linked to the use of ephedra or ephedrine and in which no other contributing factors were identified.

The FDA recently issued a set of warning letters to companies that market dietary supplements containing ephedra explaining that all the claims they make for their product (e.g., its athletic performance enhancement capabilities) must be substantiated and must not be misleading. The letters strongly warn these companies of the regulatory steps that the FDA may take against them if they make false or misleading claims about their product.

Eating Disorders and Illicit Drug Use

Bulimia nervosa is the eating disorder most strongly linked to illicit drug abuse. Bulimics are likelier to abuse a wider variety of drugs than anorexics. In a study comparing anorexic women with bulimic women, women with bulimia nervosa were more likely to have abused amphetamines, barbiturates, marijuana, tranquilizers, and cocaine. The heaviest illicit drug use is found among those who binge and then purge (e.g., by vomiting or taking pills) to compensate for the binge eating. Indeed, some bulimics report that they use heroin to help them vomit.

Women with eating disorders may use cocaine and other stimulants as a means to control or lose weight by suppressing appetite and increasing metabolism. Anorexics and bulimics may be drawn to cocaine because it is an appetite suppressant that makes them not want to eat and gives them an enhanced sense of power or control. In a study of male and female cocaine abusers, almost half of the women and 13% of the men used cocaine as a weight control measure. In another study, cocaine abusers with an eating disorder were significantly likelier to use diet pills and laxatives for weight loss than were cocaine abusers without a diagnosed eating disorder.

Health Consequences of Eating Disorders

The behaviors associated with eating disorders—fasting, excessive exercising, bingeing, self-induced vomiting, and ingesting laxatives, diuretics, or other substances—are extremely dangerous and can lead to a host of medical problems. A severe eating disorder essentially can destabilize and impair all body systems, including the digestive, cardiovascular, skeletal, muscular, endocrine, dermatological, and reproductive systems.

Pregnancy can exacerbate conditions associated with eating disorders, such as potentially fatal liver, kidney, and cardiac damage. During pregnancy, women with anorexia or bulimia experience higher rates of miscarriage. Babies of eating disordered women can be born prematurely and may be slower to develop physically, mentally, and emotionally.

Anorexia Nervosa

Individuals with anorexia nervosa can suffer from acute hair loss, malnutrition, severe dehydration, osteoporosis, and muscle atrophy. Anorexics may begin to grow a downy layer of body hair as their bodies attempt to keep warm. Perhaps most alarming, the death rate among young women with anorexia is up to 12 times higher than that of other women of the same age. Premature death most commonly results from organ failure or cardiac arrest due to starvation as well as from suicide. A severe substance use disorder further increases the risk of death among anorexics; one study of women with eating disorders found that one of the strongest predictors of death among anorexics is a severe alcohol use disorder.

Bulimia Nervosa

Bulimia nervosa can cause tooth decay, bowel irregularity, peptic ulcers, pancreatitis, gastric ruptures during bingeing, and rupture of the esophagus during vomiting. It is not uncommon for bulimics to experience electrolyte imbalances that may lead to arrhythmia and possible heart failure.

Binge Eating Disorder

Binge eating disorder often is associated with obesity and the health risks involved include high blood pressure and cholesterol levels, heart disease, secondary diabetes, and gall bladder disease.

Who Is at Risk?

Although teenage girls are at the greatest risk for the development of eating disorders, the prevalence of these disorders among males, particularly gay males, is on the rise. Young people involved in certain forms of athletics also face a higher risk of eating disorders. Whereas black girls traditionally have had the lowest rates of eating disorders compared to other racial/ethnic groups, they too are facing increasing risk.

168

Teenage Girls Are Particularly Vulnerable

Teenage girls are significantly likelier than boys than boys to be on diets and to engage in unhealthy weight-control behaviors. Girls are likelier (62.3% vs. 28.8%), dieting (58.6% vs. 28.2%) and exercising (68.4% vs. 51.0%) to lose weight or avoid gaining weight. They also are likelier to report engaging in unhealthy weight-control measures such as fasting (19.1% vs. 7.6%), using diet pills, powders, or liquids (12.6% vs. 5.5%) and purging by vomiting or taking laxatives (7.8% vs. 2.9%).

Although the risk for disordered dieting behaviors is particularly elevated in high school, many elementary school aged children also are overly concerned about their body shapes. Children as young as six years old believe that being fat is undesirable. Forty percent of girls (25% of boys) in grades one through five report that they are trying to lose weight. By the fourth grade, an overwhelming 40% of girls report dieting behavior. Among sixth graders, twice as many girls as boys report that they prefer to be thinner than they actually are.

Poor body image and unhealthy eating and dieting behaviors increase markedly during adolescence for girls. These are precisely the same years when girls are at high risk for engaging in substance use.

CASA's analysis of data from the *2001 Youth Risk Behavior Survey (YRBS)* found that female high school students with eating disorder symptoms are approximately twice as likely to report current smoking, drinking, or drug use as those without eating disorder symptoms. Specifically, smoking (45.6% vs. 21.6%), drinking (63.9% vs. 38.6%), binge drinking (43.0% vs. 20.8%) and marijuana (31.5% vs. 16.1%), inhalant (9.2% vs. 2.4%), or cocaine (8% vs. 2.2%) use are likelier among girls who report disordered weight-control behaviors than among girls who do not.

Conversely, female high school students who report current smoking, drinking or drug use are two or more times likelier to report past month eating disorder symptoms as girls who are not current substance users. Specifically, girls who smoke (43.3% vs. 20.0%), drink (37.4% vs. 17.5%), binge drink (42.9% vs. 20.7%) or use marijuana (41.7% vs. 22.9%), inhalants (57.8% vs. 25.2%), or cocaine (57.4% vs. 25.7%) are significantly likelier to report disordered weight-control behaviors than girls who do not use these substances.

Puberty Is a Risky Time for Girls

Puberty, or the transition from childhood to adolescence, poses a particular risk for the development of eating disorders like anorexia, especially among girls. While males may be at decreased risk for the development of eating disorders at this time because, for them, puberty is accompanied by a desirable increase in muscle mass, puberty among females is accompanied by weight gain from fat tissue, which is considered by many girls to be undesirable.

There also is a strong link between puberty, particularly early puberty, and the onset of substance use among girls. Girls who experience early puberty are at increased risk of engaging in substance use earlier, more often, and in greater quantities than their peers whose physical maturity occurs later. The desire to maintain one's prepubertal appearance can lead girls to smoke or use certain prescription or illicit drugs to help them fight natural weight gain.

Athletes Are at High Risk for Disordered Weight-Control Behaviors

Eating disorders are common in the athletic population, particularly among females. One study found that 35% of female and 10% of male college athletes were at risk for anorexia nervosa and 58% of female and 38% of male college athletes were at risk for bulimia nervosa; these rates are significantly higher than those in the general college population.

Athletes are at high risk of resorting to certain forms of substance abuse—including the abuse of diuretics, ephedrine, or other stimulants—to help maintain a preferred body weight.

Although athletes generally are at greater risk for disordered weight control behaviors than nonathletes, the degree of risk varies by sport and by the professional level of the athlete. Among dancers and the most elite college athletes, particularly those engaged in sports that emphasize a lean physique (e.g., gymnastics, figure skating) or weight restriction (e.g., wrestling, rowing), the prevalence of eating disorders is even higher. Athletes involved in sports for fun, fitness, or social interaction may be at reduced risk for disordered eating, in large part because of the self-esteem enhancing qualities of involvement in these sports.

Gender and Racial / Ethnic Differences in Eating Disorders

Although the classic portrait of an individual with an eating disorder is one of an upper middle class white teenage girl or young women, eating disorders are by no means limited to this group. A substantial number of males suffer from eating disorders, as do increasing numbers of minority group members.

Males. As many as one million men suffer from eating disorders and more males are seeking treatment for eating disorders than in the past. Males account for 5% to 10% of anorexics and 10% to 15% of bulimics. The onset of eating disorders in males tends to be later than in females but the characteristics of males with eating disorders are similar to those seen in females with eating disorders. Anorexic males are more similar to anorexic females, in terms of their body image and weight concerns, than they are to bulimic males. Like girls, adolescent boys with disordered eating patterns express greater body dissatisfaction, perfectionism, and depression than other boys.

Sexual orientation is an important factor in the occurrence of eating disorders. Compared to heterosexual males, gay and bisexual males are at increased risk for developing eating disorders, with reported prevalence rates ranging from 9% to 27%. Gay men are likelier than heterosexual men to be dissatisfied with their body weight and to value physical appearance as more important to their sense of self.

Racial/Ethnic Minorities. There are significant racial/ethnic differences in disordered eating attitudes and behaviors. White girls generally report greater dissatisfaction with their bodies than black girls and a greater drive to be thin. Compared to white and Hispanic teenage girls, black girls are less likely to report that in the past month they exercised to lose weight (53.4% vs. 72.5% and 66.2%), dieted (40.2% vs. 63.1% and 56.5%), fasted (15.2% vs. 19.7% and 23.1%), took diet pills (7.5% vs. 13.6% and 13.5%), or purged (4.2% vs. 8.2% and 10.8%) to lose weight or avoid gaining weight. It is important to note that Hispanic girls have caught up with and, in some cases, surpassed white girls when it comes to certain weight-control behaviors.

There is some evidence that rates of disordered eating attitudes and dieting behaviors are increasing among black girls and women. One study found that although black girls generally are not as concerned about being thin, they are likelier than white girls to demonstrate signs of perfectionism and fear of maturity—factors also associated with eating disorders. Black girls are especially vulnerable to developing eating disorders with binge eating is the core clinical feature (i.e., binge eating disorder and bulimia nervosa), whereas white girls are more vulnerable to eating disorders that involve restriction of food intake.

A variety of factors, including socioeconomic status, cultural norms, and inconsistent or inaccurate medical diagnoses may contribute to observed variations in eating disorder prevalence among different racial/ethnic groups. Lower socioeconomic status (SES) is associated with lower rates of anorexia and bulimia nervosa but not binge eating disorder. The more socialized or assimilated a racial/ethnic minority group member is to American/Western culture, the greater her risk for developing an eating disorder. In contrast, the more a racial/ethnic minority group member has a sense of ethnic pride and remains involved in a supportive racial/ethnic subculture, the lower the risk. A study of Cuban-American women found that decreased involvement in traditional Cuban culture increased the risk of eating disorders while continuing identification with and participation in Cuban culture seemed to protect against the development of eating disorders. It also is possible that the rates of eating disorders among different racial/ethnic groups actually are rather similar, but minority group members are less likely to be diagnosed with an eating disorder because of the widespread belief among health care providers that such disorders are not common among them.

Which Comes First: Substance Abuse or Eating Disorders?

The temporal order or causal relationship between eating disorders and substance use disorders is not yet well understood. Individuals with eating disorders may use certain substances as tools to help them reduce their weight or as a means of self-medicating the often-distressing psychological symptoms associated with eating disorders (e.g., low self-esteem, need for control, obsessions, and compulsions). Conversely, excessive smoking drinking and certain forms of drug use, which suppress the appetite or replace food intake, often precipitate the development of an eating disorder. In addition, withdrawal from tobacco, alcohol, and drugs may increase the risk that one will overeat to compensate for the lost stimulation to the pleasure centers in the brain.

Individuals whose eating disorder precedes their substance use disorder appear to have higher rates of obsessive-compulsive disorder (OCD), panic disorder, and social phobia in comparison to patients with eating disorders only or those whose eating disorder was preceded by a substance abuse disorder. Patients whose substance abuse occurs prior to their eating disorders typically are dependent on more substances and are more likely to have developed their dependency at an early age.

Explaining the Co-Occurrence: Common Personal, Social, and Societal Risks

Eating disorders and substance use disorders have much in common. Both are long-term, difficult-to-treat and life threatening disorders that may require ongoing and intensive therapy. Eating- and substance-related behaviors both operate on similar reinforcing and rewarding motivational systems in the brain. Both disorders involve an obsessive preoccupation with a substance (drugs or food), craving, and compulsive behavior characterized by a loss of control. They often include ritualistic behaviors, which may involve a specific way of cutting a line of cocaine or slicing into a piece of food.

Engaging in either of the disordered behaviors—whether abusing drugs or restricting, bingeing or purging—can have mood altering effects, particularly feelings of calm or numbness. Individuals with these disorders often use drugs or engage in disordered food-related behaviors as a method of coping and both groups continue to engage in the disordered behavior despite negative consequences. Other parallels, particularly between bulimia nervosa and substance use problems, include impulsive behavior, secretiveness of the behavior, low self-esteem, the experience of social isolation that often accompanies the disorder, resistance to treatment and high risk of relapse.

The risk for developing each disorder is determined by a variety of common factors within an individual's brain chemistry, personality, family, peer group, and social environment.

Common Brain Chemistry

Drugs of abuse appear to achieve their rewarding effects by activating the same brain circuits that are responsible for natural rewarding or pleasurable activities, including eating. For example, nicotine and alcohol suppress appetite by activating the same reward mechanisms in the brain that otherwise would trigger the experience of pleasure from food.

Both substance use disorders and certain forms of disordered eating (i.e., bulimia nervosa and binge eating disorder) are related to the common actions of a particular brain chemical—the neurotransmitter dopamine—that produces feelings of pleasure or reward. Low levels of dopamine stimulate the urge to eat or ingest psychoactive drugs, whereas higher doses inhibit those urges. Just as certain drugs of abuse initially trigger a rush of dopamine and then, over time, render dopamine receptors less responsive to stimulation, a similar

173

effect is produced with food. Perpetual bingeing or overeating ultimately inhibits the experience of dopamine-related reward, with increasing doses (of food or a drug) needed to achieve a pleasurable effect.

Eating disorders (particularly bulimia) and substance use disorders also may be related to another brain chemical—the neurotransmitter serotonin, which is partly responsible for regulating mood as well as appetite. For example, cocaine increases serotonin levels in the brain and, in so doing, also inhibits appetite and eating.

Common Family History

A family history of either substance abuse or eating disorders may increase the risk for the development of the other disorder. One study found that female teenage children of alcohol-abusers were significantly likelier than other teenagers to have a poor body image and to engage in binge eating, dieting, and vomiting. Conversely, an increased risk for substance use problems has been found among individuals with eating disorders and their relatives; this is especially true of those with bulimia nervosa and those with anorexia nervosa who engage in bingeing and purging behaviors. However, a recent study found no significant link between parents' substance use and daughters' disordered eating or parents' eating disorders and daughters' substance use.

Common Personal Risks

Both substance use and certain forms of eating disorders may represent ways for people with particular personality types (e.g., impulsive) or mental health problems (e.g., anxiety, depression) to deal with these conditions. For example, the strong association between substance abuse and bulimia nervosa may be due, at least in part, to the shared tendency in individuals with these disorders to behave impulsively and to have difficulty controlling their appetites. One study that compared bulimic women with alcohol and drug-abusing women found that the two groups had similar psychological profiles, displaying depression, anxiety, impulsivity, anger, rebelliousness, and social withdrawal.

Anxiety and Depression

Bulimics tend to be more vulnerable to feelings of anxiety, which is related to alcohol abuse. Depressed individuals may develop either an eating disorder (particularly bulimia) or a substance use problem when attempting to self-medicate their depression.

Low Self-Esteem

Low self-esteem is a common characteristic of individuals who have eating disorders and/or substance use problems. People who are low in self-esteem may be less able to resist peer pressure—increasing their risk for substance use, or may be more likely to engage in behaviors that superficially (and unhealthily) enhance their image or appearance—increasing their risk for eating disorders. Low self-esteem may pose a greater risk for the development of eating disorders among females than males, perhaps because females are likelier to base their self-esteem on the degree to which others approve of them rather than on self-approval.

Stress and Coping

Stressful events can provoke the onset of either substance use or eating disorders, particularly among those who have difficulty coping with life problems. In one study, 58% of anorexics and 77% of bulimics experienced a stressful event or difficulty that precipitated the eating disorder. Another study found that women with eating disorders are more likely to try to avoid or escape from their problems and less likely to seek support or try to solve their problems compared to women without eating disorders. Similar poor coping styles are employed by substance abusers.

Childhood Abuse

More than one in five (21%) high school girls report having been physically (17%) or sexually (12%) abused. Females who report childhood abuse, particularly sexual abuse, are at increased risk for both substance use and eating disorders. Girls who have been sexually or physically abused are twice as likely to smoke, drink, or use drugs as those who were not abused and childhood sexual abuse is associated with an approximate three-fold increase in the risk for alcohol and other drug dependence. Sexual abuse has been reported in up to 65% of women with eating disorders. Anorexics have a comparatively lower rate of sexual abuse history than bulimics.

Rates of sexual abuse are highest among people with bulimia nervosa and a lifetime history of substance dependence disorder.

Some estimate that approximately one-fourth of the women in the United States with bulimia would likely not engage in disordered eating had they not been sexually abused as children. The psychological effects of sexual or physical abuse often contribute to dangerous body image distortions. Survivors of sexual abuse may deliberately try to make themselves unattractive in order to avoid further abuse. Furthermore, women who have been abused are at increased risk of suffering from post-traumatic stress disorder (PTSD), which increases the risk both of eating disorders and of substance abuse disorders.

Common Links to Other Psychiatric Disorders

Approximately 65% of females with a clinical diagnosis of substance abuse or dependence have an additional psychiatric diagnosis. Certain psychiatric disorders in addition to posttraumatic stress disorder—particularly obsessive-compulsive disorder, mood disorders and personality disorders—frequently are found among those with eating disorders, with estimates ranging from 42% to 75%.

Obsessive-Compulsive Disorder. Considerable research demonstrates a strong link between eating disorders and obsessive-compulsive disorder (OCD). Up to 69% of patients with anorexia nervosa have a coexisting diagnosis of OCD and up to 33% of patients with bulimia nervosa also have OCD. One study found that patients with a previous history of eating disorders had an earlier onset of obsessive-compulsive symptoms than other OCD patients and that early onset OCD may increase the risk of eating disorders. Patients with eating disorders and OCD display significantly more disturbed weight-related attitudes and behaviors than do patients without OCD.

Research also suggests a relationship between OCD and substance use disorders. One study found that 24% of teenagers with OCD were dependent on alcohol and 19% were dependent on marijuana. Substance abuse, particularly cocaine and concurrent use of marijuana, increases the risk for the development of OCD. Patients with OCD may engage in substance use as a means of self-medicating their distressing psychiatric symptoms.

One explanation for why eating disorders and substance abuse co-occur with OCD is that the three disorders have similar obsessional and compulsive qualities. The food- and body image-related thoughts associated with anorexia and bulimia and the drug-seeking thoughts associated with substance abuse often are described as obsessional.

An anorexic's drive to exercise excessively and a bulimic's or substance abuser's drive to binge on food or alcohol often are described as compulsions.

Mood Disorders. Anorexia nervosa and bulimia nervosa are related to depression, bipolar disorder, and other mood disorders. Major depression has been reported in about 50% of women with anorexia nervosa and in about one-half to two-thirds of bulimic patients. In fact, bulimia was originally regarded as a type of mood disorder. Mood disorders also are found in approximately 35% of people with substance abuse problems.

Depression appears to be an important component of the link between eating disorders and substance abuse. Depression, depressive symptoms, and a family history of depression are found both among patients with eating disorders and among those with substance use disorders. Individuals with eating disorders who have high rates of depression also tend to have high rates of substance use disorders.

The link between depression and both eating disorders and substance use disorders also can be seen in the effectiveness of antidepressant medications in treating both types of disorders. Specifically, because nicotine serves an antidepressant function (at least initially), the use of antidepressant medications (e.g., Bupropion) in smoking cessation has proven promising. Likewise, the use of such medications in treating certain types of eating disorders, particularly bulimia nervosa, has proven promising as well.

Personality Disorders. Patients with eating disorders frequently suffer from personality disorders such as histrionic, obsessive-compulsive, avoidant, dependent, or borderline personality disorders. Likewise, there is a high rate of co-occurrence of personality disorders—particularly antisocial personality disorder and borderline personality disorder—and substance use disorders both in the general population and in clinical settings.

Common Family Characteristics

Certain features of the parent-child relationship, particularly parents' modeling of unhealthy behaviors, limited parental monitoring of children's behaviors and familial conflict, lack of warmth or support, and poor communication all increase the risk of substance use and eating disorders.

Modeling of Substance Use and Disordered Eating Behaviors

One of the most important risk factors for substance use is parental modeling of substance use behaviors. Children seem to form their beliefs about substances more on the basis of their parents' actions than on the basis of their parents' words. Likewise, children of mothers who are overly concerned about their weight are at increased risk for modeling their unhealthy attitudes and behaviors. Mothers of girls with eating disorders, compared to mothers of noneating-disordered girls, tend to have more pathological eating behaviors and attitudes and longer dieting histories.

Some eating disorder behaviors may be learned, in part, through modeling of parental behaviors or may arise from direct parental (usually maternal) pressure on daughters to lose weight. If weight and appearance are consistently held up as highly significant indicators of one's attractiveness and self-worth, children in such households may begin to internalize these messages and act accordingly. Typically, familial characteristics of women with eating disorders include a family environment in which perfection and control are the norms and in which discussion of weight and appearance are common.

Parental Monitoring of Children's Behaviors

A key risk for the development of substance use and eating disorders is low parental involvement in a child's life. Children whose parents monitor their behaviors are less likely to engage in high-risk behaviors. The normal transition to adolescence and the distancing from parents and reduced parental monitoring that typically accompany this transition can precipitate greater health risk behaviors, such as substance use and unhealthy eating or excessive exercise. With greater independence, adolescents tend to eat fewer meals with their parents, skip meals more often, and indulge in more "junk" food. Parents who eat with their children can monitor their children's eating habits as well as their substance use behaviors.

Parent-Child Relationship

The nature of the parent-child relationship is an important factor in youth substance use. People who grow up in caring and supportive family environments, in which parents have high, yet realistic expectations of their children are less likely to use or abuse substances.

Open parent-child communication, support, flexibility, and bonding all reduce the risk of substance abuse. According to CASA's teen survey, *Back to School 1999—National Survey of American Attitudes on Substance Abuse V: Teens and Their Parents*, teens with an excellent relationship with either parent had risk scores for substance abuse that were 25% lower than the average teen; those with excellent relationships with both parents had risk scores 40% lower.

Unhealthy parent-child relationships also can be seen in some individuals with eating disorders. Typical family dynamics implicated in eating disorders include ineffective conflict resolution, communication difficulties, lack of warmth, and less time spent with parents during early adolescence. Often, in this body of research, mothers are described as demanding, hypercritical, jealous, intrusive, nonresponsive, withdrawn, passive, dependent, or preoccupied with weight and appearance. Fathers often are described as either authoritative and strict or distant and uninvolved. Children might rebel against critical and coercive parents by asserting personal control over their own bodies and environments by engaging in disordered weight-control behaviors.

Peers and the Social Environment

Unhealthy social norms and pressures to conform to peers' high-risk behaviors increase the risk of developing substance use or eating disorders. People with friends who smoke, drink, or use drugs are likelier to do so as well. Peers play an important role in establishing the attitudes, beliefs and group norms for substance use behavior.

Social pressures also play a significant role in the development of eating disorders. Members of the same social group tend to be relatively similar in their attitudes and behaviors, making those who stray from the norm subject to pressure and ridicule. Social groups, such as athletic teams, cheerleading squads and sororities or fraternities, develop social norms about what is appropriate behavior for each of their members and tend to exert subtle and overt pressure on their group members to conform to those behavioral standards. Deviation from these norms can result in rejection by the group. One study found that in a sorority group, binge eating levels of group members were strongly related to the binge eating levels of their friends, suggesting the considerable power of peer influence on disordered eating behaviors.

Part Three

Drugs of Abuse

Chapter 18

Cocaine

Cocaine, the most potent stimulant of natural origin, is extracted from the leaves of the coca plant (*Erythroxylon*). It was originally used in South America in the mid-19th century by natives of the region to relieve fatigue. Pure cocaine (cocaine hydrochloride) was first used as a local anesthetic for surgeries in the 1880s and was the main stimulant drug used in tonics and elixirs for treatment of various illnesses in the early 1900s. Crack, the freebase form of cocaine, derives its name from the crackling sound made when heating the sodium bicarbonate (baking soda) or ammonia used during production. Crack became popular in the mid-1980s because of its immediate high and its inexpensive production cost.

Cocaine most often appears as a white crystalline powder or an off-white chunky material. Powder cocaine is commonly diluted with other substances such as lactose, inositol, mannitol, and local anesthetics such as lidocaine to increase the volume of the substance and the profits of the drug dealer. Powder cocaine is usually snorted or dissolved in water and injected. Crack, or "rock," is most often smoked.

Effects

The effects of cocaine normally occur immediately after ingestion and can last from a few minutes to a few hours. The duration of the drug's effects depends on how it is ingested. Snorting cocaine produces

Fact Sheet NCJ 198582, Office of National Drug Control Policy (ONDCP), Drug Policy Information Clearinghouse, November 2003.

a slow onset of effects that can last from 15 to 30 minutes, while the effects of smoking cocaine last from 5 to 10 minutes and produce a more intense high. Cocaine produces euphoric effects by building up dopamine in the brain, causing the continuous stimulation of neurons.

Users often feel euphoric, energetic, talkative, and mentally alert after taking small amounts of cocaine. Cocaine use can also temporarily lessen a user's need for food or sleep. Short-term physiological effects include constricted blood vessels, dilated pupils, and increased temperature, heart rate, and blood pressure. Ingesting large amounts of cocaine can intensify the user's high, but can also lead to bizarre, erratic, and violent behavior. Users who ingest large amounts may experience tremors, vertigo, muscle twitches, and paranoia. Other possible effects of cocaine use include irritability, anxiety, and restlessness.

Cocaine is a powerfully addictive drug. A tolerance is often developed when a user, seeking to achieve the initial pleasure received from first use, increases the dosage to intensify and prolong the euphoric effects.

Prevalence Estimates

During 2000, there were an estimated 2,707,000 chronic cocaine users and 3,035,000 occasional cocaine users in the United States.

According to *What America's Users Spend on Illegal Drugs*, users spent $35.3 billion on cocaine in 2000, a decrease from the $69.9 billion spent in 1990. Americans consumed 259 metric tons of cocaine in 2000, a decrease from the 447 metric tons consumed in 1990.

The U.S. Department of Health and Human Services' *Results from the 2002 National Survey on Drug Use and Health: National Findings* found that more than 33 million people age 12 and older (14.4%) in 2002 reported that they had used cocaine at least once in their lifetime (see Table 18.1). More than 8 million Americans (3.6%) age 12 and older had used crack cocaine at least once in their lifetime (see Table 18.2).

According to the University of Michigan's Monitoring the Future Study, in 2002, 3.6% of 8th graders, 6.1% of 10th graders, and 7.8% of 12th graders surveyed reported using cocaine at least once during their lifetime (see Table 18.3). Of the students surveyed, 2.5% of 8th graders, 3.6% of 10th graders, and 3.8% of 12th graders reported using crack within their lifetime (see Table 18.4).

The study also showed that, in 2002, 8.2% of college students and 13.5% of young adults (ages 19 to 28) reported using cocaine during their lifetime. Almost 2% of college students and 4.3% of young adults reported using crack cocaine during their lifetime.

Table 18.1. Percentage of Americans Reporting Lifetime Use of Cocaine, by Age Group, 2002.

Age Group	Lifetime	Past Year	Past Month
12–17	2.7%	2.1%	0.6%
18–25	15.4	6.7	2.0
26 and older	15.9	1.8	0.7
Total population	14.4	2.5	0.9

Source: National Survey on Drug Use and Health.

Table 18.2. Percentage of Americans Reporting Lifetime Use of Crack, by Age Group, 2002.

Age Group	Lifetime	Past Year	Past Month
12–17	0.7%	0.4%	0.1%
18–25	3.8	0.9	0.2
26 and older	3.9	0.7	0.3
Total population	3.6	0.7	0.2

Source: National Survey on Drug Use and Health.

Table 18.3. Percentage of Students Reporting Cocaine Use, 2001–2002.

	Lifetime		**Past Year**		**Past Month**	
Grade	2001	2002	2001	2002	2001	2002
8th grade	4.3%	3.6%	2.5%	2.3%	1.2%	1.1%
10th grade	5.7	6.1	3.6	4.0	1.3	1.6
12th grade	8.2	7.8	4.8	5.0	2.1	2.3

Source: Monitoring the Future Study.

Table 18.4. Percentage of Students Reporting Crack Use, 2001–2002.

	Lifetime		**Past Year**		**Past Month**	
Grade	2001	2002	2001	2002	2001	2002
8th grade	3.0%	2.5%	1.7%	1.6%	0.8%	0.8%
10th grade	3.1	3.6	1.8	2.3	0.7	1.0
12th grade	3.7	3.8	2.1	2.3	1.1	1.2

Source: Monitoring the Future Study.

In another study, among the high school students surveyed in 2001 as part of the Youth Risk Behavior Surveillance System, 9.4% reported using cocaine in their lifetime and 4.2% reported using cocaine in the 30 days before the survey. Hispanic students reported the highest percentage of lifetime cocaine use (14.9%), followed by white students (9.9%), and black students (2.1%). Male students (10.3%) were more likely than female students (8.4%) to report lifetime cocaine use.

Regional Observations

According to *Pulse Check: Trends in Drug Abuse*, during the first half of 2002 powder and crack cocaine were widely to somewhat available in the 20 Pulse Check sites across the United States. Among powder cocaine users, the predominant group consisted of white males who were older than 30 and lived in the central city. Crack cocaine users tended to be young adults between the ages of 18 and 30 who lived in the central city and were usually from low socioeconomic backgrounds. Blacks were twice as likely as whites to be reported as the predominant crack cocaine user group by Pulse Check sites.

In December 2002, the 21 Community Epidemiology Work Group (CEWG) sites reported that cocaine/crack indicators showed mixed patterns of stabilization or decline in 10 sites, while 8 sites remained stable, 1 reported an increase, and 2 reported decreases.

The Arrestee Drug Abuse Monitoring (ADAM) Program collects data on male arrestees testing positive for cocaine at the time of arrest in 36 ADAM sites. According to preliminary 2002 data, the percentage of adult male arrestees testing positive ranged from 9.1% in Honolulu to 49.4% in Atlanta. Of the 23 ADAM sites collecting female-arrestee data, the percentage of female arrestees testing positive for cocaine at the time of arrest ranged from 7.4% in Honolulu to 55.2% in Indianapolis.

Availability

Production and Trafficking

According to the National Drug Intelligence Center's *National Drug Threat Assessment 2003*, cocaine is the primary drug threat in the United States because of its high demand and availability, its expanding distribution to new markets, the high rate of overdose associated with it, and its relation to violence. Cocaine consumed in the United States originates from coca plants grown in South America. In 2002, there was the potential for 550 metric tons of cocaine production. Some 352 metric tons of export-quality cocaine was available in U.S. markets.

Approximately 75% of the coca cultivated for processing into cocaine is currently grown in Colombia, and Colombian drug trafficking organizations (DTOs) are responsible for most of the cocaine production, transportation, and distribution. Bahamian, Dominican, Haitian, Jamaican, and Puerto Rican criminal groups transport cocaine, usually under the supervision of Colombian DTOs. Mexican DTOs are involved in wholesale cocaine distribution in the United States. Gangs control retail distribution of powder and crack cocaine in urban areas, while local independent dealers are the primary distributors in suburban and rural areas.

Of the cocaine that enters the United States, 72% passes through the Mexico/Central America corridor. Another 27% moves through the Caribbean and 1% comes directly from South America. Cocaine is readily available in most major cities in the United States. Powder cocaine is typically shipped to one of six main transportation hubs— Central Arizona (Phoenix/Tulsa), El Paso, Houston, Los Angeles, Miami, and Puerto Rico. New York City also is becoming a main transportation hub. Powder cocaine is then distributed through one of the primary distribution centers—Atlanta, Chicago, Dallas, Detroit, New York City, and Philadelphia.

Crack cocaine is not usually transported in large quantities or over long distances due to the more severe mandatory sentencing for possession and distribution of the drug. Retail distributors often convert powder cocaine into crack closer to the marketing areas.

Price and Purity

In 2001, the wholesale price for powder cocaine ranged from $10,000 to $36,000 per kilogram, $400 to $1,800 per ounce, and $20 to $200 per gram. Prices for crack cocaine ranged from $3 to $50 per rock, with prices usually ranging from $10 to $20. In 2001, the average nationwide purity of powder cocaine was 69% for kilogram quantities and 56% for gram quantities.

Enforcement

Arrests

The Federal Bureau of Investigation (FBI) estimates that, during 2001, cocaine and heroin and their derivatives accounted for 9.7% of drug abuse violation arrests for sale and manufacturing and 23.1% for possession arrests (estimates of cocaine arrests alone are not available).

From October 1, 2000, to September 30, 2001, there were 12,457 federal drug arrests for cocaine, representing 37% of all federal drug arrests. Of those arrested by federal agents for cocaine, 40% were white and 59% were black.

Seizures

According to the Federal-wide Drug Seizure System (FDSS), U.S. federal law enforcement authorities seized 105,885 kilograms of cocaine in 2001 and 60,874 kilograms from January to September 2002. FDSS consolidates information about drug seizures made within the jurisdiction of the United States by DEA, the FBI, and U.S. Customs and Border Protection, as well as maritime seizures made by the U.S. Coast Guard. FDSS eliminates duplicate reporting of seizures involving more than one federal agency.

According to U.S. Customs and Border Protection, more than 171,000 pounds of cocaine were seized nationally during fiscal year (FY) 2002. Large amounts of cocaine were seized at the Southwest border and in South Florida—a total of more than 30,000 pounds at each location.

Adjudication

During FY 2001, 5,356 federal drug offenders were convicted of committing an offense involving powder cocaine and 4,999 were convicted of committing a crack cocaine offense. Of those convicted of a federal drug offense for powder cocaine, 50.2% were Hispanic, 30.5% were black, 18.1% were white, and 1.2% were of another race. Of those convicted of a federal drug offense involving crack cocaine, 82.8% were black, 9.3% were Hispanic, 7% were white, and 0.9% fell into another race category.

Corrections

Federal drug offenders received longer sentences for crack cocaine than for any other drug. In FY 2001, the average length of sentence received by federal crack cocaine offenders was 115 months, compared with 88.5 months for methamphetamine offenders, 77 months for powder cocaine offenders, 63.4 months for heroin offenders, 38 months for marijuana offenders, and 41.1 months for other drug offenders. According to a 1997 Bureau of Justice Statistics survey of federal and state prisoners, approximately 65.5% of federal and 72.1% of state drug offenders were incarcerated for a cocaine offense.

Consequences of Use

Cocaine use can lead to medical complications such as cardiovascular effects (disturbances in heart rhythm, heart attacks), respiratory failure, neurological effects (strokes, seizure, and headaches), and gastrointestinal complications such as abdominal pain and nausea. Cocaine use has been linked to heart disease, has been found to trigger ventricular fibrillation (chaotic heart rhythms), can accelerate a user's heart beat and breathing, and can increase a user's blood pressure and body temperature. Additional physical symptoms of cocaine use include blurred vision, fever, muscle spasms, convulsions, and coma. In rare instances, sudden death can occur on the first use of cocaine or unexpectedly thereafter. Cocaine-related deaths are often a result of cardiac arrest or seizures followed by respiratory arrest.

Other medical complications are related to the method of ingestion. For example, users who snort cocaine may lose their sense of smell, have nosebleeds, have problems swallowing, and have an overall irritation of their nasal septum that leads to a chronic runny nose.

Combined cocaine and alcohol use converts in the body to cocaethylene and causes a longer duration of effects in the brain that is more toxic than each drug used alone. This mixture results in more drug-related deaths than any other combination of drugs.

Although the effects of prenatal cocaine exposure are not completely understood, scientific studies have shown that such afflicted babies are often born prematurely, have low birth weights and smaller head circumferences, and are shorter in length. Originally thought to suffer irreversible neurological damage, these "crack babies" now appear to recover from the drug exposure. This is not to underestimate the many subtle but significant effects such babies later experience because of their exposure to cocaine, including impairment in behaviors that are crucial to concentrating in school.

Table 18.5. Number of Emergency Department Mentions of Cocaine, 1995–2002.

1995	1996	1997	1998	1999	2000	2001	2002
135,711	152,420	161,083	172,011	168,751	174,881	193,034	199,198

Source: Drug Abuse Warning Network.

According to emergency department (ED) data collected by the Drug Abuse Warning Network (DAWN), there were 135,711 reported mentions of cocaine in 1995 (see Table 18.5). A drug mention refers to a substance that was recorded (mentioned) during a visit to the ED. This number increased to 199,198 in 2002.

According to DAWN's 2001 mortality data, of the 42 metropolitan areas studied, 14 reported a decrease in cocaine mentions and 14 saw an overall increase since 2000. The remaining metropolitan areas had stable cocaine mentions.

Treatment

Medications to treat cocaine addiction are not available, although researchers are working to identify and test new options. The most promising experimental medication is selegiline, which still needs an appropriate method of administration. Disulfiram, a medication that has been used to treat alcoholism, has been shown to be effective in treating cocaine abuse in clinical trials. Antidepressants are usually prescribed to deal with mood changes that come with cocaine withdrawal. Medical treatments are also being developed to deal with cocaine overdose.

Treatments such as cognitive-behavioral coping skills have been shown to be effective in addressing cocaine addiction but are a short-term approach that focuses on the learning processes. Behavioral treatment attempts to help patients recognize, avoid, and cope with situations in which they are most likely to use cocaine.

According to the Treatment Episode Data Set, cocaine was the third most common illicit drug responsible for treatment admissions in 2000, accounting for 13.6% of all drug treatment admissions. There were 158,524 total admissions for smoked cocaine, accounting for 9.9% of all drug treatment admissions (73% of all cocaine admissions), and 59,787 total admissions for nonsmoked cocaine, accounting for 3.7% of all drug treatment admissions.

Those admitted for smoking crack cocaine were predominantly black (59%), followed by whites (32%) and Hispanics (6.3%). Approximately 42% of those admitted for smoking crack were female. Of all individuals admitted for smoking crack, most (59%) did not use the drug until age 21 or older and 41% reported daily use.

Those admitted for nonsmoked cocaine were predominantly white males (29%), followed by black males (23%), white females (18%), and black females (12%). More than 40% of those admitted for nonsmoked cocaine reported first using the drug by the age of 18. The more common form of nonsmoked cocaine ingestion was by inhalation (70%), followed by injection (15%).

Scheduling and Legislation

Cocaine was first controlled in the United States under the Harrison Narcotic Act of 1914. Currently, cocaine falls under Schedule II of the Controlled Substances Act. A Schedule II Controlled Substance has a high potential for abuse, is currently accepted for medical use in treatment in the United States, and may lead to severe psychological or physical dependence. Currently, cocaine can be administered by a doctor for legitimate medical uses, such as for a local anesthetic for some eye, ear, and throat surgeries.

Chapter 19

Crack

Overview

Pure cocaine was first used in the 1880s as a local anesthetic in eye, nose, and throat surgeries because of its ability to provide anesthesia as well as to constrict blood vessels and limit bleeding. Many of its therapeutic applications are now obsolete due to the development of safer drugs.[1]

Approximately 100 years after cocaine entered into use, a new variation of the substance emerged. This substance, crack, became enormously popular in the mid-1980s due in part to its almost immediate high and the fact that it is inexpensive to produce and buy.[2]

Crack is a highly addictive form of cocaine that is typically smoked. The term "crack" refers to the crackling sound heard when the substance is heated, presumably from the sodium bicarbonate that is used in the production of crack.[3]

While nearly always smoked, there are reports of users injecting crack in a few Pulse Check cities (Baltimore, Boston, Sioux Falls, and Washington, D.C.). In some cases, when users cannot find powder cocaine to inject, they inject crack instead.[4]

Prevalence Estimates

According to the *2002 National Survey on Drug Use and Health*, approximately 8.4 million Americans ages 12 and older reported trying

Drug Facts, Office of National Drug Control Policy (ONDCP), February 2004.

crack at least once during their lifetimes, representing 3.6% of the population ages 12 and older. Approximately 1.6 million (0.7%) reported past year crack cocaine use and 567,000 (0.2%) reported past month crack use.[5]

Among high school students surveyed as part of the 2003 Monitoring the Future Study, 2.5% of eighth graders, 2.7% of 10th graders, and 3.6% of 12th graders reported using crack cocaine at least once during their lifetimes. In 2002, these percentages were 2.5%, 3.6%, and 3.8%, respectively.[6]

Table 19.1. Percent of Students Reporting Crack Cocaine Use, 2003.

Student Crack Use	8th Grade	10th Grade	12th Grade
Past month use	0.7%	0.7%	0.9%
Past year use	1.6	1.6	2.2
Lifetime use	2.5	2.7	3.6

Regarding the ease by which one can obtain crack cocaine, 22.5% of eighth graders, 29.6% of 10th graders, and 35.3% of 12th graders surveyed in 2003 reported that crack cocaine was "fairly easy" or "very easy" to obtain.[7]

Nearly 49% of eighth graders, 58% of 10th graders, and 47% of 12th graders reported that using crack cocaine once or twice was a "great risk."[8]

Table 19.2. Percent of Students Reporting Risk of Using Crack Cocaine, 2003.

Percent Saying "Great Risk"	8th Grade	10th Grade	12th Grade
Try crack once or twice	48.7%	57.6%	47.3%
Use crack occasionally	70.3	76.4	64.0

During 2002, 1.9% of college students and 4.3% of young adults (ages 19–28) reported using crack cocaine at least once during their lifetimes. Approximately 0.4% of college students and 1.0% of young adults reported past year use of crack cocaine, and 0.3% of college students and young adults reported past month use of crack cocaine.[9]

According to preliminary data from the Arrestee Drug Abuse Monitoring (ADAM) Program, a median of 30.4% of adult male arrestees and 30.7% of adult female arrestees tested positive for cocaine (all varieties) at arrest in 2002. The adult male samples were compiled from 36 U.S. sites and the adult female samples were compiled from 23 sites. A median of 18.3% of adult male arrestees and 26.2% of adult female arrestees reported using crack cocaine at least once in the year before being arrested.[10]

Table 19.3. Past Crack Cocaine Use by Arrestees, 2002.

Past Crack Cocaine Use by Arrestees	Male	Female
Used in past 7 days	12.2%	18.2%
Used in past 30 days	14.4	19.8
Used in past year	18.3	26.2
Average number of days used in past 30 days	7.8	10.7

Consequences of Use

Cocaine is a strong central nervous system stimulant. Physical effects of cocaine use, including crack, include constricted blood vessels and increased temperature, heart rate, and blood pressure. Users may also experience feelings of restlessness, irritability, and anxiety.[11]

Smoking crack delivers large quantities of the drug to the lungs, producing effects comparable to intravenous injection. These effects are felt almost immediately after smoking, are very intense, but do not last long.[12] For example, the high from smoking cocaine may last from 5 to 10 minutes, while the high from snorting the drug can last for 15 to 20 minutes.[13]

Evidence suggests that users who smoke or inject cocaine may be at even greater risk of causing harm to themselves than those who snort the substance. Cocaine smokers may suffer from acute respiratory problems including coughing, shortness of breath, and severe chest pains with lung trauma and bleeding.[14] Smoking crack cocaine can also cause particularly aggressive paranoid behavior in users.[15]

An added danger of cocaine use is when cocaine and alcohol are consumed at the same time. When these substances are mixed, the human liver combines cocaine and alcohol and manufactures a third substance, cocaethylene. This intensifies cocaine's euphoric effects, while also possibly increasing the risk of sudden death.[16] Most cocaine-related deaths are a result of cardiac arrest or seizures followed by respiratory arrest.[17]

Cocaine is a powerfully addictive drug. Compulsive cocaine use seems to develop more rapidly when the substance is smoked rather than snorted. A tolerance to the cocaine high may be developed and many addicts report that they fail to achieve as much pleasure as they did from their first cocaine exposure.[18]

Table 19.4. Definitions.

Drug Episode: A drug-related ED episode is an ED visit that was in-duced by or related to the use of drug(s).

Drug Mention: A drug mention refers to a substance that was recorded during an ED episode. Because up to four drugs can be reported for each drug abuse episode, there are more mentions than episodes.

During 2002, emergency departments (ED) nationwide reported 42,146 crack mentions to the Drug Abuse Warning Network. Crack accounted for 21% of the total cocaine mentions during the year. The number of crack ED mentions has increased from 33,789 in 1995, but has decreased from 46,964 in 2001.[19]

Treatment

From 1992–2000, the number of admissions to treatment in which crack cocaine was the primary drug of abuse decreased from 183,282 in 1992 to 158,524 in 2000. The crack admissions repre-sented 12% of the total drug/alcohol treatment admissions during 1992 and 9.9% of the admissions during 2000. The average age of those admitted to treatment for crack cocaine during 2000 was 35.7 years.[20]

Arrests and Adjudication

The Drug Enforcement Administration (DEA) made 11,836 cocaine-related arrests (includes crack) during fiscal year (FY) 2002, representing 40% of the total arrests made by the DEA during the year.[21]

During FY 2000, the DEA made 6,734 arrests involving crack co-caine. More than 3,000 of those arrested by the DEA for crack-related offenses were between the ages of 21 and 30.[22]

In FY 2001, 41.2% of the federal defendants nationwide were charged with committing drug offenses. Cocaine was involved in 5,358 (22.1%) of the cases and crack cocaine was involved in 4,941 (20.4%) of the federal drug cases.[23]

Table 19.5. Street Terminology.[29]

Common Terms Associated with Crack

Term	Definition	Term	Definition
Bingers	Crack addicts	**Oolies**	Marijuana laced with crack
Geeker	Crack user	**Rooster**	Crack
Jelly beans	Crack	**Tornado**	Crack
Moonrock	Crack mixed with heroin	**Wicky stick**	PCP, marijuana, and crack

Production, Trafficking, and Distribution

Crack is cocaine that has been processed from cocaine hydrochloride to a free base for smoking. Crack cocaine is processed with ammonia or sodium bicarbonate (baking soda) and water. It is then heated to remove the hydrochloride producing a form of cocaine that can be smoked.[24]

The majority of law enforcement and epidemiologic/ethnographic Pulse Check sources consider crack to be widely available in their communities. Most of the crack available in Pulse Check cities is processed locally, either by users or by local distributors. Crack rocks tend to be sold in sizes of approximately 0.1 to 0.2 grams, which sell for approximately $10 and $20, respectively.[25]

Legislative History

Cocaine (all forms) was first federally regulated in December 1914 with the passage of the Harrison Act. This act banned the non-medical use of cocaine; prohibited its importation; imposed the same criminal penalties for cocaine users as for opium, morphine, and heroin users; and required a strict accounting of medical prescriptions for cocaine. As a result of the Harrison Act and the emergence of cheaper, legal substances such as amphetamines, cocaine became scarce in the United States. However, use began to rise again in the 1960s, prompting Congress to classify it as a Schedule II substance in 1970.[26]

Schedule II substances have a high potential for abuse, a currently accepted medical use in treatment in the United States with severe restrictions, and may lead to severe psychological or physical dependence.[27] While cocaine can currently be administered by a doctor for legitimate medical uses, such as a local anesthetic for some eye, ear, and throat surgeries, there are currently no medical uses for crack cocaine.[28]

Notes

1. Drug Enforcement Administration, *Drugs of Abuse*, February 2003.

2. National Institute on Drug Abuse, *Cocaine Abuse and Addiction*, May 1999.

3. National Institute on Drug Abuse, *Infofax: Crack and Cocaine*, October 2001.

4. Office of National Drug Control Policy, *Pulse Check: Trends in Drug Abuse, July–December 2001 Reporting Period*, April 2002.

5. Substance Abuse and Mental Health Services Administration, *Results from the 2002 National Survey on Drug Use and Health: National Findings*, September 2003.

6. National Institute on Drug Abuse and University of Michigan, *Monitoring the Future 2003 Data from In-School Surveys of 8th-, 10th-, and 12th-Grade Students*, December 2003.

7. Ibid.

8. Ibid.

9. National Institute on Drug Abuse and University of Michigan, *Monitoring the Future National Survey Results on Drug Use, 1975–2002, Volume II: College Students & Adults Ages 19–40* (PDF), 2003.

10. National Institute of Justice, *Preliminary Data on Drug Use & Related Matters Among Adult Arrestees & Juvenile Detainees, 2002* (PDF), 2003.

11. National Institute on Drug Abuse, *Infofax: Crack and Cocaine*, October 2001.

12. Drug Enforcement Administration Web site, Drug Descriptions: Cocaine.

13. National Institute on Drug Abuse, *Infofax: Crack and Cocaine*, October 2001.

14. Drug Enforcement Administration Web site, Drug Descriptions: Cocaine.

15. National Institute on Drug Abuse, *Infofax: Crack and Cocaine*, October 2001.

16. National Institute on Drug Abuse, *Infofax: Crack and Cocaine*, October 2001.

17. National Institute on Drug Abuse, *Infofax: Crack and Cocaine*, October 2001.

18. National Institute on Drug Abuse, *Infofax: Crack and Cocaine*, October 2001.

19. Substance Abuse and Mental Health Services Administration, *Emergency Department Trends from the Drug Abuse Warning Network, Final Estimates 1995–2002*, July 2003.

20. Substance Abuse and Mental Health Services Administration, *Treatment Episode Data Set (TEDS): 1992–2001*, December 2003.

21. Drug Enforcement Administration, Defendant Statistical System, as reported in *Sourcebook of Criminal Justice Statistics*.

22. Bureau of Justice Statistics, *Compendium of Federal Justice Statistics, 2000*, August 2002.

23. U.S. Sentencing Commission, *FY 2001 Federal Sentencing Statistics*.

24. National Institute on Drug Abuse, *Infofax: Crack and Cocaine*, October 2001.

25. Office of National Drug Control Policy, *Pulse Check: Trends in Drug Abuse, July–December 2001 Reporting Period*, April 2002.

26. U.S. Department of Justice, *CIA-Contra-Crack Cocaine Controversy, Appendix C*.

27. Drug Enforcement Administration, *Drugs of Abuse*, February 2003.

28. National Institute on Drug Abuse, *Cocaine: Abuse and Addiction* (PDF), May 1999.

29. Office of National Drug Control Policy, Drug Policy Information Clearinghouse, *Street Terms: Drugs and the Drug Trade*, Crack cocaine section.

Chapter 20

Dextromethorphan (DXM)

If you think your home is free of addictive drugs, you might want to think again. The potential for drug abuse could lie as near as the cough syrup or cough caplets in your family medicine cabinet. You may be surprised to find that these medicines contain a drug that can produce dissociation (a sense of disconnection from the body and surrounding environment), sensory enhancement, and hallucinatory effects when taken in sufficient quantity. Its name is Dextromethorphan, or DXM.

This Food and Drug Administration (FDA)-approved and presumably safe substance is being scrutinized by parents, health care professionals, and community leaders in light of scientific studies of abuse in Houston and Minneapolis, St. Paul, as well as recent incidents involving abuse in Plano, TX, and the hospitalization of four teenagers in Newark, NJ, and an incident in Pennsylvania involving four teenage girls who entered the hospital with complaints of short breath and racing hearts after taking the drug.

Less publicized and more easily obtained than the more well-known drug ecstasy, DXM's legal status and familiarity may lure some kids into taking it, despite the dangers it poses of addiction, injury, and death. "It's not an ugly drug. It's much less intimidating than snorting a powder or injecting a strange substance," said William Bobo, M.D., a psychiatrist who, along with Shannon Miller, M.D., is conducting an exhaustive review of the scientific literature on DXM.

"Convenience-Store High: How Ordinary Cough Medicine Is Being Abused for Its Mind-Altering Effects," by Lee Burcham, National Clearinghouse for Alcohol and Drug Information (NCADI), June 2001.

Anyone, including minors, can buy these medicines at a local convenience mart or drugstore. And since the FDA approves DXM for sale in over-the-counter medicines, those seeking a high, and especially teens, may assume it's "safe." "It's a very familiar substance, in short," said Bobo, and thus "it is felt to be benign by abusers."

This underestimation of the drug's dangers and abuse potential is not limited to abusers, explained Miller. "Many clinicians simply aren't asking these questions—and certainly when they are faced with someone using it, they tend to minimize it."

Familiar Sources

Dextromethorphan is a semisynthetic narcotic related to opium and found in many over-the-counter cough suppressants in the United States and most countries. DXM is contained in any drug whose name includes "DM" or "Tuss."

The drug comes in various forms. Most common are cough suppressants in caplet or liquid form, including Robitussin, Vicks Formula 44, Drixoral, Delsym, Pertussin, and several generic brands. (Not all medicines under these brands contain the drug since most brands put out several formulations.)

A Risky High

DXM is related to opiates in its make-up, and it produces mind-altering highs. Those hoping to achieve a high often exceed the recommended safe dosage, a daunting prospect for anyone who's ever gagged on a mere two tablespoons of cough syrup. Misuse of the drug creates both depressant and mild hallucinogenic effects. It also acts as a dissociative anesthetic, similar to PCP and ketamine. Sought-after effects include:

- Hallucinations

- Dissociation

- Euphoria

- Mania-like symptoms such as thoughts racing

- Heightened perceptual awareness

- Lethargy

- Perceptual distortion

Depending on the dose, DXM's effects vary. Users report "a set of distinct dose-dependent 'plateaus' ranging from a mild stimulant effect with distorted visual perceptions at low doses...to a sense of complete dissociation from one's body," reports the *National Institute on Drug Abuse Research Report Series: Hallucinogens and Dissociative Drugs*. The high, however, presents distinct risks to health. Adverse effects are many:

- Confusion
- Impaired judgment and mental performance
- Blurred vision
- Slurred speech
- Loss of coordination
- Rigid motor tone and involuntary muscle movement
- Tremor
- Dizziness
- Nausea, abdominal pain, vomiting, vomiting of blood
- Dysphoria (sadness)
- Paranoia
- Headache
- Decreased ability to regulate body temperature
- Excessive sweating
- Reduced sweating and increased body temperatures, or hot flashes
- Irregular heartbeat
- High blood pressure
- Numbness of fingers or toes
- Redness of face
- Loss of consciousness
- Dry mouth and loss of body fluid, from the anti-cholinergic effect of the drug
- Dry itchy skin and occasional patches of flaky skin
- Death (rarely)

A phenomenon that is sometimes called "rave-related heat stroke" occurs when DXM is "taken in a dance-club setting, accompanied by vigorous physical activity (dancing, etc.) and poor air circulation," according to the Indiana Prevention Resource Center Factline on Non-Medical Use of Dextromethorphan.

Emergency rooms increasingly report DXM overdoses and DXM-related crises. In the rare cases where DXM overdose has resulted in death, the precise cause of death is unclear, but respiratory failure appears to be a good candidate in several instances.

Associated Health Risks

Another major concern is the risk incurred when abusers get high and engage in activities requiring reasonable judgment and quick reactions, like driving or swimming. The effects induced by overdose of DXM can make these activities deadly. The story told by one teen-ager illustrates the profound disconnection with reality and inability to exercise caution caused by this drug. This teenage boy got high on DXM, spent most of the night being half-carried, half-dragged by friends through the woods, while drifting in and out of consciousness, and woke at home the next day to discover over 100 ant bites on his body. Apparently, he had fallen into an ant bed the previous night and not even noticed.

DXM is not the only danger in the over-the-counter cough preparations taken for the DXM in them. Abusers may experience toxic side effects due to other ingredients in these preparations. They may contain combinations of drugs, including acetaminophen (an analgesic pain reliever used in the popular brands Tylenol and Panadol), guaifenesin (an expectorant), ephedrine (an appetite suppressant and stimulant) and/or pseudoephedrine (an antihistamine with stimulant-like properties), and chlorpheniramine maleate (an antihistamine with anticholinergic (drying) and sedative side effects), reports the Indiana Prevention Resource Center Factline. Of particular concern is the ingredient acetaminophen, which can result in severe liver damage when taken in excessive quantities. The risk of these side effects escalates as users exceed the dosage recommendations on the medicine package.

In spite of these serious potential adverse effects of DXM, the dangerous behavior it induces, and the ingredients ingested along with DXM-containing cough medicines, abusers keep returning because of the drug's legal status and easy access. But the drug is not taken in a social vacuum. Abusers introduce other abusers to it, and they do so most often where teenagers gather, mingle, and take illicit drugs like ecstasy.

DXM and the Club Drug Culture

While DXM can be abused by anyone at any age or station in life, it is an emerging problem among school-aged youth and young adults in the United States. Its use is becoming more prevalent in dance clubs and at dance events called "raves," where it is sometimes used as an alternative for the more well-known drug ecstasy. Adolescent youth easily can obtain the drug because stores sell it over the counter, with no prescription required. Its street names include:

- DXM
- Robo
- Skittles
- Vitamin D
- Dex
- Tussin

Users are sometimes called "syrup heads." Swallowing large doses of cough syrup is known as "robodosing" or "robo-tripping." The staggering gait caused by the drug is known as the "robo-walk," and users speak of the groggy feeling it often induces as feeling "drippy."

A growing subculture has developed around the use and glorification of DXM, with several music groups such as Nightchild, Dr. Max, and Oedipus Complex producing music purportedly made under the drug's influence, and multiple Web sites devoted to perpetuating DXM use.

The imaginative scenarios and distortionary colors and graphics found on these sites often mimic the mental and sensory effects produced by DXM. Here, users and sellers can also obtain information about purchase, production, levels of dosage amounts and levels of dosage-dependent intoxication, or "plateaus." One such Web site features detailed descriptions of each "plateau"—how to attain it, its subjective characteristics, the activities compatible and incompatible with that level (such as socializing, dancing, and swimming), the adverse effects, and even the risks involved.

Many sites supply information about the ready availability of DXM in bulk powder form directly from manufacturers—since the drug is not regulated—and techniques for making it into tablets or caplets of various attractive shapes and colors, which are then handed out at raves and dance clubs. But the clandestine labs that produce these often have no quality control, making accurate dosing to unsuspecting patrons impossible.

Potential Addictive Properties

While scientific debate continues over the subject, the chemical and mental reactions caused by ingestion of DXM highlight its potential for addiction and abuse. They can be placed into three categories:

- Chemicals involved. Two main chemicals are involved: dextromethorphan (DXM), and dextrorphan. Only DXM is ingested into the body. Dextrorphan, by contrast, is a metabolite, or bodily derivative, that the body creates as it processes DXM.

- Interaction with bodily receptors. Chemically and structurally, DXM is related to the opiates, particularly codeine, and it is active at sigma-type opiate receptors in the body. However it is Dextrorphan, said Dr. Miller, that carries the real punch and that may cause addiction. "We have good, hard scientific studies showing that on the molecular level, on the receptor level, it does similar things that PCP does," he said, and it may also have "the specific chemical qualities that put it at higher risk of turning on the addiction neurobiology in the brain."

- Mental effects. Dextromethorphan (DXM) has sedative-like qualities, and Dextrorphan has hallucinogenic and dissociative qualities. These dissociative effects experienced by the mind— separate from how the drug interacts with the bodily receptors as discussed above—also illustrate the drug's similarity to addictive drugs such as PCP and ketamine.

The full potential for abuse and addiction is not yet known due to insufficient study of this relatively new drug. However, the properties discussed above strongly suggest the possibility of addictive qualities and warrant further research of DXM.

Challenged Prevention Efforts

Most states have few or no legal restrictions on DXM. The history of attempts to limit the availability of it illustrates the extreme difficulty of dealing with the abuse of a drug that is legal, and completely safe when taken in the recommended dosage.

The World Health Organization published a report in 1970 that concluded the drug needed no special monitoring and posed no concern for public health.

However, an outbreak of adolescent DXM abuse in Utah in the 1980s led that state to begin a policy of stocking medications containing DXM behind the counter so that pharmacists could exercise more discretion, especially in its sale to minors.

The Pennsylvania Drug Device and Cosmetic Board and the United States Food and Drug Administration's (FDA) Drug Advisory Committee in 1990 made inquiries into Dextromethorphan's abuse potential. Although they expressed concern about press reports of DXM abuse and official reports from several states, they ultimately found lacking the data on the problem and retained the drug's status as an over-the-counter medicine.

Education the Main Tool

This difficulty in limiting the drug's availability, combined with the lack of data on abuse in the population, makes the standard prevention-based method of treatment much more difficult. What's more, although testing can detect the drug, the standard tests for illicit drugs administered by most corporations, institutions and drug treatment facilities don't target it. Bobo and Miller therefore suggest a two-pronged approach. First, traditional treatment programs can play a limited role, but they should observe several precautions:

- The addiction treatment professional should be fully educated about the drug's nature, mechanism, and history.

- The addiction treatment professional and facility should actively test for the drug since standard drug tests don't screen for it.

- The patient should make the selected sponsor aware that their problem is with DXM and that it is a rather unconventional drug of abuse.

However, because the abuser of DXM will so seldom appear in the traditional treatment environment, the second prong of the approach is the more important. Education about the problem is needed for all people involved, including:

- Abusers and potential abusers
- Physicians
- School personnel
- Parents
- The drug prevention and treatment community

The American Medical Association (AMA) in 1997 took up the issue and resolved, according to Miller and Bobo, that the AMA should launch a physician education process to educate doctors, particularly pediatricians and primary care physicians, on the risks of DXM abuse by young people.

Information about DXM is gradually becoming more available, particularly on the Web sites of drug abuse prevention and health-related organizations. It is crucial that all those involved be aware of the drug and become as educated as possible on its dangers, potential for abuse, symptoms of intoxication, and surrounding drug culture.

The most important knowledge for everyone is simply to be aware that the problem exists. Parents should look for signs of abuse such as a child bringing home his or her own box, or an unexplained dwindling of the family's stock. Doctors can look for signs of abuse and send patients to treatment providers. Treatment providers need to be aware of the special considerations outlined above. And abusers should know that the drug is dangerous and has addictive properties.

The legal status and easy availability of DXM challenge efforts to detect its misuse, let alone deal with it. As Bobo said, when most people think of cough syrup they probably think of "your mom spooning it into your mouth and taking care of you as a kid." We should not let that innocent image block our view of the reality of the drug's abuse.

Chapter 21

Ecstasy (MDMA)

Background Information

MDMA (3-4 methylenedioxymethamphetamine) or "ecstasy" is a synthetic drug with both psychedelic and stimulant effects. The drug was created by a German company in 1912 to be used as a possible appetite suppressant. In the past, some therapists in the United States used the drug to facilitate psychotherapy. In 1988, however, MDMA became a Schedule I substance under the Controlled Substances Act.

In response to the Ecstasy Anti-Proliferation Act of 2000, the U.S. Sentencing Commission increased the guideline sentences for trafficking ecstasy. The new amendment, which became effective May 1, 2001, on an emergency basis, increases the sentence for trafficking 800 pills (approximately 200 grams) of ecstasy by 300%, from 15 months to five years. It also increases the penalty for trafficking 8,000 pills by almost 200%, from 41 months to 10 years. This new increase will affect the upper-middle-level distributors. The amendment became permanent on November 1, 2001.

Currently, MDMA is predominantly a "club drug" and is commonly used at all-night dance parties known as "raves." However, recent research indicates that the use of MDMA is moving to settings other than nightclubs, such as private homes, high schools, college dorms, and shopping malls.

"MDMA (Ecstasy)," a fact sheet produced by the Office of National Drug Control Policy (ONDCP), Drug Policy Information Clearinghouse, April 2002.

Effects

MDMA is a stimulant that has psychedelic effects that can last between 4 and 6 hours and is usually taken orally in pill form. The psychological effects of MDMA include confusion, depression, anxiety, sleeplessness, drug craving, and paranoia. Adverse physical effects include muscle tension, involuntary teeth clenching, nausea, blurred vision, feeling faint, tremors, rapid eye movement, and sweating or chills. There is also an extra risk involved with MDMA ingestion for people with circulatory problems or heart disease because of MDMA's ability to increase heart rate and blood pressure.

Rave party attendees who ingest MDMA are also at risk of dehydration, hyperthermia, and heart or kidney failure. These risks are due to a combination of the drug's stimulant effect, which allows the user to dance for long periods of time, and the hot, crowded atmosphere of rave parties. The combination of crowded all-night dance parties and MDMA use has been reported to cause fatalities.

Research conducted in 2001 by the National Institute of Mental Health supports earlier data showing that MDMA causes damage to the parts of the brain that are critical to thought and memory. The 2001 research found that MDMA damages neurons (nerve cells) that use serotonin to communicate with other neurons in the brain. Additional research indicates that MDMA also affects other neurotransmitters, such as dopamine and acetylcholine.

In addition to the dangers associated with MDMA itself, users are also at risk of being given a substitute drug. For example, PMA (paramethoxyamphetamine) is an illicit, synthetic hallucinogen that has stimulant effects similar to MDMA. However, when users take PMA thinking they are really ingesting MDMA, they often think they have taken weak ecstasy because PMA's effects take longer to appear. They then ingest more of the substance to attain a better high, which can result in overdose death.

Adulterants may be added to ecstasy without the user's knowledge. For example, in a few cities (Chicago, New York, and Washington, D.C.), heroin has been mentioned anecdotally as an adulterant to MDMA. Additional adulterants that have been reported across the country include caffeine, methamphetamine, and ephedrine.

In 1994, hospitals participating in the Drug Abuse Warning Network (DAWN) program reported 253 mentions of MDMA. These mentions refer to the number of times a reference to MDMA was made during a drug-related emergency department (ED) visit. By 2000, the number of MDMA ED mentions reported during the year reached

4,511 out of more than 1 million total drug mentions. This is a 58% increase over the 2,850 MDMA mentions reported in 1999. Preliminary data for January to June 2001 indicate that there were 2,385 ED MDMA mentions during that time.

During 2000, approximately 82% of the ED MDMA mentions were attributed to ED patients age 25 and under. MDMA overdose, was cited in 1,742 MDMA-related ED visits and was the most frequently mentioned reason for going to the ED after using MDMA.

During 1999, MDMA was mentioned in 42 of the drug abuse deaths reported to DAWN by 139 medical examiner (ME) facilities in 40 metropolitan areas across the United States. This is up from nine MDMA ME mentions in 1998. The total number of ME drug mentions for all drugs during 1999 was 29,106.

DAWN's 2000 medical examiner report was completely redesigned from its previous format. The 2000 mortality report now includes information on "club drugs" as a group, combining all mentions of MDMA, ketamine, GHB (gamma hydroxybutyrate), GBL (gamma butyrolactone), and flunitrazepam (Rohypnol). In nearly all of the cases during 2000, club drugs were reported in combination with at least one other substance such as marijuana or cocaine.

As in previous years, club drugs accounted for very few deaths in any of the DAWN metropolitan areas. Out of the 43 total metropolitan areas studied during 2000, only 10 cities reported more than five mentions of club drugs in drug-related deaths.

Prevalence Estimates

According to studies measuring drug use in the United States, MDMA use is heaviest among youth and young adults. The U.S. Department of Health and Human Services' National Household Survey on Drug Abuse found that 9.7% of 18- to 25-year-olds surveyed in 2000 had used MDMA at least once in their lifetimes. More than 6.4 million people age 12 and older reported that they had used MDMA at least once during their lifetimes. This is up from 5.1 million lifetime users in 1999.

The University of Michigan's Monitoring the Future Study found that MDMA use among high school students continued to increase in 2001. Among 10th and 12th graders surveyed in 1996, annual prevalence of MDMA use (use in the past year) was 4.6% in both grades. By 2001, annual prevalence was up to 6.2% among 10th graders and 9.2% among 12th graders. Annual use among 8th graders also rose in 2001 to 3.5%, up from 3.1% in 2000. The study also showed that 11.7% of high school seniors surveyed in 2001 had used MDMA at least once in their lifetimes, up from 11% in 2000.

While no one individual grade showed a statistically significant increase in MDMA use, all have shown a continuing increase in both lifetime and annual prevalence. Taken across all three grades combined, this 1-year increase is statistically significant.

The Monitoring the Future Study also measured perceived harmfulness and disapproval of use by high school seniors and the availability of MDMA to these students. The study found that 45.7% of seniors in 2001 thought that trying MDMA once or twice was a great risk. This is up from 37.9% in 2000. A majority (79.5%) of high school seniors in 2001 disapproved of trying MDMA. More than half (61.5%) of high school seniors in 2001 said MDMA was fairly easy or very easy to obtain, up from 40.1% in 1999 and 51.4% in 2000.

Table 21.1. Percentage of Lifetime MDMA Use among U.S. Population by Age Group, 1996–2000.

Age Group	1996	1997	1998	1999*	2000
12–17	1.1%	1.3%	1.6%	1.8%	2.6%
18–25	4.2	4.6	5.0	7.6	9.7
26–34**	2.5	3.1	2.6	1.5**	1.8**
35 and older**	0.7	0.5	0.5	–**	–**
Total population	1.5	1.5	1.5	2.3	2.9

*Beginning with 1999, new methodology was used. Comparisons cannot be made with previous years.

**For 1999 and 2000, the groups used to collect the data were ages 12 to 17, 18 to 25, and 26 and older. The 1.5% listed for 1999 and 1.8% for 2000 are for ages 26 and older, not just ages 26 to 34.

Source: U.S. Department of Health and Human Services.

Table 21.2. Percentage of High School Seniors Using MDMA by Frequency of Use, 2000–2001

Frequency	2000	2001	% Change
Lifetime	11.0%	11.7%	+0.7
Annual	8.2	9.2	+1.0
30 days	3.6	2.8	-0.9

Source: University of Michigan.

Table 21.3. Percentage of College Students and Young Adults Using MDMA by Frequency of Use, 1999–2000

	College Students			Young Adults		
Frequency	1999	2000	% Change	1999	2000	% Change
Lifetime	8.4%	13.1%	+4.7*	7.1%	11.6%	+4.6**
Annual	5.5	9.1	+3.6*	3.6	7.2	+3.6**
30 Days	2.1	2.5	+0.4	1.3	1.9	+0.5

*Level of significance of difference is .05.

**Level of significance of difference is .001.

Note: Any apparent inconsistency between the change estimate and the prevalence estimates is due to rounding.

Source: University of Michigan.

Data on MDMA use by college students and young adults 19 to 28 years old was also captured in the study. In 2000, 13.1% of college students had tried MDMA at least once in their lifetimes. Among young adults, the percentage who had tried MDMA was 11.6% in 2000.

More than 80% of law enforcement, epidemiologic, and ethnographic respondents in the 20 Pulse Check cities across the country report that the availability of ecstasy increased between 1999 and 2000.

These sources indicate that ecstasy is frequently used in combination with other substances, especially other club drugs, a practice often referred to as "cafeteria-style use." According to DAWN, more than 70% of 1999 ED visits involving club drugs such as MDMA also involved other drugs. In different cities around the country, ecstasy is sometimes combined with LSD ("candy flipping"), psilocybin mushrooms ("hippie flipping"), methamphetamine ("up ecstasy"), and heroin ("down ecstasy"). It is also reportedly combined with cocaine, diverted pharmaceuticals, cough syrup, Rohypnol, and antidepressants.

Raves

MDMA is often found at nightclubs and raves. Raves first appeared in the United States in the late 1980s in cities such as San Francisco and Los Angeles. By the early 1990s, rave parties and clubs were present in most American metropolitan areas.

Raves are characterized by high entrance fees, extensive drug use, and overcrowded dance floors. Club owners often seem to promote the use of MDMA at their clubs. They sell overpriced bottled water and sports drinks to try to manage the hyperthermia and dehydration effects of MDMA use; pacifiers to prevent involuntary teeth clenching (another MDMA effect); and menthol nasal inhalers and neon glowsticks to enhance some of the other effects of MDMA.

Raves often are promoted as alcohol-free events, which gives parents a false sense of security that their children will be safe attending these parties. In reality, raves may actually be havens for the illicit sale and abuse of club drugs.

Production, Trafficking, and Enforcement

MDMA is most often manufactured clandestinely in Western Europe, primarily in the Netherlands and Belgium. These countries produce 80% of the MDMA consumed worldwide. This is primarily because of the availability of precursor and essential chemicals and international transportation hubs in this area of the world.

In the United States, the Drug Enforcement Administration's (DEA's) Chemical Control Program is working to disrupt the production of MDMA and other controlled substances by preventing the diversion of the precursor chemicals used to produce these substances. DEA registration, record keeping, and suspicious order reporting requirements apply to those who import, export, manufacture, and distribute the chemicals being watched by DEA.

The United States also works with other countries to prevent the diversion of precursor chemicals. As a result of the 1988 United Nations Drug Convention, parties to the convention became obligated to control their chemical commerce and to cooperate with each other in their efforts to prevent chemical diversion. The United States and other governments use the annual meetings of the United Nations Commission on Narcotic Drugs to promote international acceptance of chemical control and to highlight emerging chemical control concerns. During 1999, the International Criminal Police Organization (Interpol) reported several seizures of precursor chemicals in areas such as Spain, the Slovak Republic, and the Netherlands.

The majority of the MDMA produced in other countries is trafficked to the United States by Israeli and Russian organized crime syndicates that forged relationships with Western European drug traffickers and gained control over most of the European market. These groups recruit American, Israeli, and Western European nationals as couriers. In addition, traffickers also use express mail services, commercial flights, and airfreight shipments to deliver their merchandise. All major airports in Europe act as shipping points for MDMA destined for the United States. Currently, Los Angeles, Miami, and New York are the major gateway cities for the influx of MDMA from abroad.

Domestically, DEA seized 196 MDMA tablets in 1993, 174,278 tablets in 1998, more than 1 million in 1999, and more than 3 million in 2000. The U.S. Customs Service (USCS) has also reported a large increase in the number of MDMA tablets seized. USCS seized approximately 3.5 million MDMA tablets in 1999 and 9.3 million tablets in 2000. From January to May 2001, USCS had already seized more than 4 million MDMA tablets.

According to Interpol, more than 14.1 million MDMA tablets were seized in Europe during 1999. This is nearly triple the amount seized in 1998 (5 million tablets). During the first half of 2000, more than 8.4 million MDMA tablets were seized in Europe. In 1999, global MDMA seizures totaled approximately 22 million, up from 5.6 million in 1998.

Conclusion

The synthetic drug MDMA is commonly found at rave parties, nightclubs, and more recently, other settings frequented by youth and young adults such as schools, malls, and private homes. The damaging effects of the drug can be long lasting and are possible after a small number of uses. The trafficking of MDMA is increasing at an alarming rate, and multiple agencies have reported large seizures of the drug.

For additional information on MDMA and other club drugs, visit the NCJRS (National Criminal Justice Reference Service) Spotlight on Club Drugs at www.ncjrs.org/club_drugs/club_drugs.html. There you will find information on:

- Training and technical assistance
- Grants and funding
- Related resources
- Consequences of use
- Enforcement
- Research

In recent years, some initiatives have been developed to curb the use of MDMA and other club drugs and reduce the number of raves.

For example, in 1999, the National Institute on Drug Abuse (NIDA) and its partners (American Academy of Child and Adolescent Psychiatry, Community Anti-Drug Coalitions of America, Join Together, and National Families in Action) launched a national research and education initiative to combat the increased use of club drugs. Through this initiative, "Club Drugs: Raves, Risks, and Research," NIDA increased the funding for club drug research and launched a multimedia public education strategy to alert teens, young adults, parents, educators, and others about the dangers associated with MDMA and other club drugs.

As part of ONDCP's National Youth Anti-Drug Media Campaign, a nationwide radio and Internet initiative was launched in August 2000 that focuses specifically on MDMA. This initiative was designed to educate people about MDMA's dangers and change the misconception that MDMA is a harmless drug.

Also, cities and communities throughout the United States have made attempts to reduce the number of raves in their areas and have tried to curb the use of club drugs in these raves. For example, several cities have passed new ordinances designed to regulate rave activity. Other cities have reduced rave activity through enforcement of juvenile curfews, fire codes, health and safety ordinances, liquor laws, and licensing requirements for large public gatherings.

Chapter 22

Foxy

What is foxy?

Foxy and foxy methoxy are common names for a synthetic drug with the chemical name 5-methoxy-N, N-diisopropyltryptamine (5-MeO-DIPT). Abused for the hallucinogenic effects it produces, foxy belongs to a class of chemical compounds known as tryptamines. (Other hallucinogenic tryptamines include psilocybin and psilocyn.)

What does foxy look like?

Foxy is typically available as a powder, capsule, or tablet. (Generally the powder is placed into capsules or pressed into tablets before it is sold to users.) Some capsules and tablets contain foxy powder mixed with blue, green, red, purple, tan, orange, gray, or pink powders. The tablets sometimes are embossed with logos such as a spider or an alien head.

How is foxy used?

Foxy is typically consumed orally in 6- to 20-milligram dosages, although dosage amounts vary widely. The drug also may be administered via smoking or snorting. Typically, users begin to feel the drug's effects 20 to 30 minutes after administration. The hallucinogenic effects peak

"Foxy Fast Facts: Questions and Answers," National Drug Intelligence Center (NDIC), a component of the U.S. Department of Justice, September 2003.

after approximately 60 to 90 minutes and generally last for three to six hours.

Who abuses foxy?

Foxy typically is abused by teenagers and young adults. The drug often is used at raves, nightclubs, and other venues where the use of club drugs, particularly MDMA (3-4 methylenedioxymethamphetamine; also known as "ecstasy"), is well-established. In order to capitalize on the popularity of MDMA and other club drugs, dealers sell foxy and other noncontrolled synthetic substances in these environments. However, the Drug Enforcement Administration (DEA) made foxy a controlled substance through emergency scheduling in April 2003.

What are the risks?

Foxy produces a variety of negative physical and psychological effects in users. The physical effects include dilated pupils, visual and auditory disturbances and distortions, nausea, vomiting, and diarrhea. The psychological effects associated with the use of foxy include hallucinations, talkativeness, and emotional distress. Foxy also diminishes user inhibitions, often resulting in high-risk sexual activity.

In addition, foxy is a dose-dependent drug. This means that increasing the dose results in a corresponding increase in the intensity of the drug's effects. Doubling a 6-milligram dose, for instance, may produce effects similar to those associated with LSD.

Is foxy illegal?

Yes, foxy is illegal. In April 2003 DEA temporarily designated foxy a Schedule I substance under the Controlled Substances Act. Schedule I drugs, which include heroin and MDMA, have a high potential for abuse and serve no legitimate medical purpose in the United States.

Chapter 23

Gamma Hydroxybutyrate (GHB)

Background

Gamma hydroxybutyrate (GHB) is a powerful, rapidly acting central nervous system depressant. It was first synthesized in the 1920s and was under development as an anesthetic agent in the 1960s. GHB is produced naturally by the body in small amounts but its physiological function is unclear.

GHB was sold in health food stores as a performance enhancing additive in bodybuilding formulas until the Food and Drug Administration (FDA) banned it in 1990. It is currently marketed in some European countries as an adjunct to anesthesia. GHB is abused for its ability to produce euphoric and hallucinogenic states and for its alleged function as a growth hormone that releases agents to stimulate muscle growth. GHB became a Schedule I Controlled Substance in March 2000.

In the United States, GHB is produced in clandestine laboratories with no guarantee of quality or purity, making its effects less predictable and more difficult to diagnose. GHB can be manufactured with inexpensive ingredients and using recipes on the Internet. Gamma butyrolactone (GBL) and 1,4-butanediol are analogs of GHB that can be substituted for it. Once ingested, these analogs convert to GHB and produce identical effects. GBL, an industrial solvent, is used as an immediate precursor in the clandestine production of GHB. The FDA

Fact Sheet #NCJ 194881, Office of National Drug Control Policy (ONDCP), Drug Policy Information Clearinghouse, November 2002.

has issued warnings for both GBL and 1,4-butanediol, stating that the drugs have a potential for abuse and are a public health danger.

Effects

GHB is usually taken orally. It is sold as a light-colored powder that easily dissolves in liquids or as a pure liquid packaged in vials or small bottles. In liquid form, it is clear, odorless, tasteless, and almost undetectable when mixed in a drink. GHB is typically consumed by the capful or teaspoonful at a cost of $5 to $10 per dose. The average dose is 1 to 5 grams and takes effect in 15 to 30 minutes, depending on the dosage and purity of the drug. Its effects last from 3 to 6 hours.

Consumption of less than 1 gram of GHB acts as a relaxant, causing a loss of muscle tone and reduced inhibitions. Consumption of 1 to 2 grams causes a strong feeling of relaxation and slows the heart rate and respiration. At this dosage level, GHB also interferes with blood circulation, motor coordination, and balance. In stronger doses, 2 to 4 grams, pronounced interference with motor and speech control occurs. A coma-like sleep may be induced, requiring intubation to wake the user. When mixed with alcohol, the depressant effects of GHB are enhanced. This can lead to respiratory depression, unconsciousness, coma, and overdose.

Side effects associated with GHB may include nausea, vomiting, delusions, depression, vertigo, hallucinations, seizures, respiratory distress, loss of consciousness, slowed heart rate, lowered blood pressure, amnesia, and coma. GHB can become addictive with sustained use.

Patients with a history of around-the-clock use of GHB (every 2 to 4 hours) exhibit withdrawal symptoms including anxiety, insomnia, tremors, and episodes of tachycardia (abnormally fast heart rates), and may progress to delirium and agitation. Because GHB has a short duration of action and quickly leaves the user's system, withdrawal symptoms may occur within 1 to 6 hours of the last dose. These symptoms may last for many months.

According to the Drug Abuse Warning Network (DAWN), GHB emergency department (ED) mentions have increased from 56 in 1994 to 3,340 in 2001 (see Table 23.1).

Table 23.1. Estimated Number of Emergency Department GHB Mentions, 1994–2001.

1994	1995	1996	1997	1998	1999	2000	2001
56	145	638	762	1,282	3,178	4,969	3,340

Source: Drug Abuse Warning Network.

GHB-related deaths have occurred in several Community Epidemiology Work Group (CEWG) sites. In 1999, there were three reported deaths involving GHB in Texas and two in Minnesota. Missouri has reported five GHB-related deaths and two near deaths in which GHB was used to facilitate rapes. In Florida, during 2000, GHB was detected in 23 deaths and identified as the cause of death in 6 cases. Since 1990, the U.S. Drug Enforcement Administration (DEA) has documented more than 15,600 overdoses and law enforcement encounters and 72 deaths relating to GHB.

Prevalence Estimates

GHB is often ingested with alcohol by young adults and teens at nightclubs and parties. It is used as a pleasure enhancer that depresses the central nervous system and induces intoxication. It also can be used as a sedative to reduce the effects of stimulants (cocaine, methamphetamine, ephedrine) or hallucinogens (LSD, mescaline) and to prevent physical withdrawal symptoms.

Since 2000, GHB has been included in the University of Michigan's Monitoring the Future Survey questionnaire. Survey results indicate that annual GHB use by secondary school students in 2000 ranged from 1.1% among 10th graders to 1.2% among 8th graders and 1.9% among 12th graders. In 2001, estimates of annual GHB use ranged from 1.0% among 10th graders to 1.1% among 8th graders and 1.6% among 12th graders.

Regional Observations

According to CEWG, as of 2001, 15 CEWG areas reported increases in GHB indicators. They were Boston, Chicago, Dallas/Houston, Denver, Los Angeles, Miami, Minneapolis/St. Paul, Newark, New York, Philadelphia, Phoenix, St. Louis, San Diego, San Francisco, and Seattle. Atlanta, Baltimore, and Washington, D.C., reported stable GHB indicators. Only two CEWG sites, Detroit and New Orleans, reported declines in GHB indicators. Most CEWG areas report that GHB is frequently used in combination with alcohol, causing users to overdose.

In 2000, according to the National Drug Intelligence Center (NDIC), GHB availability was stable or increasing in nearly every DEA Field Division and High Intensity Drug Trafficking Area. Many areas reported that the increased availability of GHB occurred in concert with a rise in rave activity. Law enforcement also reported increases in the number of cases involving GHB analogs.

According to *Pulse Check: Trends in Drug Abuse*, GHB users and sellers tend to be between the ages of 18 and 30. Most users are middle-class white males. GHB is typically packaged in plastic bottles (mostly water or sports drink bottles) and distributed by the capful for $5 to $20 per dose. Additional packaging includes eyedropper bottles, glass vials, and mouthwash bottles.

Drug-Facilitated Rape

Drug-facilitated rape is defined as sexual assault made easier by the offender's use of an anesthetic-type drug that renders the victim physically incapacitated or helpless and unable to consent to sexual activity. Whether the victim is unwittingly administered the drug or willingly ingests it for recreational use is irrelevant— the person is victimized because of their inability to consciously consent to sexual acts.

According to NDIC, GHB has surpassed Rohypnol (flunitrazepam) as the most common substance used in drug-facilitated sexual assaults. GHB can mentally and physically paralyze an individual, and these effects are intensified when the drug is combined with alcohol. To date, DEA has documented 15 sexual assaults involving 30 victims who were under the influence of GHB. Of the 711 drug-positive urinalysis samples submitted from victims of alleged sexual assault, 48 tested positive for GHB.

It is difficult to estimate the incidence of drug-facilitated rape involving GHB. Victims may not seek help until days after the assault, in part because the drug impairs their memory and in part because they may not identify signs of sexual assault. GHB is only detectable in a person's system for a limited amount of time and, if the victim does not seek immediate help, the opportunity to detect the drug can quickly pass. Also, law enforcement agencies may not be trained to gather necessary evidence and may not be using equipment that is sensitive enough to test for the drug.

Scheduling and Legislation

In response to the use of drugs in sexual assaults, Congress passed the Drug-Induced Rape Prevention and Punishment Act of 1996 to combat drug-facilitated crimes of violence, including sexual assaults. The act imposes harsh penalties for distribution of a controlled substance to an individual without the individual's knowledge and consent with intent to commit a crime of violence, including rape.

On February 18, 2000, the Hillory J. Farias and Samantha Reid Date-Rape Prevention Act of 2000 (Public Law 106-72) became law. It made GBL a List I chemical subject to the criminal, civil, and administrative sanctions of the Federal Controlled Substances Act of 1970. As a result of the law, GHB became a Schedule I Controlled Substance. A Schedule I drug has a high potential for abuse, is not currently accepted for medical use in treatment in the United States, and lacks accepted safety for use under medical supervision.

On March 20, 2001, the Commission on Narcotic Drugs placed GHB in Schedule IV of the 1971 Convention of Psychotropic Substances. This placement affects international drug control laws with which countries that are a part of the convention must comply. Schedule IV mandates international requirements on licensing for manufacture, trade, and distribution of the drug. It also requires parties to comply with prohibition of and restrictions on export and import of the drug and to adopt measures for the repression of acts contrary to these laws and regulations.

On July 17, 2002, Xyrem, a drug with an active ingredient of sodium oxybate or GHB, was approved by the FDA to treat cataplexy attacks in patients with narcolepsy. Cataplexy is a condition characterized by weak or paralyzed muscles. Xyrem, when used as medically prescribed, is a Schedule III Controlled Substance. A Schedule III Controlled Substance has less potential for abuse than Schedule I and II categories, is currently accepted for medical use in treatment in the United States, and may lead to moderate or low physical dependence. Illicit use of Xyrem is subject to Schedule I penalties.

Chapter 24

Heroin

Heroin was first synthesized in 1874 from morphine, a naturally occurring substance extracted from the seed pod of certain varieties of poppy plants. It was commercially marketed in 1898 as a new pain remedy and became widely used in medicine in the early 1900s until it became a controlled substance in 1914 under the Harrison Narcotic Act. Heroin is a highly addictive drug and is considered the most abused and most rapidly acting opiate.

Heroin comes in various forms, but pure heroin is a white powder with a bitter taste. Most illicit heroin comes in powder form in colors ranging from white to dark brown. The colors are due to the impurities left from the manufacturing process or the presence of additives. "Black tar" is another form of heroin that resembles roofing tar or is hard like coal. Color varies from dark brown to black.

Effects

Heroin can be injected, smoked, or snorted. Intravenous injection produces the greatest intensity and most rapid onset of euphoria. Effects are felt in 7 to 8 seconds. Even though effects for sniffing or smoking develop more slowly, beginning in 10 to 15 minutes, sniffing or smoking heroin has increased in popularity because of the availability of high-purity heroin and the fear of sharing needles. Also,

Fact Sheet #NCJ 197335, Office of National Drug Control Policy (ONDCP), Drug Policy Information Clearinghouse, June 2003.

users tend to mistakenly believe that sniffing or smoking heroin will not lead to addiction.

After ingestion, heroin crosses the blood-brain barrier. While in the brain, heroin converts to morphine and binds rapidly to opioid receptors. Users tend to report feeling a "rush" or a surge of pleasurable sensations. The feeling varies in intensity depending on how much of the drug was ingested and how rapidly the drug enters the brain and binds to the natural opioid receptors. The rush is usually accompanied by a warm flushing of the skin, dry mouth, and a heavy feeling in the user's arms and legs. The user may also experience nausea, vomiting, and severe itching. Following the initial effects, the user will be drowsy for several hours with clouded mental function and slow cardiac function. Breathing is slowed, possibly to the point of death.

Repeated heroin use produces tolerance and physical dependence. Physical dependence causes the user's body to adapt to the presence of the drug and withdrawal symptoms occur if use is reduced. Withdrawal symptoms begin within a few hours of last use and can include restlessness, muscle and bone pain, insomnia, diarrhea, vomiting, cold flashes with goose bumps, and involuntary leg movements. These symptoms peak between 24 and 48 hours after the last dose and subside after about a week, but may persist for up to a month. Heroin withdrawal is not usually fatal in an otherwise healthy adult, but can cause death to the fetus of a pregnant addict.

Prevalence Estimates

Although it is difficult to obtain an exact number of heroin users because of the transient nature of this population, several surveys have attempted to provide estimates. A rough estimate of the hardcore addict population in the United States places the number between 750,000 and 1,000,000 users.

The U.S. Department of Health and Human Services' *National Household Survey on Drug Abuse* found that, in 2001, approximately 3.1 million Americans (1.4%) 12 years old and older had used heroin at least once in their lifetime. Persons ages 18 to 25 reported the highest percentage of lifetime heroin use with 1.6% in 2001 (see Table 24.1).

According to the University of Michigan's Monitoring the Future Study in 2002, 1.6% of 8th graders, 1.8% of 10th graders, and 1.7% of 12th graders surveyed reported using heroin at least once during their lifetime. That study also showed that 0.9% of 8th graders, 1.1% of 10th graders, and 1% of 12th graders reported using heroin in the past year.

Among college students surveyed in 2001, 1.2% reported using heroin during their lifetime and 0.1% reported using heroin in the 30 days before being surveyed. Of those young adults surveyed between ages 19 and 28, 2% reported using heroin during their lifetime and 0.3% reported using heroin within the 30 days before being surveyed.

In another study, of those high school students surveyed in 2001 as part of the Youth Risk Behavior Surveillance System, 3.1% reported using heroin at least once during their lifetime. Male students (3.8%) were more likely than female students (2.5%) to report lifetime heroin use.

Table 24.1. Percentage of Americans Reporting Lifetime Use of Heroin, by Age Group, 1999–2001.

Age	1999	2000	2001
12–17	0.4%	0.4%	0.3%
18–25	1.8	1.4	1.6
26–34	1.3	1.1	1.3
35 and older	1.5	1.4	1.5
Total population	1.4	1.2	1.4

Source: National Household Survey on Drug Abuse.

Regional Observations

According to *Pulse Check: Trends in Drug Abuse*, during the first half of 2002, heroin was perceived to be the drug associated with the most serious consequences (medical, legal, and societal) in 15 of the 20 Pulse Check sites across the United States. Heroin users are predominantly white males, over age 30, who live in central city areas. Most heroin sellers tend to be young adults between the ages of 18 and 30.

The different forms of heroin vary in availability across the Pulse Check sites in the United States. High-purity, South American (Colombian) white heroin is widely available across the Northeast, South, and Midwest. Mexican black tar, a less pure form of heroin, is more commonly found in the West. Southeast Asian heroin is considered widely available in New Orleans, Portland, Maine, and Washington, D.C., and Southwest Asian heroin (the least common form of heroin) is only considered widely available in Chicago and New Orleans.

According to the Community Epidemiology Work Group (CEWG), as of December 2002, heroin use indicators increased in four CEWG sites, decreased in one, were stable in seven, and were mixed in nine. Despite mixed patterns, heroin abuse indicators remain high in many CEWG areas. The sites where heroin indicators increased were Atlanta, Boston, Detroit, and Washington, D.C.

The Arrestee Drug Abuse Monitoring Program (ADAM) collects data on male arrestees testing positive for opiates at the time of arrest in 36 ADAM sites. During 2002, the percentage of adult male arrestees testing positive ranged from 0% in Woodbury, Iowa, to 26% in Chicago. Of the 28 ADAM sites collecting female arrestee data, the percentage of female arrestees testing positive for opiates at the time of arrest ranged from 0% in Woodbury, Iowa, to 18% in Portland, Oregon, and Washington, D.C. The ADAM program also collects data on reported drug use by arrestees in the past 30 days. For adult male arrestees during 2002, the average number of days that arrestees reported using heroin ranged from 0.7 days in Omaha to 21.5 days in Woodbury, Iowa. The average number of days reported by adult female arrestees ranged from zero days in Woodbury, Iowa, to 16 days in New York City.

Availability

According to *What America's Users Spend on Illegal Drugs*, heroin expenditures were an estimated $22 billion in 1990, and decreased to $10 billion in 2000. During 1990, Americans consumed 13.6 metric tons of heroin. Current estimates of heroin consumption remain relatively unchanged and show that 13.3 metric tons of heroin were consumed in 2000.

Production and Trafficking

According to the *National Drug Intelligence Center's National Drug Threat Assessment 2003*, heroin is cultivated from opium poppies in four source areas: South America, Mexico, and Southeast and Southwest Asia. Opium cultivation decreased from 5,082 metric tons during 2000 to 1,255 metric tons during 2001. This led to a reduction in heroin production from 482.2 metric tons during 2000 to 109.3 metric tons during 2001.

South American heroin is the most prevalent type of heroin in the United States. Colombian criminal groups, operating independently of major cocaine cartels, dominate the smuggling of South

American heroin into the United States. Others involved in the transportation of South American heroin include Bahamian, Dominican, Guatemalan, Haitian, Jamaican, and Puerto Rican criminal groups.

Heroin is smuggled into the United States through the air, sea, land, and mail services. Once in the United States, heroin is distributed at the wholesale level, most frequently by Colombian, Dominican, Mexican, Nigerian, and Chinese criminal groups described as small, independent, and loosely structured. Retail- or street-level distribution of heroin is handled by a larger array of criminal groups. Gangs also are involved in the wholesale and retail distribution of heroin. Many members of national gangs, such as the Gangster Disciples, Vice Lords, and Latin Kings, keep links to heroin traffickers to guarantee a constant supply of the drug.

Price and Purity

During 2001, wholesale prices for South American heroin ranged from $50,000 to $250,000 per kilogram. Southeast and Southwest Asian heroin wholesale prices ranged from $35,000 to $120,000 per kilogram, and Mexican heroin ranged from $15,000 to $65,000 per kilogram. Street-level heroin usually sells for $10 per dose, although prices vary throughout the country.

According to the Drug Enforcement Administration (DEA), during 2000, retail purity levels of heroin ranged from 48.1% for South American heroin, to 34.6% for Southwest Asian heroin, to 20.8% for Mexican heroin. The national average purity for retail heroin from all sources was 36.8%.

Enforcement

Arrests

The Federal Bureau of Investigation (FBI) estimates that, during 2001, heroin or cocaine and their derivatives accounted for 9.7% of drug arrests for sale and manufacturing and 23.1% of drug arrests for possession (estimates of heroin arrests alone are not available).

From October 1, 1999, to September 30, 2000, there were 3,557 arrests by DEA for opiates out of 38,411 total drug arrests. These figures represent only DEA's portion of heroin arrests nationwide during 2000.

Seizures

According to the Federal-wide Drug Seizures System (FDSS), 1,587 kilograms of heroin were seized from January to September 2002 by U.S. federal law enforcement authorities, a decline from 2,493 kilograms in 2001. FDSS comprises information about drug seizures made within the jurisdiction of the United States by DEA, the FBI, the U.S. Customs Service, and the U.S. Border Patrol, as well as maritime seizures made by the U.S. Coast Guard. FDSS eliminates duplicate reporting of seizures involving more than one federal agency.

Adjudication

During fiscal year (FY) 2001, 1,757 federal drug offenders were convicted of committing an offense involving heroin. Of those convicted of a federal drug offense for heroin, 61.3% were Hispanic, 23% were black, 14% were white, and 1.7% were of another race.

Corrections

In FY 2001, the average length of sentence received by federal heroin offenders was 63.4 months, compared to 115 months for crack cocaine offenders, 88.5 months for methamphetamine offenders, 77 months for powder cocaine offenders, 38 months for marijuana offenders, and 41.1 months for other drug offenders. According to a 1997 Bureau of Justice Statistics survey of federal and state prisoners, approximately 10% of federal and 12.8% of state drug offenders were incarcerated for an offense involving heroin or other opiates.

Consequences of Use

Chronic heroin use can lead to medical consequences such as scarred and/or collapsed veins, bacterial infections of the blood vessels and heart valves, abscesses and other soft-tissue infections, and liver or kidney disease. Poor health conditions and depressed respiration from heroin use can cause lung complications, including various types of pneumonia and tuberculosis.

Addiction is the most detrimental long-term effect of heroin use because it is a chronic, relapsing disease characterized by compulsive drug seeking and use, as well as neurochemical and molecular changes in the brain.

Long-term effects of heroin use also can include arthritis and other rheumatologic problems and infection of bloodborne pathogens such as HIV/AIDS and hepatitis B and C (which are contracted by sharing and reusing syringes and other injection paraphernalia). It is estimated that injection drug use has been a factor in one-third of all HIV and more than half of all hepatitis C cases in the United States.

Heroin use by a pregnant woman can result in a miscarriage or premature delivery. Heroin exposure in utero can increase a newborns' risk of SIDS (sudden infant death syndrome).

Street heroin is often cut with substances such as sugar, starch, powdered milk, strychnine and other poisons, and other drugs. These additives may not dissolve when injected in a user's system and can clog the blood vessels that lead to the lungs, liver, kidneys, or brain, infecting or killing patches of cells in vital organs. In addition, many users do not know their heroin's actual strength or its true contents and are at an elevated risk of overdose or death.

Table 24.2. Number of Emergency Department Mentions of Heroin, 1994–2001.

1994	1995	1996	1997	1998	1999	2000	2001
63,158	69,556	72,980	70,712	75,688	82,192	94,804	93,064

Source: Drug Abuse Warning Network.

According to Drug Abuse Warning Network (DAWN) emergency department (ED) data, there were 93,064 reported mentions of heroin in 2001, an increase of 47.4% since 1994 (see Table 24.2). Preliminary ED data for the first half of 2002 revealed that there were 42,571 mentions of heroin. A drug mention refers to a substance that was recorded (mentioned) during a visit to the ED. Heroin represented 15% of 638,484 total ED episodes in 2001. Approximately 56% of heroin ED mentions were for people ages 35 and older. Almost half (43%) of heroin ED mentions were for whites.

According to DAWN's 2001 mortality data, of the 42 metropolitan areas studied, 19 areas saw a decrease in the number of heroin/morphine mentions, while 9 areas reported an increase in heroin/morphine mentions.

Treatment

According to Treatment Episode Data Set, heroin accounted for 15.2% of all treatment admissions in 2000 (243,523 admissions). Males accounted for 66.9% of heroin treatment admissions. Treatment admissions by race/ethnicity ranged from 47.3% white, to 24.7% Hispanic, to 24.2% black.

Eighty-one percent of heroin treatment admissions reported daily use of the drug. Almost 80% of heroin admissions had been in treatment before the current episode and 25% had been in treatment five or more times. Methadone treatment was planned to be used for 40% of primary heroin admissions.

Methadone has been used to treat opioid addiction for more than 30 years. This synthetic narcotic suppresses opioid withdrawal symptoms for 24 to 36 hours. Although the patient remains physically dependent on the opioid, the craving from heroin use is reduced and the highs and lows are blocked. This permits the patient to be free from the uncontrolled, compulsive, and disruptive behavior associated with heroin addiction.

Table 24.3. Street Terms for Heroin

Al Capone	Golden Girl	Ogoy
Antifreeze	Good horse	Old Steve
Ballot	Hard candy	Orange line
Bart Simpson	Hazel	P-dope
Big bag	Hero	Pangonadalot
Big H	Hombre	Peg
Brown sugar	Horse	Perfect high
Capital H	HRN	Poison
Cheese	Isda	Pure
Chip	Jee gee	Rawhide
Crank	Joy	Ready rock
Dead on arrival	Junk	Salt
Dirt	Lemonade	Sweet dreams
Dr. Feelgood	Mexican brown	Train
Ferry dust	Nice and easy	White boy
George smack	Noise	Zoquete

Other pharmaceutical approaches to heroin treatment include detoxification, naloxone and naltrexone, LAAM (levo-alpha-acetyl-methadol), and buprenorphine.

Detoxification relieves the withdrawal symptoms experienced when substance use is discontinued. Detoxification is not a treatment for addiction, although it can be used to aid in the transition to long-term treatment.

Naloxone and naltrexone are medications that inhibit the effects of opiates such as morphine and heroin. LAAM, a synthetic opiate similar to methadone, is used to treat heroin addiction. This treatment's long duration of action (up to 72 hours) allows patients to administer their dosage three times a week instead of daily. Buprenorphine, another opiate treatment, causes weaker opiate effects and is not as likely to cause overdose. Buprenorphine creates a lower level of physical dependence and makes it easier for patients to discontinue medication.

Scheduling and Legislation

Heroin was first controlled in the United States under the Harrison Narcotic Act of 1914. Currently, heroin falls under Schedule I of the Controlled Substances Act. A Schedule I Controlled Substance has a high potential for abuse, is not currently accepted for medical use in treatment in the United States, and lacks accepted safety for use under medical supervision.

Chapter 25

Inhalants

The term "inhalants" refers to more than a thousand household and commercial products that can be abused by inhaling them through one's mouth or nose for an intoxicating effect. These products are composed of volatile solvents and substances commonly found in commercial adhesives, lighter fluids, cleaning solvents, and paint products. Their easy accessibility, low cost, and ease of concealment make inhalants one of the first substances abused.

Inhalant users can ingest substances in various ways that include inhaling directly from containers for products such as rubber cement or correction fluid, sniffing fumes from plastic bags held over the mouth and nose, or sniffing a cloth saturated with the substance. The substance may be inhaled directly from an aerosol can or out of an alternative container such as a balloon filled with nitrous oxide. Some volatile substances release intoxicating vapors when heated.

Prevalence Estimates

Typical first use of inhalants occurs between late childhood and early adolescence. According to the *National Household Survey on Drug Abuse (NHSDA)*, there were an estimated 979,000 new inhalant users in 2000, up from 410,000 in 1985. During 2001, more than 18 million (8.1%) persons ages 12 and older reported using an inhalant at least once in their lifetime (see Table 25.1). The 2002 Monitoring the

Fact Sheet #NCJ 197105, Office of National Drug Control Policy (ONDCP), Drug Policy Information Clearinghouse, February 2003.

Future Study from the University of Michigan reported that 7.7% of eighth graders, 5.8% of 10th graders, and 4.5% of 12th graders used inhalants in the past year (see Table 25.2). The study also showed that 3.8% of eighth graders, 2.4% of 10th graders, and 1.5% of 12th graders used inhalants in the past month (see Table 25.3).

Table 25.1. Percentage of People Ages 12 and Older Reporting Inhalant Use, 1999–2001.

	Past Month	Past Year	Lifetime
1999	0.3	0.9	7.8
2000	0.3	0.9	7.5
2001	0.2	0.9	8.1

Source: National Household Survey on Drug Abuse.

This study also showed that in 2001, 2.8% of college students reported using inhalants in the past year and 0.4% reported using inhalants in the 30 days before being surveyed. Of those young adults between the ages of 19 and 28, 1.7% reported using inhalants in the past year and 0.4% reported using inhalants in the 30 days before being surveyed.

Table 25.2. Percentage of Students Reporting Past Year Inhalant Use, 1996–2002.

	1996	1997	1998	1999	2000	2001	2002
8th graders	12.2	11.8	11.1	10.3	9.4	9.1	7.7
10th graders	9.5	8.7	8.0	7.2	7.3	6.6	5.8
12th graders	7.6	6.7	6.2	5.6	5.9	4.5	4.5

Source: Monitoring the Future Study.

Table 25.3. Percentage of Students Reporting Past Month Inhalant Use, 1996–2002.

	1996	1997	1998	1999	2000	2001	2002
8th graders	5.8	5.6	4.8	5.0	4.5	4.0	3.8
10th graders	3.3	3.0	2.9	2.6	2.6	2.4	2.4
12th graders	2.5	2.5	2.3	2.0	2.2	1.7	1.5

Source: Monitoring the Future Study.

According to the 2001 Youth Risk Behavior Surveillance Survey, 14.7% of high school students nationwide have sniffed glue, breathed the contents of aerosol spray cans, or inhaled paints or spray to get high at least once during their lifetime. Some 4.7% of high school students reported using inhalants in the 30 days preceding the survey.

Effects

The effects of inhalant use resemble alcohol inebriation. Upon inhalation, the body becomes starved of oxygen, forcing the heart to beat more rapidly in an attempt to increase blood flow to the brain. The user initially experiences stimulation, a loss of inhibition, and a distorted perception of reality and spatial relations. After a few minutes, the senses become depressed and a sense of lethargy arises as the body attempts to stabilize blood flow to the brain, usually referred to as a "head rush." Users can become intoxicated several times over a few hours because of a chemical's short-acting, rapid-onset effect. Many users also experience headaches, nausea, vomiting, slurred speech, loss of coordination, and wheezing.

Heavy or sustained use of inhalants can cause tolerance and physical withdrawal symptoms within several hours to a few days after use. Withdrawal symptoms may include sweating, rapid pulse, hand tremors, insomnia, nausea, vomiting, physical agitation, anxiety, hallucinations, and grand mal seizures. Indicators of inhalant abuse include paint or stains on the body or clothing, spots or sores around the mouth, red or runny eyes and nose, chemical odor on the breath, a drunken or dazed appearance, loss of appetite, excitability, and/or irritability.

Table 25.4. Commonly Abused Commercial Products.

Adhesives:	Model airplane glue, rubber cement, household glue.
Aerosols:	Spray paint, hair spray, air freshener, deodorant, fabric protector.
Anesthetics:	Nitrous oxide, ether, chloroform.
Cleaning agents:	Dry cleaning fluid, spot remover, degreaser.
Food products:	Vegetable cooking spray, "whippets" (nitrous oxide).
Gases:	Nitrous oxide, butane, propane, helium.
Solvents and gases:	Nail polish remover, paint thinner, typing correction fluid and thinner, toxic markers, pure toluene, toluol, cigar lighter fluid, gasoline.

Source: National Inhalant Prevention Coalition.

Consequences of Use

There is a common link between inhalant abuse and problems in school such as failing grades, memory loss, learning problems, chronic absences, and general apathy. Inhalant users tend to be disruptive, deviant, or delinquent because of the early onset of use, the user's lack of physical and emotional maturation, and the physical consequences of extended use.

According to Drug Abuse Warning Network (DAWN) emergency department (ED) data, in 1994 there were 1,511 reported mentions of inhalants. This number increased to 2,225 in 1997 and sharply declined to 676 in 2001 (see Table 25.5). Preliminary data for the first half of 2002 showed that there were 559 reported mentions of inhalants.

During 2001, approximately 47% of ED inhalant mentions were for people 35 years old or older. Unexpected reaction was cited in 41% of inhalant-related ED visits and was the most frequently mentioned reason for visiting the emergency department after using an inhalant.

During 1999, 129 inhalant abuse deaths were reported to DAWN by 139 medical examiner facilities in 40 metropolitan areas across the United States. This was up from 103 inhalant abuse deaths in 1998.

DAWN's 2000 medical examiner report was redesigned from its previous format and presents only regional data without national totals. Out of the 43 metropolitan areas studied during 2000, only the cities of Dallas, Louisville, Oklahoma City, and St. Louis reported more than 4 mentions of inhalant drug-related deaths.

Table 25.5. Emergency department mentions of inhalants, 1994–2001

1994	1995	1996	1997	1998	1999	2000	2001
1,511	1,036	1,313	2,225	2,211	1,162	1,522	676

Source: Drug Abuse Warning Network

Treatment

According to the Treatment Episode Data Set, inhalants were reported as the primary substance of abuse in 1,251 (0.1%) admissions to treatment facilities in 2000. People admitted for inhalant abuse were generally under age 18 (44%), male (72%), and non-Hispanic White (66%). Twenty-eight percent of those admitted reported daily use of inhalants, and almost 26% admitted using inhalants by age 12.

Table 25.6. Damage to Body Caused by Inhalants.

Acoustic nerve and muscle:	Destruction of cells that relay sound to the brain may cause deafness.
Blood:	The oxygen-carrying capacity of the blood can be inhibited.
Bone marrow:	Components containing benzene have been shown to cause leukemia.
Brain:	Damage is also caused to the cerebral cortex and the cerebellum, resulting in personality changes, memory impairment, hallucinations, loss of coordination, and slurred speech.
Heart:	Sudden sniffing death (SSD) syndrome,* an unexpected disturbance in the heart's rhythm, may cause fatal cardiac arrhythmias (heart failure).
Kidneys:	The kidney's ability to control the amount of acid in the blood may be impaired. Kidney stones may develop after use is terminated.
Liver:	Gathering of fatty tissue may cause liver damage.
Lungs:	Damaged lungs and impaired breathing occurs with repeated use.
Muscle:	Chronic use can lead to muscle wasting and reduced muscle tone and strength.
Peripheral nervous system:	Damage to the nerves may result in numbness, tingling, and paralysis.
Skin:	A severe rash around the nose and mouth, referred to as "glue sniffer's rash," may result.

*SSD syndrome may result when a user deeply inhales a chemical for the effect of intoxication. This causes a decrease in available oxygen in the body. If the user becomes startled or engages in sudden physical activity, an increased flow of adrenalin from the brain to the heart induces cardiac arrest and death occurs within minutes.

Source: National Inhalant Prevention Coalition.

Legislation

Most of the common household and commercial products abused as inhalants are not regulated under the Controlled Substances Act. Consequently, many state legislatures have attempted to deter youth from abusing them by placing restrictions on their sale to minors.

According to the National Conference of State Legislatures, 38 states have adopted laws preventing the sale, use, and/or distribution of various products commonly abused as inhalants to minors. Some states have introduced fines, incarceration, or mandatory treatments for the sale, distribution, use, and/or possession of inhalable chemicals.

Chapter 26

Ketamine

What is ketamine?

Ketamine is an anesthetic that is abused for its hallucinogenic properties. Its predominant legitimate use is as a veterinary anesthetic; however, it has been approved for use with both animals and humans. Abuse of the drug gained popularity when users discovered that it produced effects similar to those associated with PCP. Because of its anesthetic properties, ketamine also reportedly has been used by sexual predators to incapacitate their intended victims.

What does ketamine look like?

Ketamine generally is sold as either a colorless, odorless liquid or as a white or off-white powder.

How is ketamine abused?

In either its powder or liquid forms, ketamine is mixed with beverages or added to smokable materials such as marijuana or tobacco. As a powder the drug is snorted or pressed into tablets—often in combination with other drugs such as 3,4-methylenedioxymethamphetamine (MDMA, also known as ecstasy). As a liquid, ketamine is injected; it often is injected intramuscularly.

"Ketamine Fast Facts: Questions and Answers," National Drug Intelligence Center (NDIC), a component of the U.S. Department of Justice, June 2003.

Who uses ketamine?

Teenagers and young adults represent the majority of ketamine users. According to the Drug Abuse Warning Network, individuals aged 12 to 25 accounted for 74% of the ketamine emergency department mentions in the United States in 2000.

Ketamine use among high school students is a particular concern. Nearly 3% of high school seniors in the United States used the drug at least once in the past year, according to the University of Michigan's Monitoring the Future Survey.

What are the risks?

Ketamine causes users to have distorted perceptions of sight and sound and to feel disconnected and out of control. Use of the drug can impair an individual's senses, judgment, and coordination for up to 24 hours after the drug is taken even though the drug's hallucinogenic effects usually last for only 45 to 90 minutes.

Use of ketamine has been associated with serious problems—both mental and physical. Ketamine can cause depression, delirium, amnesia, impaired motor function, high blood pressure, and potentially fatal respiratory problems.

In addition to the risks associated with ketamine itself, individuals who use the drug may put themselves at risk of sexual assault. Sexual predators reportedly have used ketamine to incapacitate their intended victims—either by lacing unsuspecting victims' drinks with the drug or by offering ketamine to victims who consume the drug without understanding the effects it will produce.

What is ketamine called?

The most common names for ketamine are K, special K, cat valium, and vitamin K.

Is ketamine illegal?

Yes, it is illegal to abuse ketamine. Ketamine is a controlled substance. Specifically, it is a Schedule III substance under the Controlled Substances Act. Schedule III drugs, which include codeine and anabolic steroids, have less potential for abuse than Schedule I (heroin) or Schedule II (cocaine) drugs. However, abuse of Schedule III substances may lead to physical or psychological dependence on the drug.

Chapter 27

Khat

What is khat?

Khat (*Catha edulis*) is a flowering shrub native to northeast Africa and the Arabian Peninsula. Individuals chew khat leaves because of the stimulant effects, which are similar to but less intense than those caused by abusing cocaine or methamphetamine.

What does khat look like?

When fresh, khat leaves are glossy and crimson-brown in color, resembling withered basil. Khat leaves typically begin to deteriorate 48 hours after being cut from the shrub on which they grow. Deteriorating khat leaves are leathery and turn yellow-green in color.

How is khat used?

Khat typically is ingested by chewing the leaves—as is done with loose tobacco. Dried khat leaves can be brewed in tea or cooked and added to food. After ingesting khat, the user experiences an immediate increase in blood pressure and heart rate. The effects of the drug generally begin to subside between 90 minutes and three hours after ingestion; however, they can last up to 24 hours.

"Khat Fast Facts: Questions and Answers," National Drug Intelligence Center (NDIC), a component of the U.S. Department of Justice, July 2003.

Who uses khat?

The use of khat is accepted within the Somali, Ethiopian, and Yemeni cultures, and in the United States khat use is most prevalent among immigrants from those countries. Abuse levels are highest in cities with sizable populations of immigrants from Somalia, Ethiopia, and Yemen, including Boston, Columbus, Dallas, Detroit, Kansas City, Los Angeles, Minneapolis, Nashville, New York, and Washington, D.C. In addition, there is evidence to suggest that some nonimmigrants in these areas have begun abusing the drug.

What are the risks?

Individuals who abuse khat typically experience a state of mild depression following periods of prolonged use. Taken in excess khat causes extreme thirst, hyperactivity, insomnia, and loss of appetite (which can lead to anorexia).

Frequent khat use often leads to decreased productivity because the drug tends to reduce the user's motivation. Repeated use can cause manic behavior with grandiose delusions, paranoia, and hallucinations. (There have been reports of khat-induced psychosis.) The drug also can cause damage to the nervous, respiratory, circulatory, and digestive systems.

Is khat illegal?

Yes, khat is illegal. Fresh khat leaves contain cathinone—a Schedule I drug under the Controlled Substances Act. Schedule I drugs, which include heroin and LSD, have a high potential for abuse and serve no legitimate medical purpose. When khat leaves are no longer fresh (typically after 48 hours), their chemical composition breaks down. At that point the leaves contain cathine, a Schedule IV substance. Schedule IV drugs are considered to have a lower potential for abuse but still can lead to limited physical or psychological dependence.

Chapter 28

Lysergic Acid Diethylamide (LSD)

Overview

LSD, commonly referred to as "acid," was discovered in 1938 when a chemist working for Sandoz Laboratories in Switzerland synthesized the drug. It was developed initially as a circulatory and respiratory stimulant. In the 1940s, interest in the drug was revived when it was thought to be a possible treatment for schizophrenia. During the early 1960s, the first group of casual LSD users evolved and expanded into a subculture.[1]

LSD (lysergic acid diethylamide) is manufactured from lysergic acid, which is found in ergot, a fungus that grows on rye and other grains. It is sold on the street in tablets, capsules, and, occasionally, in liquid form. LSD is an odorless and colorless substance, which has a slightly bitter taste and is usually ingested orally. It is often added to absorbent paper, such as blotter paper, and divided into small decorated squares, with each square representing one dose.[2]

The Drug Enforcement Administration (DEA) reports that the strength of LSD samples obtained currently from illicit sources ranges from 20 to 80 millionths of a gram (micrograms) of LSD per dose. This is much less than the levels reported during the 1960s and early 1970s, when the dosage ranged from 100 to 200 micrograms, or higher, per unit.[3] Generally, the dosage level that will produce a hallucinogenic effect in humans is 25 micrograms.[4]

"LSD," Drug Facts, Office of National Drug Control Policy (ONDCP), March 2004.

Prevalence Estimates

According to the National Survey on Drug Use and Health, 112,000 Americans aged 12 and older were current LSD users during 2002. Of those surveyed, 10.4% indicated using LSD at least once in their lifetime. Almost 3% of those surveyed between the ages of 12 and 17 (2.7%), reported the use of LSD at least once in their lifetime, whereas 15.9% of those surveyed between the ages of 18 and 25 reported lifetime LSD use.[5]

According to data from the Monitoring the Future Study, the annual prevalence of LSD use among U.S. high school students has remained below 10% for the last 25 years. In 2003, lifetime prevalence of LSD for eighth, 10th, and 12th graders was 2.1%, 3.5%, and 5.9%, respectively.[6]

Table 28.1. Percentage of High School Students Reporting LSD Use, 2003.

Grade	Lifetime	Annual	Past 30 Days
8th grade	2.1%	1.3%	0.6%
10th grade	3.5	1.7	0.6
12th grade	5.9	1.9	0.6

Reported availability of LSD by 12th graders has varied quite a bit over the years. It fell considerably from 1975–1983, remained level for a few years, and then began a substantial rise after 1986, reaching a peak in 1995 with 53.8% of 12th graders reporting it as fairly easy to obtain. LSD availability also rose among eighth and 10th graders in the early '90s, reaching a peak in 1995 and 1996. There has been some falloff in availability among all eighth, 10th, and 12th graders since those peak years.[7]

During 2002, 8.6% of college students reported having used LSD within their lifetime, compared to 15.1% of young adults between the ages of 19 to 28 who reported lifetime use of LSD.[8]

Table 28.2. Percentage of College Students and Young Adults Reporting LSD Use, 2002.

	Lifetime	Annual	Past 30 Days
College students	8.6%	2.1%	0.2%
Young adults	15.1	1.8	0.3

According to *Pulse Check: Trends in Drug Abuse*, the use of LSD in combination with Ecstasy was mentioned in numerous location, including Boston, Chicago, Denver, Los Angeles, and St. Louis.[9]

Consequences of Use

LSD, although commonly perceived as harmless, can lead to many consequences for users. Powerful hallucinations can lead to acute panic reactions when the mental effects of LSD cannot be controlled and when the user wishes to end the drug-induced state. While these panic reactions, more often than not, are resolved successfully over time, prolonged anxiety and psychotic reactions have been reported. The mental effects can cause psychotic crises and add to existing psychiatric problems.[10]

The effects of LSD are unpredictable. They depend on the amount taken; the user's personality, mood, and expectations; and the surroundings in which the drug is used. Usually, the user feels the first effects of the drug within 30 to 90 minutes of ingestion. These experiences last for extended periods of time and typically begin to clear after about 12 hours. The physical effects include dilated pupils, higher body temperature, increased heart rate and blood pressure, sweating, loss of appetite, sleeplessness, dry mouth, and tremors. If taken in a large enough dose, the drug produces delusions and visual hallucinations. The user's sense of time and self changes. Sensations may seem to "cross over," giving the user the feeling of hearing colors and seeing sounds. These changes can be frightening and can cause panic.[11]

Many LSD users experience flashbacks, recurrences of certain aspects of a person's experience, without the user having taken the drug again. A flashback occurs suddenly, often without warning, and may occur within a few days or more than a year after LSD use. LSD users may manifest relatively long-lasting psychoses, such as schizophrenia or severe depression.[12]

Most users of LSD voluntarily decrease or stop its use over time. LSD is not considered an addictive drug since it does not produce compulsive drug-seeking behavior as do cocaine, amphetamine, heroin, alcohol, and nicotine. However, like many of the addictive drugs, LSD produces tolerance, so some users who take the drug repeatedly must take progressively higher doses to achieve the state of intoxication that they had previously achieved.[13]

Death related to LSD abuse has occurred as a result of the panic reactions, hallucinations, delusions, and paranoia experienced by users. The cause of most LSD-related problems is the intense visual illusions that seem real and become overpowering, prompting the user to want to withdraw from the drug state immediately. Initially, at lower dosage levels, the visual images are intensified and color or flashes of light are seen. The visual images progress to brightly colored geometric designs and become distorted. At higher dosages, images appear as distortions of reality or as completely new visual images and can be seen with the eyes open or closed. Hallucinations also take other forms: thoughts become dreamlike or free-flowing, perception of time can become slowed or distorted, and out-of-body experiences or the perception that one's body has merged with another person or object may occur.[14]

Table 28.3. Definitions.

Drug Episode: A drug-related ED episode is an ED visit that was induced by or related to the use of drug(s).

Drug Mention: A drug mention refers to a substance that was recorded during an ED episode. Because up to four drugs can be reported for each drug abuse episode, there are more mentions than episodes.

According to the Drug Abuse Warning Network (DAWN) emergency department (ED) data for 2002, there were 891 mentions of LSD in emergency departments reporting to DAWN. This was a decrease from the 5,682 LSD mentions in 1995. During 2002, the age group in which LSD was most frequently mentioned was the 18- to 25-year-olds at 506 mentions. The race/ethnic group and gender accounting for the most LSD mentions was white with 670 mentions, and males with 776 mentions.[15]

More than 300 of those going to the ED because of LSD where there because of an unexpected reaction to the drug.[16]

Table 28.4. Reason for LSD-Related Emergency Department Contact, 2002.

Reason	Number of Visits
Unexpected reaction	349
Overdose	147
Chronic effects	-
Withdrawal	-
Seeking detoxification	119
Accident/injury	8
Other	44
Unknown	-

Table 28.5. Reason for LSD Use as Reported by LSD-Related Emergency Department Contacts, 2002.

Reason	Number of Visits
Psychic effects	421
Dependence	352
Suicide	49
Unknown motive for drug use	65

Arrests and Sentencing

Large amounts of LSD have been seized by drug law enforcement authorities during the last several years, and numerous distributors have been arrested and convicted. Penalties for Federal trafficking depend on the number of prior offenses and quantity of the drug confiscated. Penalties can range from monetary fines to incarceration.[17]

Production, Trafficking, and Distribution

LSD is available in retail quantities in almost every state. Since the 1960s, LSD has been manufactured illegally within the United States. It is reportedly produced on the West Coast, particularly in San Francisco, northern California, the Pacific Northwest, and recently the Midwest. The production of LSD is a time-consuming and complex procedure that requires a high degree of chemical expertise. There have been few LSD laboratory seizures in the United States because of infrequent and irregular production cycles. Chemists do not usually sell the drug, but instead distribute it to trusted associates.[18]

LSD is produced in crystal form that is converted to liquid and distributed primarily in the form of squares of blotter paper saturated with the liquid. Distribution of LSD is unique within the drug culture. An abundance of mail order sales has created a marketplace for sellers to remain virtually unknown to the buyers, which gives the drug traffickers a level of protection from drug law enforcement operations. Rock concerts continue to be favorite distribution sites for LSD traffickers; however, distribution at raves throughout the United States is becoming more popular.[19]

LSD is relatively inexpensive. The average price is approximately $5 per retail dosage unit and less than $1 per dosage unit in wholesale lots of 1,000 or more. Pure, high-potency LSD is a clear or white, odorless crystalline material that is soluble in water. Variations in the manufacturing process or the presence of precursors or by-products can cause LSD to range in color from clear or white, to tan or black, indicating poor quality or degradation. To mask product differences, distributors often apply LSD to off-white, tan, or yellow paper to disguise discoloration.[20]

Legislation

LSD is a Schedule I substance, meaning it has a high potential for abuse, there is no currently accepted medical use in treatment in the United States, and there is a lack of accepted safety for use of the substance under medical supervision.[21]

Lysergic acid and lysergic acid amide, substances used in the production of LSD, are both classified in Schedule III of the Controlled Substances Act (CSA). Ergotamine tartrate another item often used in LSD production, is regulated under the Chemical Diversion and Trafficking Act.[22]

Notes

1. Drug Enforcement Administration, *LSD in the United States*, October 1995.

2. National Institute on Drug Abuse, *Infofax-LSD*, January 2003.

3. Drug Enforcement Administration, *LSD in the United States*, October 1995.

4. National Institute on Drug Abuse, *Infofax-LSD*, January 2003.

5. Substance Abuse and Mental Health Services Administration, *Results from the 2002 National Survey on Drug Use and Health: National Findings*, September 2003.

6. National Institute on Drug Abuse and University of Michigan, *Monitoring the Future 2003 Data from In-School Surveys of 8th-, 10th-, and 12th-Grade Students*, December 2003.

7. Ibid.

8. National Institute on Drug Abuse and University of Michigan, *Monitoring the Future National Survey Results on Drug Use, 1975-2002, Volume II: College Students & Adults Ages 19–40* (PDF), 2003.

9. Office of National Drug Control Policy, *Pulse Check: Trends in Drug Abuse*, November 2002.

10. Drug Enforcement Administration, *LSD in the United States*, October 1995.

11. Ibid.

12. Ibid.

13. Ibid.

14. Ibid.

15. Substance Abuse and Mental Health Services Administration, *Emergency Department Trends from the Drug Abuse Warning Network, Final Estimates 1995–2002*, July 2003.

16. Ibid.

17. Drug Enforcement Administration, *LSD in the United States*, October 1995.

18. Ibid.

19. Ibid.

20. Ibid.

21. Drug Enforcement Administration, Controlled Substances Act.

22. Drug Enforcement Administration, *LSD in the United States*, October 1995.

Chapter 29

Marijuana

Marijuana is the most commonly used illicit drug in the United States. A dry, shredded green/brown mix of flowers, stems, seeds, and leaves of the hemp plant Cannabis sativa, it usually is smoked as a cigarette (joint, nail), or in a pipe (bong). It also is smoked in blunts, which are cigars that have been emptied of tobacco and refilled with marijuana, often in combination with another drug. Use also might include mixing marijuana in food or brewing it as a tea. As a more concentrated, resinous form it is called hashish and, as a sticky black liquid, hash oil. Marijuana smoke has a pungent and distinctive, usually sweet-and-sour odor. There are countless street terms for marijuana including pot, herb, weed, grass, widow, ganja, and hash, as well as terms derived from trademarked varieties of cannabis, such as Bubble Gum®, Northern Lights®, Juicy Fruit®, Afghani #1®, and a number of Skunk varieties.

The main active chemical in marijuana is THC (delta-9-tetra-hydrocannabinol). The membranes of certain nerve cells in the brain contain protein receptors that bind to THC. Once securely in place, THC kicks off a series of cellular reactions that ultimately lead to the high that users experience when they smoke marijuana.

Extent of Use

In 2001, over 12 million Americans age 12 and older used marijuana at least once in the month prior to being surveyed. That is more

NIDA InfoFacts, National Institute on Drug Abuse (NIDA), October 2002.

than three quarters (76%) of the total number of Americans who used any illicit drug in the past month in 2001. Of the 76%, more than half (56%) consumed only marijuana; 20% used marijuana and another illicit drug; and the remaining 24% used an illicit drug or drugs other than marijuana.[1]

Although marijuana is the most commonly used illicit drug in the United States, among students in the eighth, 10th, and 12th grades nationwide its use remained stable from 1999 through 2001.[2] Among eighth graders, however, past year use has decreased, from 18.3% in 1996 to 15.4% in 2001. Also in 2001, more than half (57.4%) of 12th graders believed it was harmful to smoke marijuana regularly and 79.3% disapproved of regular marijuana use. Since 1975, 83% to 90% of every 12th grade class surveyed has found it "fairly easy" or "very easy" to obtain marijuana.[3]

Data for drug-related hospital emergency department visits in the continental United States recently showed a 15% increase in the number of visits to an emergency room that were induced by or related to the use of marijuana (referred to as mentions), from 96,426 in 2000 to 110,512 in 2001. The 12 to 34 age range was involved most frequently in these mentions. For emergency room patients in the 12 to 17 age range, the rate of marijuana mentions increased 23% between 1999 and 2001 (from 55 to 68 per 100,000 population) and 126% (from 30 to 68 per 100,000 population) since 1994.[4]

Effects on the Brain

Scientists have learned a great deal about how THC acts in the brain to produce its many effects. When someone smokes marijuana, THC rapidly passes from the lungs into the bloodstream, which carries the chemical to organs throughout the body, including the brain.

In the brain, THC connects to specific sites called cannabinoid receptors on nerve cells and influences the activity of those cells. Some brain areas have many cannabinoid receptors; others have few or none. Many cannabinoid receptors are found in the parts of the brain that influence pleasure, memory, thought, concentration, sensory and time perception, and coordinated movement.[5]

The short-term effects of marijuana use can include problems with memory and learning; distorted perception; difficulty in thinking and problem solving; loss of coordination; and increased heart rate. Research findings for long-term marijuana use indicate some changes in the brain similar to those seen after long-term use of other major drugs of abuse. For example, cannabinoid (THC or synthetic forms of THC) withdrawal in chronically exposed animals leads to an increase in the activation of the stress-response system[6] and changes in the activity of nerve cells containing dopamine.[7] Dopamine neurons are involved in the regulation of motivation and reward, and are directly or indirectly affected by all drugs of abuse.

Effects on the Heart

One study has indicated that a user's risk of heart attack more than quadruples in the first hour after smoking marijuana.[8] The researchers suggest that such an effect might occur from marijuana's effects on blood pressure and heart rate and reduced oxygen-carrying capacity of blood.

Effects on the Lungs

A study of 450 individuals found that people who smoke marijuana frequently but do not smoke tobacco have more health problems and miss more days of work than nonsmokers.[9] Many of the extra sick days among the marijuana smokers in the study were for respiratory illnesses.

Even infrequent use can cause burning and stinging of the mouth and throat, often accompanied by a heavy cough. Someone who smokes marijuana regularly may have many of the same respiratory problems that tobacco smokers do, such as daily cough and phlegm production, more frequent acute chest illness, a heightened risk of lung infections, and a greater tendency to obstructed airways.[10]

Cancer of the respiratory tract and lungs may also be promoted by marijuana smoke.[11] A study comparing 173 cancer patients and 176 healthy individuals produced strong evidence that smoking marijuana increases the likelihood of developing cancer of the head or neck, and the more marijuana smoked the greater the increase.[12] A statistical analysis of the data suggested that marijuana smoking doubled or tripled the risk of these cancers.

Marijuana use has the potential to promote cancer of the lungs and other parts of the respiratory tract because it contains irritants and carcinogens.[13] In fact, marijuana smoke contains 50% to 70% more carcinogenic hydrocarbons than does tobacco smoke.[14] It also produces high levels of an enzyme that converts certain hydrocarbons into their carcinogenic form—levels that may accelerate the changes that ultimately produce malignant cells.[15] Marijuana users usually inhale more deeply and hold their breath longer than tobacco smokers do, which increases the lungs' exposure to carcinogenic smoke. These facts suggest that, puff for puff, smoking marijuana may increase the risk of cancer more than smoking tobacco.

Other Health Effects

Some of marijuana's adverse health effects may occur because THC impairs the immune system's ability to fight off infectious diseases and cancer. In laboratory experiments that exposed animal and human cells to THC or other marijuana ingredients, the normal disease-preventing reactions of many of the key types of immune cells were inhibited.[16] In other studies, mice exposed to THC or related substances were more likely than unexposed mice to develop bacterial infections and tumors.[17, 18]

Effects of Heavy Marijuana Use on Learning and Social Behavior

Depression[19], anxiety[20], and personality disturbances[21] are all associated with marijuana use. Research clearly demonstrates that marijuana use has potential to cause problems in daily life or make a person's existing problems worse. Because marijuana compromises the ability to learn and remember information, the more a person uses marijuana the more he or she is likely to fall behind in accumulating intellectual, job, or social skills. Moreover, research has shown that marijuana's adverse impact on memory and learning can last for days or weeks after the acute effects of the drug wear off.[22, 23]

Students who smoke marijuana get lower grades and are less likely to graduate from high school, compared to their non-smoking peers.[24, 25, 26, 27] In one study, researchers compared marijuana-smoking and non-smoking 12th-graders' scores on standardized tests of verbal and mathematical skills. Although all of the students had scored equally well in 4th grade, the marijuana smokers' scores were significantly lower in 12th grade.[28]

A study of 129 college students found that, for heavy users of marijuana (those who smoked the drug at least 27 of the preceding 30 days), critical skills related to attention, memory, and learning were significantly impaired even after they had not used the drug for at least 24 hours.[29] The heavy marijuana users in the study had more trouble sustaining and shifting their attention and in registering, organizing, and using information than did the study participants who had used marijuana no more than 3 of the previous 30 days. As a result, someone who smokes marijuana once daily may be functioning at a reduced intellectual level all of the time.

More recently, the same researchers showed that the ability of a group of long-term heavy marijuana users to recall words from a list remained impaired for a week after quitting, but returned to normal within 4 weeks.[30] An implication of this finding is that some cognitive abilities may be restored in individuals who quit smoking marijuana, even after long-term heavy use.

Workers who smoke marijuana are more likely than their coworkers to have problems on the job. Several studies associate workers' marijuana smoking with increased absences, tardiness, accidents, workers' compensation claims, and job turnover. A study of municipal workers found that those who used marijuana on or off the job reported more "withdrawal behaviors"—such as leaving work without permission, daydreaming, spending work time on personal matters, and shirking tasks—that adversely affect productivity and morale.[31]

Effects on Pregnancy

Research has shown that babies born to women who used marijuana during their pregnancies display altered responses to visual stimuli, increased tremulousness, and a high-pitched cry, which may indicate problems with neurological development.[32] During infancy and preschool years, marijuana-exposed children have been observed to have more behavioral problems and poorer performance on tasks of visual perception, language comprehension, sustained attention, and memory.[33, 34] In school, these children are more likely to exhibit deficits in decision-making skills, memory, and the ability to remain attentive.[35, 36, 37]

Addictive Potential

Long-term marijuana use can lead to addiction for some people; that is, they use the drug compulsively even though it often interferes with family, school, work, and recreational activities. Drug craving and withdrawal symptoms can make it hard for long-term marijuana smokers to stop using the drug. People trying to quit report irritability, sleeplessness, and anxiety.[38] They also display increased aggression on psychological tests, peaking approximately one week after the last use of the drug.[39]

Genetic Vulnerability

Scientists have found that whether an individual has positive or negative sensations after smoking marijuana can be influenced by heredity. A 1997 study[40] demonstrated that identical male twins were more likely than non-identical male twins to report similar responses to marijuana use, indicating a genetic basis for their response to the drug. (Identical twins share all of their genes.)

It also was discovered that the twins' shared or family environment before age 18 had no detectable influence on their response to marijuana. Certain environmental factors, however, such as the availability of marijuana, expectations about how the drug would affect them, the influence of friends and social contacts, and other factors that differentiate experiences of identical twins were found to have an important effect.

Treating Marijuana Problems

The latest treatment data indicate that, in 1999, marijuana was the primary drug of abuse in about 14% (223,597) of all admissions to treatment facilities in the United States. Marijuana admissions were primarily male (77%), white (58%), and young (47% under 20 years old). Those in treatment for primary marijuana use had begun use at an early age; 57% had used it by age 14 and 92% had used it by 18.[41]

One study of adult marijuana users found comparable benefits from a 14-session cognitive-behavioral group treatment and a 2-session individual treatment that included motivational interviewing and advice on ways to reduce marijuana use. Participants were mostly men in their early thirties who had smoked marijuana daily for more than 10 years. By increasing patients' awareness of what triggers their marijuana use, both treatments sought to help patients devise avoidance strategies. Use, dependence symptoms, and psychosocial problems decreased for at least 1 year following both treatments; about 30% of users were abstinent during the last 3-month follow-up period.[42]

Another study suggests that giving patients vouchers that they can redeem for goods—such as movie passes, sporting equipment, or vocational training—may further improve outcomes.[43]

Although no medications are currently available for treating marijuana abuse, recent discoveries about the workings of the THC receptors have raised the possibility of eventually developing a medication that will block the intoxicating effects of THC. Such a medication might be used to prevent relapse to marijuana abuse by lessening or eliminating its appeal.

Notes

1. These data are from the annual *National Household Survey on Drug Abuse*, funded by the Substance Abuse and Mental Health Services Administration, U.S. Department of Health and Human Services (DHHS). The latest data (2001) are available at (800) 729-6686 or online at www.samhsa.gov.

2. These data are from the Monitoring the Future Survey, funded by National Institute on Drug Abuse, National Institutes of Health, DHHS, and conducted by the University of Michigan's Institute for Social Research. The survey has tracked 12th graders' illicit drug use and related attitudes since 1975; in 1991, eighth and 10th graders were added to the study. The latest data (2001) are online at www.drugabuse.gov.

3. Ibid.

4. These data are from the annual Drug Abuse Warning Network, funded by the Substance Abuse and Mental Health Services Administration, DHHS. The survey provides information about emergency department visits that are induced by or related to the use of an illicit drug or the nonmedical use of a legal drug. The latest data (2001) are available at (800) 729-6686 or online at www.samhsa.gov.

5. Herkenham M, Lynn A., Little MD, Johnson MR, et al: Cannabinoid receptor localization in the brain. *Proc Natl Acad Sci*, USA 87:1932-1936, 1990.

6. Rodriguez de Fonseca F, et al: Activation of cortocotropin-releasing factor in the limbic system during cannabinoid withdrawal. *Science* 276(5321):2050-2064, 1997.

7. Diana M, Melis M, Muntoni AL, et al: Mesolimbic dopaminergic decline after cannabinoid withdrawal. *Proc. Natl. Acad. Sci* 95:10269-10273, 1998.

8. Mittleman MA, Lewis RA, Maclure M, et al: Triggering myocardial infarction by marijuana. *Circulation* 103:2805-2809, 2001.

9. Polen M R, Sidney S, Tekawa IS, et al: Health care use by frequent marijuana smokers who do not smoke tobacco. *West J Med* 158:596-601, 1993.

10. Tashkin DP: Pulmonary complications of smoked substance abuse. *West J Med* 152:525-530, 1990.

11. Ibid.

12. Zhang ZF, Morgenstern H, Spitz MR, et al: Marijuana use and increased risk of squamous cell carcinoma of the head and neck. *Cancer Epidemiology, Biomarkers & Prevention* 6:1071-1078, 1999.

13. Sridhar KS, Raub WA, Weatherby, NL Jr, et al: Possible role of marijuana smoking as a carcinogen in the development of lung cancer at a young age. *Journal of Psychoactive Drugs* 26(3):285-288, 1994.

14. Hoffman D, Brunnemann KD, Gori GB, et al: On the carcinogenicity of marijuana smoke. In: VC Runeckles, ed, *Recent Advances in Phytochemistry*. New York. Plenum, 1975.

15. Cohen S: Adverse effects of marijuana: selected issues. *Annals of the New York Academy of Sciences* 362:119-124, 1981.

16. Adams IB, Martin BR: Cannabis: pharmacology and toxicology in animals and humans. *Addiction* 91:1585-1614, 1996.

17. Klein TW, Newton C, Friedman H: Resistance to Legionella pneumophila suppressed by the marijuana component, tetrahydrocannabinol. *J Infectious Disease* 169:1177-1179, 1994.

18. Zhu L, Stolina M, Sharma S, et al: Delta-9 tetrahydrocannabinol inhibits antitumor immunity by a CB2 receptor-mediated, cytokine-dependent pathway. *J Immunology*, 2000, pp. 373-380.

19. Brook JS, et al: The effect of early marijuana use on later anxiety and depressive symptoms. *NYS Psychologist*, January 2001, pp. 35-39.

20. Green BE, Ritter C: Marijuana use and depression. *J Health Soc Behav* 41(1):40-49, 2000.

21. Brook JS, Cohen P, Brook DW: Longitudinal study of co-occurring psychiatric disorders and substance use. *J Acad Child and Adolescent Psych* 37:322-330, 1998.

22. Pope HG, Yurgelun-Todd D: The residual cognitive effects of heavy marijuana use in college students. *JAMA* 272(7):521-527, 1996.

23. Block RI, Ghoneim MM: Effects of chronic marijuana use on human cognition. *Psychopharmacology* 100(1-2):219-228, 1993.

24. Lynskey M, Hall W: The effects of adolescent cannabis use on educational attainment: a review. *Addiction* 95(11):1621-1630, 2000.

25. Kandel DB, Davies M: High school students who use crack and other drugs. *Arch Gen Psychiatry* 53(1):71-80, 1996.

26. Rob M, Reynolds I, Finlayson PF: Adolescent marijuana use: risk factors and implications. *Aust NZ J Psychiatry* 24(1):45-56, 1990.

27. Brook JS, Balka EB, Whiteman M: The risks for late adolescence of early adolescent marijuana use. *Am J Public Health* 89(10):1549-1554, 1999.

28. Block RI, Ghoneim MM: Effects of chronic marijuana use on human cognition. *Psychopharmacology* 100(1-2):219 228, 1993.

29. Ibid ref 22.

30. Pope, Gruber, Hudson, et al: Neuropsychological performance in long-term cannabis users. *Archives of General Psychiatry*.

31. Lehman WE, Simpson DD: Employee substance abuse and on-the-job behaviors. *Journal of Applied Psychology* 77(3):309-321, 1992.

32. Lester, BM; Dreher, M: Effects of marijuana use during pregnancy on newborn cry. *Child Development* 60:764-771, 1989.

33. Fried, PA: The Ottawa prenatal prospective study (OPPS): methodological issues and findings-it's easy to throw the baby out with the bath water. *Life Sciences* 56:2159-2168, 1995.

34. Fried, PA: Prenatal exposure to marihuana and tobacco during infancy, early and middle childhood: effects and an attempt at synthesis. *Arch Toxicol Supp* 17:233-60, 1995.

35. Ibid ref 33.

36. Ibid ref 34.

37. Cornelius MD, Taylor PM, Geva D, et al: Prenatal tobacco and marijuana use among adolescents: effects on offspring gestational age, growth, and morphology. *Pediatrics* 95:738-743, 1995.

38. Kouri EM, Pope HG, Lukas SE: Changes in aggressive behavior during withdrawal from long-term marijuana use. *Psychopharmacology* 143:302-308, 1999.

39. Haney M, Ward AS, Comer SD, et al: Abstinence symptoms following smoked marijuana in humans. *Psychopharmacology* 141:395-404, 1999.

40. Lyons MJ, et al: *Addiction* 92(4):409-417, 1997.

41. These data from the Treatment Episode Data Set (TEDS) 1994–1999: National Admissions to Substance Abuse Treatment Services, November 2001, funded by the Substance Abuse and Mental Health Service Administration, DHHS. The latest data are available at (800) 729-6686 or online at www.samhsa.gov.

42. Stephens RS, Roffman RA, Curtin L: Comparison of extended versus brief treatments for marijuana use. *J Consult Clin Psychol* 68(5):898-908, 2000.

43. Budney AJ, Higgins ST, Radonovich KJ, et al: Adding voucher-based incentives to coping skills and motivational enhancement improves outcomes during treatment for marijuana dependence. *J Consult Clin Psychol* 68(6):1051-1061, 2000.

Chapter 30

Methadone

What is methadone?

Methadone is a synthetic (man-made) narcotic. It is used legally to treat addiction to narcotics and to relieve severe pain, often in individuals who have cancer or terminal illnesses. Although methadone has been legally available in the United States since 1947, more recently it has emerged as a drug of abuse. This trend may be driven in part by the ready availability of the drug as it increasingly is used in the treatment of narcotic addiction and to relieve chronic pain.

What does methadone look like?

Methadone is available as a tablet, oral solution, or injectable liquid.

How is methadone used?

Some methadone tablets are designed to be swallowed intact, while others are intended to be dissolved first in liquid. Likewise, methadone is available either as a ready-to-drink solution or as a concentrate, which must be mixed first with water or fruit juice. Methadone also is available as a liquid that is administered via injection.

"Methadone Fast Facts: Questions and Answers," National Drug Intelligence Center (NDIC), a component of the U.S. Department of Justice, September 2003.

When used to treat narcotic addiction, methadone suppresses withdrawal symptoms for 24 to 36 hours. Individuals who are prescribed methadone for treatment of heroin addiction experience neither the cravings for heroin nor the euphoric rush that are typically associated with use of that drug.

Who abuses methadone?

It is difficult to gauge the extent of methadone abuse in the United States because most data sources that quantify drug abuse combine methadone with other narcotics. This lack of statistical information renders it impossible to describe a typical methadone abuser. Information provided by the Treatment Episode Data Set does reveal that the number of individuals who were treated for abuse of "other opiates" (a category that includes methadone) increased dramatically from 28,235 in 2000 to 36,265 in 2001. These individuals were predominantly Caucasian; they were nearly evenly split between males and females and represented various age groups.

Methadone abuse among high school students is a concern. Nearly 1% of high school seniors in the United States abused the drug at least once in their lifetime, according to the University of Michigan's Monitoring the Future Survey.

What are the risks?

Individuals who abuse methadone risk becoming tolerant of and physically dependent on the drug. When these individuals stop using the drug they may experience withdrawal symptoms including muscle tremors, nausea, diarrhea, vomiting, and abdominal cramps.

Overdosing on methadone poses an additional risk. In some instances, individuals who abuse other narcotics (such as heroin or OxyContin) turn to methadone because of its increasing availability. Methadone, however, does not produce the euphoric rush associated with those other drugs; thus, these users often consume dangerously large quantities of methadone in a vain attempt to attain the desired effect.

Methadone overdoses are associated with severe respiratory depression, decreases in heart rate and blood pressure, coma, and death. The Drug Abuse Warning Network reports that methadone was involved in 10,725 emergency department visits in 2001—a 37% increase from the previous year.

Is abusing methadone illegal?

Yes, abusing methadone is illegal. Methadone is a Schedule II substance under the Controlled Substances Act. Schedule II drugs, which include cocaine and methamphetamine, have a high potential for abuse. Abuse of these drugs may lead to severe psychological or physical dependence.

Chapter 31

Methamphetamine and Other Amphetamines

Questions and Answers about Amphetamines

What are amphetamines?

Amphetamine, dextroamphetamine, methamphetamine, and their various salts are collectively referred to as amphetamines. In fact, their chemical properties and actions are so similar that even experienced users have difficulty knowing which drug they have taken. Methamphetamine is the most commonly abused.

What does methamphetamine look like?

- Typically meth is a white powder that easily dissolves in water.

- Another form of meth, in clear chunky crystals, called crystal meth, or ice.

- Meth can also be in the form of small, brightly colored tablets. The pills are often called by their Thai name, yaba.

This chapter begins with questions and answers from "Methamphetamine and Amphetamines," Drug Enforcement Administration (DEA), U.S. Department of Justice, 2002. "Facts about Methamphetamine" is from "Methamphetamine," Fact Sheet #NCJ 197534, Office of National Drug Control Policy (ONDCP), Drug Policy Information Clearinghouse, November 2003.

What are the methods of usage?

- Injecting
- Snorting
- Smoking
- Oral ingestion[1]

Who uses methamphetamine and amphetamines?

- During 2000, 4% of the U.S. population reported trying methamphetamine at least once in their lifetime.[2]
- Abuse is concentrated in the western, southwestern, and midwestern United States.

How do methamphetamine and amphetamines get to the United States?

- Clandestine laboratories in California and Mexico are the primary sources of supply for methamphetamine available in the United States.
- Domestic labs that produce methamphetamine are dependent on supplies of the precursor chemical pseudoephedrine, which is sometimes diverted from legitimate sources. It is smuggled from Canada, and to a lesser extent from Mexico.
- Domestic independent laboratory operators, mostly in the western, southwestern, and midwestern United States, also produce and distribute methamphetamine but on a smaller scale.
- Yaba (meth in tablet form) is most often produced in Southeast Asia and sent by mail or courier to the United States.[3]

How much do methamphetamine and amphetamines cost?

- Prices for methamphetamine vary throughout different regions of the United States.
- At the distribution level, prices range from $3,500 per pound in parts of California and Texas to $21,000 per pound in southeastern and northeastern regions of the country. Retail prices range from $400 to $3,000 per ounce.[4]

What are some consequences of methamphetamine and amphetamine use?

- Effects of usage include addiction, psychotic behavior, and brain damage.[5]

- Withdrawal symptoms include depression, anxiety, fatigue, paranoia, aggression, and intense cravings.[6]

- Chronic use can cause violent behavior, anxiety, confusion, insomnia, auditory hallucinations, mood disturbances, delusions, and paranoia.[7]

- Damage to the brain cause by meth usage is similar to Alzheimer's disease, stroke, and epilepsy.[8]

Notes

1. Drug Enforcement Administration, *The Forms of Methamphetamine*, April 2002.

2. Substance Abuse and Mental Health Services Administration, *Summary of Findings from the 2000 National Household Survey on Drug Abuse*, September 2001.

3. Drug Enforcement Administration, *Drug Trafficking in the United States*, September 2001.

4. Ibid.

5. Office of National Drug Control Policy, *Drug Facts: Methamphetamine*, May 2002.

6. Ibid.

7. Ibid.

8. National Institute on Drug Abuse, *Methamphetamine: Abuse and Addiction*, April 1998. *What Are the Effects of Methamphetamine Abuse?*

Facts about Methamphetamine

Methamphetamine, a derivative of amphetamine, is a powerful stimulant that affects the central nervous system. Amphetamines were originally intended for use in nasal decongestants and bronchial inhalers and have limited medical applications, which include the treatment of narcolepsy, weight control, and attention deficit disorder. Methamphetamine can be smoked, snorted, orally ingested, and injected. It is accessible in many different forms and may be identified by color, which ranges from white to yellow to darker colors such as red and brown. Methamphetamine comes in a powder form that resembles granulated crystals and in a rock form known as "ice," which is the smokeable version of methamphetamine that came into use during the 1980s.

Effects

Methamphetamine use increases energy and alertness and decreases appetite. An intense rush is felt, almost instantaneously, when a user smokes or injects methamphetamine. Snorting methamphetamine affects the user in approximately 5 minutes, whereas oral ingestion takes about 20 minutes for the user to feel the effects. The intense rush and high felt from methamphetamine results from the release of high levels of dopamine into the section of the brain that controls the feeling of pleasure. The effects of methamphetamine can last up to 12 hours. Side effects include convulsions, dangerously high body temperature, stroke, cardiac arrhythmia, stomach cramps, and shaking.

Chronic use of methamphetamine can result in a tolerance for the drug. Consequently, users may try to intensify the desired effects by taking higher doses of the drug, taking it more frequently, or changing their method of ingestion. Some abusers, while refraining from eating and sleeping, will binge, also known as "run," on methamphetamine. During these binges, users will inject as much as a gram of methamphetamine every two to three hours over several days until they run out of the drug or are too dazed to continue use.

Chronic methamphetamine abuse can lead to psychotic behavior including intense paranoia, visual and auditory hallucinations, and out-of-control rages that can result in violent episodes. Chronic users at times develop sores on their bodies from scratching at "crank bugs," which describes the common delusion that bugs are crawling under the skin. Long-term use of methamphetamine may result in anxiety, insomnia, and addiction.

After methamphetamine use is stopped, several withdrawal symptoms can occur, including depression, anxiety, fatigue, paranoia, aggression, and an intense craving for the drug. Psychotic symptoms can sometimes persist for months or years after use has ceased.

Table 31.1. Percentage of Lifetime Methamphetamine Use among U.S. Population by Age Group, 2002.

Age Group	Lifetime	Past Year	Past Month
12–17	1.5%	0.9%	0.3%
18–25	5.7	1.7	0.5
26 and older	5.7	0.4	0.2
Total population	5.3	0.7	0.3

Source: National Survey on Drug Use and Health.

Table 31.2. Percentage of Methamphetamine Use by Secondary School Students, by Grade, 1999–2002.

Lifetime

Grade	1999	2000	2001	2002
8th graders	4.5%	4.2%	4.4%	3.5%
10th graders	7.3	6.9	6.4	6.1
12th graders	8.2	7.9	6.9	6.7

Annual

Grade	1999	2000	2001	2002
8th graders	3.2%	2.5%	2.8%	2.2%
10th graders	4.6	4.0	3.7	3.9
12th graders	4.7	4.3	3.9	3.6

Past 30 Days

Grade	1999	2000	2001	2002
8th graders	1.1%	0.8%	1.3%	1.1%
10th graders	1.8	2.0	1.5	1.8
12th graders	1.7	1.9	1.5	1.7

Source: Monitoring the Future Study.

Prevalence Estimates

According to the U.S. Department of Health and Human Services' *Results From the 2002 National Survey on Drug Use and Health: National Findings*, more than 12 million people age 12 and older (5.3%) reported that they had used methamphetamine at least once in their lifetime (see Table 31.1). Of those surveyed, 597,000 persons age 12 and older (0.3%) reported past month use of methamphetamine.

Since 1999, methamphetamine has been included in the University of Michigan's Monitoring the Future survey questionnaire. Survey results indicate that annual methamphetamine use (use within the past year) by secondary school students in 1999 ranged from 3.2% among 8th graders, to 4.6% among 10th graders, to 4.7% among 12th graders (see Table 31.2). In 2002, estimates of annual methamphetamine use ranged from 2.2% among eighth graders, to 3.9% among 10th graders, to 3.6% among 12th graders.

The study also collected data on methamphetamine use by college students and young adults ages 19 to 28. During 1999, 3.3% of college students and 2.8% of young adults tried methamphetamine in the past year (see Table 31.3). In 2002, annual use of methamphetamine declined to 1.2% for college students and 2.5% for young adults.

According to the Centers for Disease Control and Prevention's *Youth Risk Behavior Surveillance—United States, 2001* study, 9.8% of high school students had used methamphetamine within their lifetime. Overall, white (11.4%) and Hispanic (9.1%) students were more likely than black students (2.1%) to report lifetime methamphetamine use.

Regional Observations

The widespread availability of methamphetamine is illustrated by increasing numbers of methamphetamine seizures, arrests, indictments, and sentences. According to the National Drug Intelligence Center (NDIC), methamphetamine is widely available throughout the Pacific, Southwest, and West Central regions and is increasingly available in the Great Lakes and Southeast.

Similarly, the National Institute on Drug Abuse's Community Epidemiology Work Group (CEWG) reports that, in 2002, methamphetamine indicators remained highest in West Coast areas and parts of the Southwest, as well as Hawaii. Methamphetamine abuse is spreading in areas such as Atlanta, Chicago, Detroit, St. Louis, and Texas.

Relatively low indicators were found in East Coast and Mid-Atlantic CEWG areas, although abuse is increasing.

According to the Arrestee Drug Abuse Monitoring Program sites, during 2002, methamphetamine use by adult arrestees was concentrated in the Western region of the United States. Out of 36 sites, the highest percentages of adult male arrestees testing positive for methamphetamine were located in Honolulu (44.8%), Sacramento (33.5%), San Diego (31.7%), and Phoenix (31.2%). Out of 23 sites, the highest percentages of adult female arrestees testing positive for methamphetamine were located in Honolulu (50%), San Jose (42.8%), Phoenix (41.7%), Salt Lake City (37.7%), and San Diego (36.8%).

According to *Pulse Check: Trends in Drug Abuse*, law enforcement agencies and epidemiologic/ethnographic sources surveyed in 2002 reported that methamphetamine availability increased in the following sites: Boston, Billings, Chicago, Columbia (South Carolina), Denver, Detroit, Honolulu, Los Angeles, Memphis, Miami, New York, and Sioux Falls (South Dakota). The remaining 12 Pulse Check sites reported stable methamphetamine availability. There were no reported decreases in availability.

Table 31.3. Percentage of Methamphetamine Use by College Students and Young Adults, 1999–2002.

Lifetime

Age Groups	1999	2000	2001	2002
College students	7.1%	5.1%	5.3%	5.0%
Young adults	8.8	9.3	9.0	9.1

Annual

Age Groups	1999	2000	2001	2002
College students	3.3%	1.6%	2.4%	1.2%
Young adults	2.8	2.5	2.8	2.5

Past 30 Days

Age Groups	1999	2000	2001	2002
College students	1.2%	0.2%	0.5%	0.2%
Young adults	0.8	0.7	1.0	1.0

Source: Monitoring the Future Study.

Availability

Yaba, the Thai name for a tablet form of methamphetamine mixed with caffeine, is appearing in Asian communities in California. These tablets are popular in Southeast and East Asia where they are produced. The tablets are small enough to fit in the end of a drinking straw and are usually reddish-orange or green with various logos. There are indications that methamphetamine tablets are becoming more popular in the rave scene because their appearance is similar to club drugs such as ecstasy.

Production and Trafficking

Methamphetamine trafficking and abuse have changed in the United States during the past 10 years. Mexican drug trafficking organizations have become the dominant manufacturing and distribution group in cities in the Midwest and the West. Methamphetamine production and abuse were previously controlled by independent laboratory operators, such as outlaw motorcycle gangs, which continue to operate but to a smaller extent. The Mexican criminal organizations are able to manufacture in excess of 10 pounds of methamphetamine in a 24-hour period, producing high-purity, low-cost methamphetamine.

Methamphetamine precursor chemicals usually include pseudo-ephedrine and ephedrine drug products. Mexican organizations sometimes use methylsulfonylmethane (MSM) to "cut" the methamphetamine in the production cycle. MSM is legitimately used as a dietary supplement for horses and humans. The supplement is readily available at feed/livestock stores and in health/nutrition stores. By adding MSM, the volume of methamphetamine produced is increased, which in turn increases the profits for the dealer.

Price and Purity

According to the Drug Enforcement Administration (DEA), during 2001, the price of methamphetamine ranged nationally from $3,500 to $23,000 per pound, $350 to $2,200 per ounce, and $20 to $300 per gram. The average purity of methamphetamine decreased from 71.9% in 1994 to 40.1% in 2001. International controls have reduced the availability of chemicals used to produce high-purity methamphetamine and may have contributed to the decrease in purity levels.

Enforcement

Arrests

From October 1, 2000, to September 30, 2001, there were 3,932 federal drug arrests for amphetamine/methamphetamine, representing 12% of all federal drug arrests.

Seizures

According to the Federal-wide Drug Seizure System (FDSS), 2,807 kilograms of methamphetamine were seized in 2001 by U.S. federal law enforcement authorities, down from 3,373 kilograms in 2000. FDSS consolidates information about drug seizures made within the jurisdiction of the United States by DEA, the Federal Bureau of Investigation (FBI), and U.S. Customs and Border Protection, as well as maritime seizures made by the U.S. Coast Guard. FDSS eliminates duplicate reporting of seizures involving more than one federal agency.

In addition, federal authorities seized 301,697 Southeast Asian methamphetamine tablets in U.S. Postal Service facilities in Oakland, Los Angeles, and Honolulu in 2000, representing a 656% increase from the 1999 seizures of 39,917 tablets.

According to the El Paso Intelligence Center's National Clandestine Laboratory Seizure System, 8,290 methamphetamine labs were seized in 2001. In 2001, there were 303 "superlabs" with the capacity to produce 10 or more pounds of methamphetamine in one production cycle seized in the United States.

Adjudication

During fiscal year (FY) 2001, 3,404 federal drug offenders were convicted of committing an offense involving methamphetamine. Of those convicted of a federal drug offense for methamphetamine, 59% were white, 35.2% were Hispanic, 4.2% were of another race, and 1.6% were black.

Corrections

In FY 2001, the average length of sentence received by federal methamphetamine offenders was 88.5 months, compared with 115 months for crack cocaine offenders, 77 months for powder cocaine offenders, 63.4 months for heroin offenders, 38 months for marijuana offenders, and 41.1 months for other drug offenders.

Consequences of Use

Chronic methamphetamine abuse can result in inflammation of the heart lining and, for injecting drug users, damaged blood vessels and skin abscesses. Social and occupational connections progressively deteriorate for chronic methamphetamine users. Acute lead poisoning is another potential risk for methamphetamine abusers because of a common method of production that uses lead acetate as a reagent.

Medical consequences of methamphetamine use can include cardiovascular problems such as rapid heart rate, irregular heartbeat, increased blood pressure, and stroke-producing damage to small blood vessels in the brain. Hyperthermia and convulsions can occur when a user overdoses and, if not treated immediately, can result in death. Research has shown that as much as 50% of the dopamine-producing cells in the brain can be damaged by prolonged exposure to relatively low levels of methamphetamine and that serotonin-containing nerve cells may be damaged even more extensively.

Methamphetamine abuse during pregnancy can cause prenatal complications such as increased rates of premature delivery and altered neonatal behavior patterns, such as abnormal reflexes and extreme irritability, and may be linked to congenital deformities. Methamphetamine abuse, particularly by those who inject the drug and share needles, can increase users' risks of contracting HIV/AIDS and hepatitis B and C.

Table 31.4. Number of Emergency Department Methamphetamine Mentions, 1995–2002.

1995	1996	1997	1998	1999	2000	2001	2002
15,933	11,002	17,154	11,486	10,447	13,505	14,923	17,696

Source: Drug Abuse Warning Network.

During 1995, hospitals participating in the Drug Abuse Warning Network (DAWN) reported 15,933 mentions of methamphetamine (see Table 31.4). A drug mention refers to a substance that was recorded (mentioned) during a drug-related visit to the emergency department (ED). By 1999, the number of methamphetamine ED mentions decreased to 10,447. This number increased to 17,696 in 2002.

In 2001, DAWN's mortality data for methamphetamine mentions to medical examiners remained concentrated in the Midwest and West regions of the United States. The metropolitan areas reporting the most methamphetamine mentions were Phoenix (122), San Diego (94), and Las Vegas (53). The East Coast area that reported the highest number of methamphetamine mentions was Long Island (49). Out of 42 metropolitan areas studied, 15 areas reported fewer than 5 methamphetamine mentions.

Treatment

According to the Treatment Episode Data Set, during 2000 methamphetamine treatment admissions accounted for 4.1% of total admissions or 66,052 admissions. Those admitted for methamphetamine/amphetamine were primarily white (79%) and male (53%). In 1994, there were half as many admissions for methamphetamine, 33,432 or about 2% of all admissions for treatment.

There are no pharmacological treatments for methamphetamine dependence. Antidepressant medications can be used to combat the depressive symptoms of withdrawal. The most effective treatment for methamphetamine addiction is cognitive behavioral interventions, which modify a patient's thinking, expectancies, and behavior while increasing coping skills to deal with life stressors.

Clandestine Laboratories

Methamphetamine can be easily manufactured in clandestine laboratories (meth labs) using ingredients purchased in local stores. Over-the-counter cold medicines containing ephedrine or pseudoephedrine and other materials are "cooked" in meth labs to make methamphetamine.

The manufacture of methamphetamine has a severe impact on the environment. The production of one pound of methamphetamine releases poisonous gas into the atmosphere and creates 5 to 7 pounds of toxic waste. Many laboratory operators dump the toxic waste down household drains, in fields and yards, or on rural roads.

Due to the creation of toxic waste at methamphetamine production sites, many first response personnel incur injury when dealing with the hazardous substances. The most common symptoms suffered by first responders when they raid meth labs are respiratory and eye irritations, headaches, dizziness, nausea, and shortness of breath.

Meth labs can be portable and so are easily dismantled, stored, or moved. This portability helps methamphetamine manufacturers avoid law enforcement authorities. Meth labs have been found in many different types of locations, including apartments, hotel rooms, rented storage spaces, and trucks. Methamphetamine labs have been known to be booby trapped and lab operators are often well armed.

According to DEA, in 2001 there were 12,715 methamphetamine laboratory incidents reported in 46 states. The West Coast accounted for most of the laboratory incidents. On the East Coast, the following States reported the highest incident rates: Georgia (51), North Carolina (31), and Florida (29). Nationally, the highest rate of lab activity took place in Missouri, which reported 2,207 incidents. California and Washington also had high incident rates with 1,847 and 1,477, respectively.

Scheduling and Legislation

Methamphetamine is a Schedule II drug under the Controlled Substance Act of 1970. A Schedule II Controlled Substance has high potential for abuse, is currently accepted for medical use in treatment in the United States, and may lead to severe psychological or physical dependence.

The chemicals that are used to produce methamphetamine also are controlled under the Comprehensive Methamphetamine Control Act of 1996 (MCA). This legislation broadened the restrictions on listed chemicals used in the production of methamphetamine, increased penalties for the trafficking and manufacturing of methamphetamine and listed chemicals, and expanded the controls of products containing the licit chemicals ephedrine, pseudoephedrine, and phenylpropanolamine (PPA).

The Methamphetamine Anti-Proliferation Act was passed in July 2000. The act strengthens sentencing guidelines and provides training for federal and state law enforcement officers on methamphetamine investigations and the handling of the chemicals used in clandestine meth labs. It also puts in place controls on the distribution of the chemical ingredients used in methamphetamine production and expands substance abuse prevention efforts.

Chapter 32

Methylphenidate (Ritalin)

Methylphenidate is a medication prescribed for individuals (usually children) who have an abnormally high level of activity or attention-deficit hyperactivity disorder (ADHD). According to the National Institute of Mental Health, about 3% to 5% of the general population has the disorder, which is characterized by agitated behavior and an inability to focus on tasks. Methylphenidate also is occasionally prescribed for treating narcolepsy.

Health Effects

Methylphenidate is a central nervous system (CNS) stimulant. It has effects similar to, but more potent than, caffeine and less potent than amphetamines. It has a notably calming effect on hyperactive children and a "focusing" effect on those with ADHD.

Recent research[1] at Brookhaven National Laboratory may begin to explain how methylphenidate helps people with ADHD. The researchers used positron emission tomography (PET—a noninvasive brain scan) to confirm that administering normal therapeutic doses of methylphenidate to healthy, adult men increased their dopamine levels. The researchers speculate that methylphenidate amplifies the release of dopamine, a neurotransmitter, thereby improving attention and focus in individuals who have dopamine signals that are weak, such as individuals with ADHD.

NIDA InfoFacts, National Institute on Drug Abuse (NIDA), April 2001.

When taken as prescribed, methylphenidate is a valuable medicine. Research shows that people with ADHD do not become addicted to stimulant medications when taken in the form prescribed and at treatment dosages.[2] Another study found that ADHD boys treated with stimulants such as methylphenidate are significantly less likely to abuse drugs and alcohol when they are older than are non-treated ADHD boys.[3]

Because of its stimulant properties, however, in recent years there have been reports of abuse of methylphenidate by people for whom it is not a medication. Some individuals abuse it for its stimulant effects: appetite suppression, wakefulness, increased focus/attentiveness, and euphoria. When abused, the tablets are either taken orally or crushed and snorted. Some abusers dissolve the tablets in water and inject the mixture—complications can arise from this because insoluble fillers in the tablets can block small blood vessels.

Trends in Ritalin Abuse

At their June 2000 meeting, members of NIDA's Community Epidemiology Work Group (CEWG) shared the following information.

- The abuse of methylphenidate has been reported in Baltimore, mostly among middle and high schools students; Boston, especially among middle and upper-middle class communities; Detroit; Minneapolis/St. Paul; Phoenix; and Texas.

- When abused, methylphenidate tablets are often used orally or crushed and used intranasally.

- In 1999, 165 methylphenidate-related poison calls were made in Detroit; 419 were reported in Texas, with 114 of those involving intentional misuse or abuse.

- On Chicago's South Side, some users inject methylphenidate (this is referred to as "west coast"). Also, some mix it with heroin (a "speedball") or in combination with both cocaine and heroin for a more potent effect.

Because stimulant medicines such as methylphenidate do have potential for abuse, the U.S. Drug Enforcement Administration (DEA) has placed stringent, Schedule II controls on their manufacture, distribution, and prescription. For example, DEA requires special licenses for these activities, and prescription refills are not allowed. States may impose further regulations, such as limiting the number of dosage units per prescription.

Notes

1. Nora Volkow, et al., Therapeutic Doses of Oral Methylphenidate Significantly Increase Extracellular Dopamine in the Human Brain, *The Journal of Neuroscience*, 2001, 21:RC121:1-5.

2. Nora Volkow, et al., Dopamine Transporter Occupancies in the Human Brain Induced by Therapeutic Doses of Oral Methyl-phenidate, *Am J Psychiatry* 155:1325-1331, October 1998.

3. Joseph Biederman, et al., Pharmacotherapy of Attention-deficit Hyperactivity Disorder Reduces Risk for Substance Use Disor-der, *Pediatrics* 1999 104:e20.

Chapter 33

OxyContin

What is OxyContin?

OxyContin, a trade name for the narcotic oxycodone hydrochloride, is a painkiller available in the United States only by prescription. OxyContin is legitimately prescribed for relief of moderate to severe pain resulting from injuries, bursitis, neuralgia, arthritis, and cancer. Individuals abuse OxyContin for the euphoric effect it produces—an effect similar to that associated with heroin use.

What does OxyContin look like?

OxyContin is available as a 10 milligram (mg), 20 mg, 40 mg, or 80 mg tablet. The tablets vary in color and size according to dosage. The tablets are imprinted with the letters OC on one side and the number of milligrams on the opposite side.

How is OxyContin abused?

OxyContin tablets have a controlled-release feature and are designed to be swallowed whole. In order to bypass the controlled-release feature, abusers either chew or crush the tablets. Crushed tablets can be snorted or dissolved in water and injected.

"OxyContin Fast Facts: Questions and Answers," National Drug Intelligence Center (NDIC), a component of the U.S. Department of Justice, August 2003.

Who abuses OxyContin?

Individuals of all ages abuse OxyContin—data reported in the *National Household Survey on Drug Abuse* indicate that nearly 1 million U.S. residents aged 12 and older used OxyContin nonmedically at least once in their lifetime.

OxyContin abuse among high school students is a particular problem. Four percent of high school seniors in the United States abused the drug at least once in the past year, according to the University of Michigan's Monitoring the Future Survey.

What are the risks?

Individuals who abuse OxyContin risk developing tolerance for the drug, meaning they must take increasingly higher doses to achieve the same effects. Long-term abuse of the drug can lead to physical dependence and addiction. Individuals who become dependent upon or addicted to the drug may experience withdrawal symptoms if they cease using the drug.

Withdrawal symptoms associated with OxyContin dependency or addiction include restlessness, muscle and bone pain, insomnia, diarrhea, vomiting, cold flashes, and involuntary leg movements.

Individuals who take a large dose of OxyContin are at risk of severe respiratory depression that can lead to death. Inexperienced and new users are at particular risk, because they may be unaware of what constitutes a large dose and have not developed a tolerance for the drug.

In addition, OxyContin abusers who inject the drug expose themselves to additional risks, including contracting HIV (human immunodeficiency virus), hepatitis B and C, and other blood-borne viruses.

What is OxyContin called?

The most common names for OxyContin are OCs, ox, and oxy.

Is it illegal to abuse OxyContin?

Yes, abusing OxyContin is illegal. OxyContin is a Schedule II substance under the Controlled Substances Act. Schedule II drugs, which include cocaine and methamphetamine, have a high potential for abuse. Abuse of these drugs may lead to severe psychological or physical dependence.

Chapter 34

Phencyclidine (PCP)

PCP (phencyclidine) was developed in the 1950s as an intravenous anesthetic. Its use in humans was discontinued in 1965, because patients often became agitated, delusional, and irrational
while recovering from its anesthetic effects. PCP is illegally manufactured in laboratories and is sold on the street by such names as
angel dust, ozone, wack, and rocket fuel. Killer joints and crystal
supergrass are names that refer to PCP combined with marijuana.
The variety of street names for PCP reflects its bizarre and volatile effects.

PCP is a white crystalline powder that is readily soluble in water or alcohol. It has a distinctive bitter chemical taste. PCP can
be mixed easily with dyes and turns up on the illicit drug market
in a variety of tablets, capsules, and colored powders. It is normally
used in one of three ways: snorted, smoked, or ingested. For smoking, PCP is often applied to a leafy material such as mint, parsley,
oregano, or marijuana.

Health Hazards

PCP is addictive—its use often leads to craving and compulsive
PCP-seeking behavior. First introduced as a street drug in the 1960s,
PCP quickly gained a reputation as a drug that could cause bad re-
actions and was not worth the risk. After using PCP once, many people

"PCP (Phencyclidine)," NIDA InfoFacts, National Institute on Drug Abuse
(NIDA), September 2003.

will not knowingly use it again. Others, however, use it regularly, sometimes because of its addictive properties. Others attribute their continued use to feelings of strength, power, invulnerability, and a numbing effect on the mind.

Many PCP users are brought to emergency rooms because of PCP overdose or because of the drug's unpleasant psychological effects. In a hospital or detention setting, these people often become violent or suicidal and are very dangerous to themselves and others. They should be kept in a calm setting and not be left alone.

At low to moderate doses, physiological effects of PCP include a slight increase in breathing rate and a pronounced rise in blood pressure and pulse rate. Breathing becomes shallow, and flushing and profuse sweating occur. Generalized numbness of the extremities and loss of muscular coordination also may occur. Psychological effects include distinct changes in body awareness, similar to those associated with alcohol intoxication. Adolescents who use PCP may experience interference with their learning process and with growth and development hormones.

At high doses of PCP, blood pressure, pulse rate, and respiration drop. This may be accompanied by nausea, vomiting, blurred vision, flicking up and down of the eyes, drooling, loss of balance, and dizziness. High doses of PCP can also cause seizures, coma, and death (though death more often results from accidental injury or suicide during PCP intoxication). Psychological effects at high doses can cause effects that mimic the full range of symptoms of schizophrenia, such as delusions, hallucinations, paranoia, disordered thinking, a sensation of distance from one's environment, and catatonia. Speech is often sparse and garbled.

People who use PCP for long periods report memory loss, difficulties with speech and thinking, depression, and weight loss. These symptoms can persist up to a year after stopping PCP use. Mood disorders also have been reported. PCP has sedative effects, and interactions with other central nervous system depressants, such as alcohol and benzodiazepines, can lead to coma or accidental overdose.

Extent of Use

2002 Monitoring the Future Survey (MTF)[1]

MTF data show that the percent of high school seniors who have ever used PCP remained stable at 3.1% in 2002, and past-year use remained stable at 1.1%. PCP use in the past month among 12th-graders has declined significantly in the last few years, from 1.0% in 1998 to 0.4% in 2002. Data on PCP use by eighth- and 10th-graders are not available.

2002 Drug Abuse Warning Network (DAWN)[2]

PCP mentions in emergency departments increased 28% from 1995 to 2002. There was a 42% increase from the 5,404 mentions in 2000 to 7,648 in 2002. There were significant increases in PCP mentions in Washington D.C., Newark, Philadelphia, Baltimore, and Dallas. Chicago had a decrease in mentions of PCP, declining 48% from 874 in 2001 to 459 in 2002.

2002 National Survey on Drug Use and Health (NSDUH)[3]

According to the 2002 NSDUH, 3.2% of the population aged 12 and older have used PCP at least once. Lifetime use of PCP was highest among those aged 26 or older (3.5%), compared with people aged 18 to 25 (2.7%) and those aged 12 to 17 (0.9%).

Notes

1. Conducted annually since 1975, MTF assesses drug use and attitudes among eighth-, 10th-, and 12th-graders, college students, and young adults nationwide. The survey is conducted by the University of Michigan's Institute for Social Research and is funded by NIDA. Copies of the latest published survey are available from the National Clearinghouse for Alcohol and Drug Information at (800) 729-6686 or may be downloaded from www.monitoringthefuture.org.

2. The latest data on drug abuse-related hospital emergency department (ED) visits are from the 2002 DAWN report, from the U.S. Department of Health and Human Service (HHS)'s Substance Abuse and Mental Health Services Administration. These data are from a national probability survey of 437 hospital EDs in 21 metropolitan areas in the U.S. during the year. For detailed information from DAWN, visit www.samhsa.gov/statistics/statistics.html, or call the National Clearinghouse for Alcohol and Drug Information at (800) 729-6686.

3. The 2002 NSDUH, produced by HHS's Substance Abuse and Mental Health Services Administration, creates a new baseline for future national drug use trends. The survey is

based on interviews with 68,126 respondents who were interviewed in their homes. The interviews represent 98% of the U.S. population age 12 and older. Not included in the survey are persons in the active military, in prisons, or other institutionalized populations, or who are homeless. Findings from the 2002 National Survey on Drug Use and Health are available online at www.DrugAbuseStatistics.samhsa.gov.

Chapter 35

Prescription Drugs

Commonly Prescribed Drugs Regulated under the Controlled Substances Act

Meperidine

Introduced as an analgesic in the 1930s, meperidine produces effects that are similar, but not identical, to morphine (shorter duration of action and reduced antitussive and antidiarrheal actions). Currently it is used for pre-anesthesia and the relief of moderate to severe pain, particularly in obstetrics and post-operative situations. Meperidine is available in tablets, syrups, and injectable forms under generic and brand name (Demerol®, Mepergan®, etc.) Schedule II preparations. Several analogues of meperidine have been clandestinely produced. During the clandestine synthesis of the analogue MPPP, a neurotoxic by-product (MPTP) was produced. A number of individuals who consumed the MPPP-MPTP preparation developed an irreversible Parkinsonian-like syndrome. It was later found that MPTP destroys the same neurons as those

"Commonly Prescribed Drugs Regulated under the Controlled Substances Act," includes "Meperidine," "Morphine," and "Opium," fact sheets produced by the Drug Enforcement Administration (DEA), U.S. Department of Justice, 1997; updated by David A. Cooke, M.D., April 2004. "Prescription Drugs: Abuse and Addiction," is from *Research Report*, National Institute on Drug Abuse (NIDA), NIH Pub. No. 01-4881, July 2001; available online at http://www.drug abuse.gov/PDF/RRPrescription.pdf.

damaged in the Parkinsonian-like syndrome. It was later found that MPTP destroys the same neurons as those damaged in Parkinson's disease.

Morphine

Morphine is the principal constituent of opium and can range in concentration from 4% to 21%. Commercial opium is standardized to contain 10% morphine. In the United States, a small percentage of the morphine obtained from opium is used directly (about 15 tons): the remaining is converted to codeine and other derivatives (about 120 tons). Morphine is one of the most effective drugs known for the relief of severe pain and remains the standard against which new analgesics are measured. Like most narcotics, the use of morphine has increased significantly in recent years. Since 1990, there has been about a 3-fold increase in morphine products in the United States.

Morphine is marketed under generic and brand name products including "MS-Contin®," Oramorph SR®," MSIR®," Roxanol®," Kadian®," "Avinza®," and RMS®." Morphine is used parenterally (by injection) for preoperative sedation, as a supplement to anesthesia, and for analgesia. It is the drug of choice for relieving pain of myocardial infarction and for its cardiovascular effects in the treatment of acute pulmonary edema. Traditionally, morphine was almost exclusively used by injection. Today, morphine is marketed in a variety of forms, including oral solutions, immediate and sustained-release tablets and capsules, suppositories, and injectable preparations. In addition, the availability of high-concentration morphine preparations (i.e., 20-mg/ml oral solutions, 25-mg/ml injectable solutions, and 200-mg sustained-release tablets) partially reflects the use of this substance for chronic pain management in opiate-tolerant patients.

Opium

There were no legal restrictions on the importation or use of opium until the early 1900s. In the United States, the unrestricted availability of opium, the influx of opium-smoking immigrants from East Asia, and the invention of the hypodermic needle contributed to the more severe variety of compulsive drug abuse seen at the turn of the 20th century. In those days, medicines often contained opium without any warning label. Today, there are state, federal, and international laws governing the production and distribution of narcotic substances.

Although opium is used in the form of paregoric to treat diarrhea, most opium imported into the United States is broken down into its alkaloid constituents. These alkaloids are divided into two distinct chemical classes, phenanthrenes and isoquinolines. The principal phenanthrenes are morphine, codeine, and thebaine, while the isoquinolines have no significant central nervous system effects and are not regulated under the Controlled Substances Act (CSA).

Prescription Drugs: Abuse and Addiction

What are some of the commonly abused prescription drugs?

Although many prescription drugs can be abused or misused, there are three classes of prescription drugs that are most commonly abused:

- Opioids, which are most often prescribed to treat pain;

- CNS depressants, which are used to treat anxiety and sleep disorders;

- Stimulants, which are prescribed to treat the sleep disorder narcolepsy, attention-deficit hyperactivity disorder (ADHD), and obesity.

Opioids

What are opioids?

Opioids are commonly prescribed because of their effective analgesic, or pain-relieving, properties. Medications that fall within this class—sometimes referred to as narcotics—include morphine, codeine, and related drugs. Morphine, for example, is often used before or after surgery to alleviate severe pain. Codeine, because it is less efficacious than morphine, is used for milder pain. Other examples of opioids that can be prescribed to alleviate pain include oxycodone (OxyContin), propoxyphene (Darvon), hydrocodone (Vicodin), and hydromorphone (Dilaudid), as well as meperidine (Demerol), which is used less often because of its side effects. In addition to their pain-relieving properties, some of these drugs—for example, codeine and diphenoxylate (Lomotil)—can be used to relieve coughs and diarrhea.

How do opioids affect the brain and body?

Opioids act by attaching to specific proteins called opioid receptors, which are found in the brain, spinal cord, and gastrointestinal tract. When these drugs attach to certain opioid receptors, they can block the transmission of pain messages to the brain. In addition, opioids can produce drowsiness, cause constipation, and, depending upon the amount of drug taken, depress respiration. Opioid drugs also can cause euphoria by affecting the brain regions that mediate what we perceive as pleasure.

What are the possible consequences of opioid use and abuse?

Chronic use of opioids can result in tolerance for the drugs, which means that users must take higher doses to achieve the same initial effects. Long-term use also can lead to physical dependence and addiction—the body adapts to the presence of the drug, and withdrawal symptoms occur if use is reduced or stopped. Symptoms of withdrawal include restlessness, muscle and bone pain, insomnia, diarrhea, vomiting, cold flashes with goose bumps ("cold turkey"), and involuntary leg movements. Finally, taking a large single dose of an opioid could cause severe respiratory depression that can lead to death. Many studies have shown, however, that properly managed medical use of opioid analgesic drugs is safe and rarely causes clinical addiction, defined as compulsive, often uncontrollable use of drugs. Taken exactly as prescribed, opioids can be used to manage pain effectively.

Is it safe to use opioid drugs with other medications?

Opioids are safe to use with other drugs only under a physician's supervision. Typically, they should not be used with other substances that depress the central nervous system, such as alcohol, antihistamines, barbiturates, benzodiazepines, or general anesthetics, as such a combination increases the risk of life-threatening respiratory depression.

What role to opioid medications play in the treatment of pain?

It is estimated that more than 50 million Americans suffer from chronic pain. When treating pain, health care providers have long wrestled with a dilemma: How to adequately relieve a patient's suffering while avoiding the potential for that patient to become addicted to pain medication?

Many health care providers under prescribe painkillers because they overestimate the potential for patients to become addicted to medications such as morphine and codeine. Although these drugs carry a heightened risk of addiction, research has shown that providers' concerns that patients will become addicted to pain medication are largely unfounded. This fear of prescribing opioid pain medications is known as "opiophobia."

Most patients who are prescribed opioids for pain, even those undergoing long-term therapy, do not become addicted to the drugs. The few patients who do develop rapid and marked tolerance for and addiction to opioids usually have a history of psychological problems or prior substance abuse. In fact, studies have shown that abuse potential of opioid medications is generally low in healthy, nondrug-abusing volunteers. One study found that only 4 out of about 12,000 patients who were given opioids for acute pain became addicted. In a study of 38 chronic pain patients, most of whom received opioids for four to seven years, only two patients became addicted, and both had a history of drug abuse.

The issues of under prescription of opioids and the suffering of millions of patients who do not receive adequate pain relief has led to the development of guidelines for pain treatment. These guidelines may help bring an end to under prescribing, but alternative forms of pain control are still needed. National Institute on Drug Abuse (NIDA)-funded scientists continue to search for new ways to control pain and to develop new pain medications that are effective but do not have the potential for addiction.

CNS Depressants

What are CNS depressants?

CNS depressants are substances that can slow normal brain function. Because of this property, some CNS depressants are useful in the treatment of anxiety and sleep disorders. Among the medications that are commonly prescribed for these purposes are the following:

- Barbiturates, such as mephobarbital (Mebaral) and pentobarbital sodium (Nembutal), which are used to treat anxiety, tension, and sleep disorders.

- Benzodiazepines, such as diazepam (Valium), chlordiazepoxide HCl (Librium), and alprazolam (Xanax), which can be prescribed to treat anxiety, acute stress reactions, and panic attacks; the more sedating benzodiazepines, such as triazolam (Halcion) and estazolam (ProSom), can be prescribed for short-term treatment of sleep disorders.

In higher doses, some CNS depressants can be used as general anesthetics.

How do CNS depressants affect the brain and body?

There are numerous CNS depressants; most act on the brain by affecting the neurotransmitter gamma-aminobutyric acid (GABA). Neurotransmitters are brain chemicals that facilitate communication between brain cells. GABA works by decreasing brain activity. Although the different classes of CNS depressants work in unique ways, ultimately it is through their ability to increase GABA activity that they produce a drowsy or calming effect that is beneficial to those suffering from anxiety or sleep disorders.

What are the possible consequences of CNS depressant use and abuse?

Despite their many beneficial effects, barbiturates and benzodiazepines have the potential for abuse and should be used only as prescribed. During the first few days of taking a prescribed CNS depressant, a person usually feels sleepy and uncoordinated, but as the body becomes accustomed to the effects of the drug, these feelings begin to disappear. If one uses these drugs long term, the body will develop tolerance for the drugs, and larger doses will be needed to achieve the same initial effects. In addition, continued use can lead to physical dependence and—when use is reduced or stopped—withdrawal. Because all CNS depressants work by slowing the brain's activity, when an individual stops taking them, the brain's activity can rebound and race out of control, possibly leading to seizures and other harmful consequences. Withdrawal from prolonged use of CNS depressants can have life-threatening complications. Therefore, someone who is thinking about discontinuing CNS-depressant therapy or who is suffering withdrawal from a CNS depressant should speak with a physician or seek medical treatment.

Is it safe to use CNS depressants with other medications?

CNS depressants should be used with other medications only under a physician's supervision. Typically, they should not be combined with any other medication or substance that causes CNS depression, including prescription pain medicines, some over-the-counter cold and allergy medications, or alcohol. Using CNS depressants with these other substances—particularly alcohol—can slow breathing, or slow both the heart and respiration, and possibly lead to death.

Stimulants

What are stimulants?

As the name suggests, stimulants are a class of drugs that enhance brain activity—they cause an increase in alertness, attention, and energy that is accompanied by elevated blood pressure and increased heart rate and respiration. Stimulants were used historically to treat asthma and other respiratory problems, obesity, neurological disorders, and a variety of other ailments. But as their potential for abuse and addiction became apparent, the medical use of stimulants began to wane. Now, stimulants are prescribed for the treatment of only a few health conditions, including narcolepsy, attention-deficit hyperactivity disorder, and depression that has not responded to other treatments. Stimulants may be used as appetite suppressants for short-term treatment of obesity, and they also may be used for patients with asthma.

How do stimulants affect the brain and body?

Stimulants, such as dextroamphetamine (Dexedrine) and methylphenidate (Ritalin), have chemical structures that are similar to a family of key brain neurotransmitters called monoamines, which include norepinephrine and dopamine. Stimulants increase the amount of these chemicals in the brain. This, in turn, increases blood pressure and heart rate, constricts blood vessels, increases blood glucose, and opens up the pathways of the respiratory system. In addition, the increase in dopamine is associated with a sense of euphoria that can accompany the use of these drugs.

What are the possible consequences of stimulant use and abuse?

The consequences of stimulant abuse can be dangerous. Although their use may not lead to physical dependence and risk of withdrawal, stimulants can be addictive in that individuals begin to use them compulsively. Taking high doses of some stimulants repeatedly over a short time can lead to feelings of hostility or paranoia. Additionally, taking high doses of a stimulant may result in dangerously high body temperatures and an irregular heartbeat. There is also the potential for cardiovascular failure or lethal seizures.

Is it safe to use stimulants with other medications?

Stimulants should be used with other medications only when the patient is under a physician's supervision. For example, a stimulant may be prescribed to a patient taking an antidepressant. However, health care providers and patients should be mindful that antidepressants enhance the effects of a stimulant. Patients also should be aware that stimulants should not be mixed with over-the-counter cold medicines that contain decongestants, as this combination may cause blood pressure to become dangerously high or lead to irregular heart rhythms.

Trends in Prescription Drug Abuse

Several indicators suggest that prescription drug abuse is on the rise in the United States. According to the 1999 National Household Survey on Drug Abuse, in 1998, an estimated 1.6 million Americans used prescription pain relievers nonmedically for the first time. This represents a significant increase since the 1980s, when there were generally fewer than 500,000 first-time users per year. From 1990 to 1998, the number of new users of pain relievers increased by 181%; the number of individuals who initiated tranquilizer use increased by 132%; the number of new sedative users increased by 90%; and the number of people initiating stimulant use increased by 165%. In 1999, an estimated 4 million people—almost 2% of the population aged 12 and older—were currently (use in past month) using certain prescription drugs nonmedically: pain relievers (2.6 million users), sedatives and tranquilizers (1.3 million users), and stimulants (0.9 million users).

Although prescription drug abuse affects many Americans, some trends of concern can be seen among older adults, adolescents, and women. In addition, health care professionals—including physicians, nurses, pharmacists, dentists, anesthesiologists, and veterinarians—may be at increased risk of prescription drug abuse because of ease of access, as well as their ability to self-prescribe drugs. In spite of this increased risk, recent surveys and research in the early 1990s indicate that health care providers probably suffer from substance abuse, including alcohol and drugs, at a rate similar to rates in society as a whole, in the range of 8% to 12%.

Older Adults

The misuse of prescription drugs may be the most common form of drug abuse among the elderly. Elderly persons use prescription medications approximately three times as frequently as the general population and have been found to have the poorest rates of compliance with directions for taking a medication. In addition, data from the Veterans Affairs Hospital System suggest that elderly patients may be prescribed inappropriately high doses of medications such as benzodiazepines and may be prescribed these medications for longer periods than are younger adults. In general, older people should be prescribed lower doses of medications, because the body's ability to metabolize many medications decreases with age.

An association between age-related morbidity and abuse of prescription medications likely exists. For example, elderly persons who take benzodiazepines are at increased risk for falls that cause hip and thigh fractures, as well as for vehicle accidents. Cognitive impairment also is associated with benzodiazepine use, although memory impairment may be reversible when the drug is discontinued. Finally, use of benzodiazepines for longer than 4 months is not recommended for elderly patients because of the possibility of physical dependence.

Adolescents and Young Adults

Data from the National Household Survey on Drug Abuse indicate that the most dramatic increase in new users of prescription drugs for nonmedical purposes occurs in 12- to 17-year-olds and 18- to 25-year-olds. In addition, 12- to 14-year-olds reported psychotherapeutics (for example, painkillers or stimulants) as one of two primary drugs used. The 1999 Monitoring the Future survey showed that for barbiturates, tranquilizers, and narcotics other than heroin, the general, long-term declines in use among young adults in the 1980s leveled off in the early 1990s, with modest increases again in the mid-to late 1990s. For example, the use of methylphenidate (Ritalin) among high school seniors increased from an annual prevalence (use of the drug within the preceding year) of 0.1% in 1992 to an annual prevalence of 2.8% in 1997 before reaching a plateau.

It also appears that college students' nonmedical use of pain relievers such as oxycodone with aspirin (Percodan) and hydrocodone (Vicodin) is on the rise. The 1999 Drug Abuse Warning Network, which collects data on drug-related episodes in hospital emergency departments, reported that mentions of hydrocodone as a cause for visiting an emergency room increased by 37% among all age groups from 1997 to 1999. Mentions of the benzodiazepine clonazepam (Klonopin) increased by 102% since 1992.

Gender Differences

Studies suggest that women are more likely than men to be prescribed an abusable prescription drug, particularly narcotics and anti-anxiety drugs—in some cases 48% more likely.

Overall, men and women have roughly similar rates of nonmedical use of prescription drugs. An exception is found among 12- to 17-year-olds: In this age group, young women are more likely than young men to use psychotherapeutic drugs nonmedically. In addition, research has shown that women and men who use prescription opioids are equally likely to become addicted. However, among women and men who use either a sedative, anti-anxiety drug, or hypnotic, women are almost two times more likely to become addicted.

Preventing and Detecting Prescription Drug Abuse

Although most patients use medications as directed, abuse of and addiction to prescription drugs are public health problems for many Americans. However, addiction rarely occurs among those who use pain relievers, CNS depressants, or stimulants as prescribed; the risk for addiction exists when these medications are used in ways other than as prescribed. Health care providers such as primary care physicians, nurse practitioners, and pharmacists as well as patients can all play a role in preventing and detecting prescription drug abuse.

Role of Health Care Providers

About 70% of Americans—approximately 191 million people—visit a health care provider, such as a primary care physician, at least once every two years. Thus, health care providers are in a unique position not only to prescribe needed medications appropriately, but also to identify prescription drug abuse when it exists and help the patient recognize the problem, set goals for recovery, and seek appropriate treatment when necessary. Screening for any type of substance abuse can be incorporated into routine history taking with questions about what prescriptions and over-the-counter medicines the patient is taking and why. Screening also can be performed if a patient presents with specific symptoms associated with problem use of a substance.

Table 35.1. Assessing Prescription Drug Abuse: Four Simple Questions for You and Your Physician.

- Have you ever felt the need to cut down on your use of prescription drugs?
- Have you ever felt annoyed by remarks your friends or loved ones made about your use of prescription drugs?
- Have you ever felt guilty or remorseful about your use of prescription drugs?
- Have you ever used prescription drugs as a way to "get going" or to "calm down?"

Adapted from Ewing, J.A. "Detecting Alcoholism: The CAGE Questionnaire."
Journal of the American Medical Association 252(14):1905–1907, 1984.

Over time, providers should note any rapid increases in the amount of a medication needed—which may indicate the development of tolerance—or frequent requests for refills before the quantity prescribed should have been used. They should also be alert to the fact that those addicted to prescription medications may engage in "doctor shopping," moving from provider to provider in an effort to get multiple prescriptions for the drug they abuse.

Preventing or stopping prescription drug abuse is an important part of patient care. However, health care providers should not avoid prescribing or administering strong CNS depressants and painkillers, if they are needed.

Role of Pharmacists

Pharmacists can play a key role in preventing prescription drug misuse and abuse by providing clear information and advice about how to take a medication appropriately, about the effects the medication may have, and about any possible drug interactions. Pharmacists can help prevent prescription fraud or diversion by looking for false or altered prescription forms. Many pharmacies have developed "hotlines" to alert other pharmacies in the region when a fraud is detected.

Role of Patients

There are several ways that patients can prevent prescription drug abuse. When visiting the doctor, provide a complete medical history and a description of the reason for the visit to ensure that the doctor understands the complaint and can prescribe appropriate medication. If a doctor prescribes a pain medication, stimulant, or CNS depressant, follow the directions for use carefully and learn about the effects that the drug could have, especially during the first few days during which the body is adapting to the medication. Also be aware of potential interactions with other drugs by reading all information provided by the pharmacist. Do not increase or decrease doses or abruptly stop taking a prescription without consulting a health care provider first. For example, if you are taking a pain reliever for chronic pain and the medication no longer seems to be effectively controlling the pain, speak with your physician; do not increase the dose on your own. Finally, never use another person's prescription.

Treating Prescription Drug Addiction

Years of research have shown us that addiction to any drug, illicit or prescribed, is a brain disease that can, like other chronic diseases, be effectively treated. But no single type of treatment is appropriate for all individuals addicted to prescription drugs. Treatment must take into account the type of drug used and the needs of the individual. To be successful, treatment may need to incorporate several components, such as counseling in conjunction with a prescribed medication, and multiple courses of treatment may be needed for the patient to make a full recovery.

The two main categories of drug addiction treatment are behavioral and pharmacological. Behavioral treatments teach people how to function without drugs, how to handle cravings, how to avoid drugs and situations that could lead to drug use, how to prevent relapse, and how to handle relapse should it occur. When delivered effectively, behavioral treatments—such as individual counseling, group or family counseling, contingency management, and cognitive-behavioral therapies—also can help patients improve their personal relationships and ability to function at work and in the community.

Some addictions, such as opioid addiction, can also be treated with medications. These pharmacological treatments counter the effects of the drug on the brain and behavior. Medications also can be used to relieve the symptoms of withdrawal, to treat an overdose, or to help overcome drug cravings.

Although a behavioral or pharmacological approach alone may be effective for treating drug addiction, research shows that a combination of both, when available, is most effective.

Treating Addiction to Prescription Opioids

Several options are available for effectively treating addiction to prescription opioids. These options are drawn from experience and research regarding the treatment of heroin addiction. They include medications, such as methadone and LAAM (levo-alpha-acetyl-methadol), and behavioral counseling approaches.

A useful precursor to long-term treatment of opioid addiction is detoxification. Detoxification in itself is not a treatment for opioid addiction. Rather, its primary objective is to relieve withdrawal symptoms while the patient adjusts to being drug free. To be effective, detoxification must precede long-term treatment that either requires complete abstinence or incorporates a medication, such as methadone, into the treatment plan. Methadone is a synthetic opioid that blocks the effects of heroin and other opioids, eliminates withdrawal symptoms, and relieves drug craving. It has been used successfully for more than 30 years to treat people addicted to opioids. Other medications include LAAM, an alternative to methadone that blocks the effects of opioids for up to 72 hours, and naltrexone, an opioid blocker that is often employed for highly motivated individuals in treatment programs promoting complete abstinence. Buprenorphine, another effective medication, has been recently approved by the Food and Drug Administration (FDA) for treatment of opioid addiction. Finally, naloxone, which counteracts the effects of opioids, is used to treat overdoses.

Treating Addiction to CNS Depressants

Patients addicted to barbiturates and benzodiazepines should not attempt to stop taking them on their own, as withdrawal from these drugs can be problematic, and in the case of certain CNS depressants, potentially life-threatening. Although no extensive body of research regarding the treatment of barbiturate and benzodiazepine addiction exists, patients addicted to these medications should undergo medically supervised detoxification because the dose must be gradually tapered off. Inpatient or outpatient counseling can help the individual during this process. Cognitive behavioral therapy also has been used successfully to help individuals adapt to the removal from benzodiazepines.

Often the abuse of barbiturates and benzodiazepines occurs in conjunction with the abuse of another substance or drug, such as alcohol or cocaine. In these cases of polydrug abuse, the treatment approach must address the multiple addictions.

Treating Addiction to Prescription Stimulants

Treatment of addiction to prescription stimulants, such as Ritalin, is often based on behavioral therapies proven effective for treating cocaine or methamphetamine addiction. At this time, there are no proven medications for the treatment of stimulant addiction. However, antidepressants may help manage the symptoms of depression that can accompany the early days of abstinence from stimulants.

Depending on the patient's situation, the first steps in treating prescription stimulant addiction may be tapering off the drug's dose and attempting to treat withdrawal symptoms. The detoxification process could then be followed by one of many behavioral therapies. Contingency management, for example, uses a system that enables patients to earn vouchers for drug-free urine tests. The vouchers can be exchanged for items that promote healthy living.

Another behavioral approach is cognitive-behavioral intervention, which focuses on modifying the patient's thinking, expectations, and behaviors while at the same time increasing skills for coping with various life stressors. Recovery support groups may also be effective in conjunction with behavioral therapy.

Chapter 36

Psilocybin

What is psilocybin?

Psilocybin is a hallucinogenic substance obtained from certain types of mushrooms that are indigenous to tropical and subtropical regions of South America, Mexico, and the United States. These mushrooms typically contain 0.2% to 0.4% psilocybin and a trace amount of psilocin, another hallucinogenic substance. Both psilocybin and psilocin can be produced synthetically, but law enforcement reporting currently does not indicate that this is occurring.

What does psilocybin look like?

Mushrooms containing psilocybin are available fresh or dried and have long, slender stems topped by caps with dark gills on the underside. Fresh mushrooms have white or whitish-gray stems; the caps are dark brown around the edges and light brown or white in the center. Dried mushrooms are generally rusty brown with isolated areas of off-white.

How is psilocybin abused?

Psilocybin mushrooms are ingested orally. They may be brewed as a tea or added to other foods to mask their bitter flavor. Some users coat the mushrooms with chocolate—this both masks the flavor and

This chapter contains text from the document "Psilocybin Fast Facts: Questions and Answers," National Drug Intelligence Center (NDIC), a component of the U.S. Department of Justice, August 2003.

disguises the mushrooms as candy. Once the mushrooms are ingested, the body breaks down the psilocybin to produce psilocin.

Who abuses psilocybin?

Psilocybin mushrooms are popular at raves, clubs and, increasingly, on college campuses and generally are abused by teenagers and young adults. It is difficult to gauge the extent of psilocybin use in the United States because most data sources that quantify drug use exclude psilocybin. The Monitoring the Future Survey, conducted by the University of Michigan, does reveal that 9.2% of high school seniors in the United States used hallucinogens other than LSD—a category that includes psilocybin—at least once in their lifetime. Two percent of high school seniors used hallucinogens other than LSD in the past month.

What are the risks?

Use of psilocybin is associated with negative physical and psychological consequences. The physical effects, which appear within 20 minutes of ingestion and last approximately 6 hours, include nausea, vomiting, muscle weakness, drowsiness, and lack of coordination. While there is no evidence that users may become physically dependent on psilocybin, tolerance for the drug does develop when it is ingested continuously over a short period of time.

The psychological consequences of psilocybin use include hallucinations and an inability to discern fantasy from reality. Panic reactions and psychosis also may occur, particularly if a user ingests a large dose.

In addition to the risks associated with ingestion of psilocybin, individuals who seek to abuse psilocybin mushrooms also risk poisoning if one of the many varieties of poisonous mushrooms is incorrectly identified as a psilocybin mushroom.

What is psilocybin called?

The most common names for psilocybin are magic mushroom, mushroom, and shrooms.

Is psilocybin illegal?

Yes, psilocybin is illegal. Psilocybin is a Schedule I substance under the Controlled Substances Act. Schedule I drugs, which include heroin and LSD, have a high potential for abuse and serve no legitimate medical purpose in the United States.

Chapter 37

Rohypnol (Flunitrazepam)

Rohypnol is the trade name for the drug flunitrazepam, a benzodiazepine (central nervous system depressant) like Valium, yet 10 times more potent. Outside the United States, Rohypnol is legally manufactured by Hoffman-LaRoche, Inc., and is available by prescription for the short-term treatment of severe sleep disorders. It is widely available in Europe, Mexico, and Colombia, but is neither manufactured nor approved for sale in the United States.

Illicit use of Rohypnol began in the 1970s in Europe and appeared in the United States in the early 1990s. Much of the concern surrounding Rohypnol is its abuse as a "date rape" drug. Rohypnol is a tasteless and odorless drug and, until recent manufacturer efforts, dissolved clear in liquid, which masked its presence. Rohypnol comes in pill form and is usually sold in the manufacturer's bubble packaging, which can mislead users in the United States into believing the drug is safe and legal. Since February 1999, reformulated Rohypnol tablets, which turn blue in a drink to increase visibility, have been approved and marketed in 20 countries. The old noncolored tablets are still available, however. In response to the reformulated blue tablets, people who intend to commit a sexual assault facilitated by Rohypnol are now serving blue tropical drinks and punches in which the blue dye can be disguised.

Office of National Drug Control Policy, Drug Policy Information Clearinghouse, February 2003.

Effects

Rohypnol can be ingested orally, snorted, or injected. It is often combined with alcohol or used as a remedy for the depression that follows a stimulant high. The effects of Rohypnol begin within 15 to 20 minutes of administration and, depending on the amount ingested, may persist for more than 12 hours. The drug's metabolic properties are detectable in urine for up to 72 hours after ingestion.

Under Rohypnol, individuals may experience a slowing of psychomotor performance, muscle relaxation, decreased blood pressure, sleepiness, and/or amnesia. Some of the adverse side effects associated with the drug's use are drowsiness, headaches, memory impairment, dizziness, nightmares, confusion, and tremors. Although classified as a depressant, Rohypnol can induce aggression and/or excitability.

Prevalence Estimates

Rohypnol is popular with youth because of its low cost, which is usually less than $5 per tablet. It has been used throughout the United States by high school and college students, street gang members, rave and nightclub attendees, drug addicts, and alcohol abusers. Rohypnol is used in combination with alcohol, marijuana, cocaine, heroin, ecstasy, and LSD. The predominant user age group is 13 to 30 years old and users tend to be male.

A questionnaire about Rohypnol use was included in the Monitoring the Future Survey for the first time in 1996. Lifetime Rohypnol use by secondary school students in 1996 ranged from 1.5% among eighth and 10th graders to 1.2% among 12th graders (see Table 37.1). Current estimates of lifetime Rohypnol use range from 1.1% among eighth graders, to 1.5% among 10th graders, to 1.7% among 12th graders.

Availability, Trafficking, and Seizures

Because Rohypnol is not manufactured nor approved for medical use in the United States, distributors must obtain their supply from other countries. Colombian traffickers ship Rohypnol to the United States via mail services and/or couriers using commercial airlines. Distributors also travel to Mexico to obtain supplies of the drug and smuggle it into the United States.

Table 37.1. Rohypnol Use by Secondary School Students, 1996–2001.

	1996	1997	1998	1999	2000	2001
8th grade						
Lifetime	1.5	1.1	1.4	1.3	1.0	1.1
Annual	1.0	0.8	0.8	0.5	0.5	0.7
30-day	0.5	0.3	0.4	0.3	0.3	0.4
10th grade						
Lifetime	1.5	1.7	2.0	1.8	1.3	1.5
Annual	1.1	1.3	1.2	1.0	0.8	1.0
30-day	0.5	0.5	0.4	0.5	0.4	0.2
12th grade						
Lifetime	1.2	1.8	3.0	2.0	1.5	1.7
Annual	1.1	1.2	1.4	1.0	0.8	0.9
30-day	0.5	0.3	0.3	0.3	0.4	0.3

In the late 1980s, Rohypnol abuse and distribution were occasionally reported in Florida and in the border areas of Arizona, California, and Texas. Beginning around 1993, the abuse and distribution of Rohypnol began to spread, with the vast majority of Rohypnol-related law enforcement cases occurring between January 1993 and December 1996. The two largest Rohypnol seizures occurred in February 1995. At that time, more than 52,000 tablets were seized in Louisiana and 57,000 tablets were seized in Texas. By June 1996, the Drug Enforcement Administration (DEA) had documented more than 2,700 federal, state, and local law enforcement encounters with Rohypnol.

On March 5, 1996, the U.S. Customs Service began seizing Rohypnol at United States borders on advice from DEA and the U.S. Food and Drug Administration. By December 1997, Customs Service efforts had substantially reduced the availability of the drug.

In May 2000, DEA, along with the U.S. Border Patrol, seized 900 Rohypnol tablets in Texas. In July 2000, multiagency investigations led to the closure of a pharmacy in Mexico that used the mail to distribute Rohypnol to California.

According to DEA's System to Retrieve Information from Drug Evidence (STRIDE) data, Rohypnol seizures were at their highest in 1995, with 164,534 dosage units, and have since decreased to 4,967 units in 2000.

Regional Observations

According to *Pulse Check: Trends in Drug Abuse*, Rohypnol is now the least available club drug in the United States. Nevertheless, Los Angeles and El Paso report that the drug is widely available. The remaining Pulse Check sites report it as somewhat, not very, or not at all available.

In El Paso, speedball (a combination of heroin and cocaine) users often use Rohypnol to "soften the fall when coming down." El Paso treatment centers also report clients using "roche," which is presumed to be Rohypnol smuggled in from Mexico.

According to the Community Epidemiology Work Group (CEWG), reports of Rohypnol use have been declining since recent legislation and its use is very low or nonexistent in the majority of CEWG areas. Cities that are exceptions to this decline in use include Atlanta and New Orleans. Poison control calls involving Rohypnol in combination with other drugs have increased in Atlanta where Rohypnol sells for $5 to $10 per pill. In New Orleans, Rohypnol is common in nightclubs and private rave parties.

Texas has experienced increases in poison control calls and treatment admissions for Rohypnol, especially among Hispanic youth close to the Mexican border. In the first quarter of 2000, DEA reported increases in Rohypnol seizures in Laredo, Beaumont, and Austin.

Drug-Facilitated Rape

Drug-facilitated rape can be defined as sexual assault made easier by the offender's use of an "anesthesia" type drug that can render the victim physically incapacitated or helpless and unable to give consent to sexual activity. Whether the victim is unwittingly administered the drug or willingly ingests it for recreational use is irrelevant. The person is victimized because of an inability to consciously consent to sexual acts.

Rohypnol is one of the drugs most commonly implicated in drug-facilitated rape. It can mentally and physically paralyze an individual. Effects of the drug are of particular concern in combination with alcohol and can lead to anterograde amnesia, where events that occurred during the time the drug was in effect are forgotten.

During 2000, some 261,000 rapes/sexual assaults occurred, but it is unknown how many were drug facilitated. Many factors contribute to this lack of data, including the short period of time that the drug can be detected in the victim's system. Also, victims may not seek help until days after the assault, partly because the drug impairs their memory and partly because of their inability to recognize signs of sexual assault. As with any sexual assault, survivors need help regaining a sense of control and security. Many victims rely on a support system to help them deal with the flood of emotions in the aftermath of the assault.

Scheduling and Legislation

As a result of the 1971 United Nations Convention on Psychotropic Substances, the United States placed Rohypnol under Schedule IV of the Controlled Substances Act in 1984. Rohypnol is not approved for manufacture or sale within the United States.

Table 37.2. Controlled Substances Act—Formal Scheduling

Schedule	Description
Schedule I	The drug has a high potential for abuse, is not currently accepted for medical use in treatment in the United States, and lacks accepted safety for use under medical supervision.
Schedule II	The drug has a high potential for abuse, is currently accepted for medical use in treatment in the United States, and may lead to severe psychological or physical dependence.
Schedule III	The drug has less potential for abuse than drugs in Schedule I and II categories, is currently accepted for medical use in treatment in the United States, and may lead to moderate or low physical dependence or high psychological dependence.
Schedule IV	The drug has low potential for abuse relative to other drugs, is currently accepted for medical use in treatment in the United States, and may lead to limited physical dependence or psychological dependence relative to drugs in Schedule III.
Schedule V	The drug has a low potential for abuse relative to drugs in Schedule IV, is currently accepted for medical use in treatment in the United States, and may lead to limited physical or psychological dependence relative to drugs in Schedule IV.

By March 1995, the United Nations Commission on Narcotic Drugs had transferred Rohypnol from a Schedule IV to a Schedule III drug. DEA is reviewing the possibility of reclassifying Rohypnol as a Schedule I drug. At the state level, Rohypnol already has been reclassified as a Schedule I substance in Florida, Idaho, Minnesota, New Hampshire, New Mexico, North Dakota, Oklahoma, and Pennsylvania.

In response to Rohypnol abuse and use of the drug to facilitate sexual assaults, the U.S. Congress passed the Drug Induced Rape Prevention and Punishment Act, effective October 13, 1996. The law provides for harsher penalties regarding the distribution of a controlled substance to an individual without the individual's consent and with the intent to commit a crime of violence, including rape. The law imposes a penalty of up to 20 years in prison and a fine for the importation and distribution of 1 gram or more of Rohypnol. Simple possession is punishable by 3 years in prison and a fine.

In 1997, penalties for possession, trafficking, and distribution of Rohypnol were further increased by the U.S. Sentencing Commission's Federal Sentencing Guidelines to those of a Schedule I substance because of growing abuse of the drug.

Chapter 38

Steroids

What are anabolic steroids?

"Anabolic steroids" is the familiar name for synthetic substances related to the male sex hormones (androgens). They promote the growth of skeletal muscle (anabolic effects) and the development of male sexual characteristics (androgenic effects), and also have some other effects. The term "anabolic steroids" will be used throughout this report because of its familiarity, although the proper term for these compounds is "anabolic-androgenic" steroids.

Anabolic steroids were developed in the late 1930s primarily to treat hypogonadism, a condition in which the testes do not produce sufficient testosterone for normal growth, development, and sexual functioning. The primary medical uses of these compounds are to treat delayed puberty, some types of impotence, and wasting of the body caused by HIV infection or other diseases.

During the 1930s, scientists discovered that anabolic steroids could facilitate the growth of skeletal muscle in laboratory animals, which led to use of the compounds first by bodybuilders and weightlifters and then by athletes in other sports. Steroid abuse has become so widespread in athletics that it affects the outcome of sports contests. More than 100 different anabolic steroids have been developed, but they require a prescription to be used legally in the United States. Most

"Anabolic Steroid Abuse," *Research Report,* National Institute on Drug Abuse (NIDA), April 2000.

steroids that are used illegally are smuggled in from other countries, illegally diverted from U.S. pharmacies, or synthesized in clandestine laboratories.

What are steroidal supplements?

In the United States, supplements such as dehydroepiandrosterone (DHEA) and androstenedione (street name Andro) can be purchased legally without a prescription through many commercial sources including health food stores. They are often referred to as dietary supplements, although they are not food products. They are often taken because the user believes they have anabolic effects.

Steroidal supplements can be converted into testosterone (an important male sex hormone) or a similar compound in the body. Whether such conversion produces sufficient quantities of testosterone to promote muscle growth or whether the supplements themselves promote muscle growth is unknown. Little is known about the side effects of steroidal supplements, but if large quantities of these compounds substantially increase testosterone levels in the body, they also are likely to produce the same side effects as anabolic steroids.

What is the scope of steroid abuse in the United States?

Recent evidence suggests that steroid abuse among adolescents is on the rise. The 1999 Monitoring the Future study, a National Institute on Drug Abuse (NIDA)-funded survey of drug abuse among adolescents in middle and high schools across the United States, estimated that 2.7% of eighth- and 10th-graders and 2.9% of 12th-graders had taken anabolic steroids at least once in their lives. For 10th-graders, that is a significant increase from 1998, when 2.0% of 10th-graders said they had taken anabolic steroids at least once. For all three grades, the 1999 levels represent a significant increase from 1991, the first year that data on steroid abuse were collected from the younger students. In that year, 1.9% of eighth-graders, 1.8% of 10th-graders, and 2.1% of 12th-graders reported that they had taken anabolic steroids at least once.

Few data exist on the extent of steroid abuse by adults. It has been estimated that hundreds of thousands of people aged 18 and older abuse anabolic steroids at least once a year.

Among both adolescents and adults, steroid abuse is higher among males than females. However, steroid abuse is growing most rapidly among young women.

312

Table 38.1. Commonly Abused Steroids

Oral Steroids	Injectable Steroids
• Anadrol (oxymetholone)	• Deca-Durabolin (nandrolone decanoate)
• Oxandrin (oxandrolone)	• Durabolin (nandrolone phenpropionate)
• Dianabol (methandrostenolone)	• Depo-Testosterone (testosterone cypionate)
• Winstrol (stanozolol)	• Equipoise (boldenone undecylenate)

Why do people abuse anabolic steroids?

One of the main reasons people give for abusing steroids is to improve their performance in sports. Among competitive bodybuilders, steroid abuse has been estimated to be very high. Among other athletes, the incidence of abuse probably varies depending on the specific sport.

Another reason people give for taking steroids is to increase their muscle size and/or reduce their body fat. This group includes some people who have a behavioral syndrome (muscle dysmorphia) in which a person has a distorted image of his or her body. Men with this condition think that they look small and weak, even if they are large and muscular. Similarly, women with the syndrome think that they look fat and flabby, even though they are actually lean and muscular.

Some people who abuse steroids to boost muscle size have experienced physical or sexual abuse. They are trying to increase their muscle size to protect themselves. In one series of interviews with male weightlifters, 25% who abused steroids reported memories of childhood physical or sexual abuse, compared with none who did not abuse steroids. In a study of women weightlifters, twice as many of those who had been raped reported using anabolic steroids and/or another purported muscle-building drug, compared to those who had not been raped. Moreover, almost all of those who had been raped reported that they markedly increased their bodybuilding activities after the attack. They believed that being bigger and stronger would discourage further attacks because men would find them either intimidating or unattractive.

Finally, some adolescents abuse steroids as part of a pattern of high-risk behaviors. These adolescents also take risks such as drinking and driving, carrying a gun, not wearing a helmet on a motorcycle, and abusing other illicit drugs. While conditions such as muscle dysmorphia, a history of physical or sexual abuse, or a history of engaging in high-risk behaviors may increase the risk of initiating or continuing steroid abuse, researchers agree that most steroid abusers are psychologically normal when they start abusing the drugs.

How are anabolic steroids used?

Some anabolic steroids are taken orally, others are injected intramuscularly, and still others are provided in gels or creams that are rubbed on the skin. Doses taken by abusers can be 10 to 100 times higher than the doses used for medical conditions.

Steroid abusers typically "stack" the drugs, meaning that they take two or more different anabolic steroids, mixing oral and/or injectable types and sometimes even including compounds that are designed for veterinary use. Abusers think that the different steroids interact to produce an effect on muscle size that is greater than the effects of each drug individually, a theory that has not been tested scientifically.

Often, steroid abusers also "pyramid" their doses in cycles of six to 12 weeks. At the beginning of a cycle, the person starts with low doses of the drugs being stacked and then slowly increases the doses. In the second half of the cycle, the doses are slowly decreased to zero. This is sometimes followed by a second cycle in which the person continues to train but without drugs. Abusers believe that pyramiding allows the body time to adjust to the high doses and the drug-free cycle allows the body's hormonal system time to recuperate. As with stacking, the perceived benefits of pyramiding and cycling have not been substantiated scientifically.

What are the health consequences of steroid abuse?

Anabolic steroid abuse has been associated with a wide range of adverse side effects ranging from some that are physically unattractive, such as acne and breast development in men, to others that are life threatening, such as heart attacks and liver cancer. Most are reversible if the abuser stops taking the drugs, but some are permanent.

Most data on the long-term effects of anabolic steroids on humans come from case reports rather than formal epidemiological studies. From the case reports, the incidence of life-threatening effects appears to be low, but serious adverse effects may be under-recognized or under-reported. Data from animal studies seem to support this possibility. One study found that exposing male mice for one-fifth of their lifespan to steroid doses comparable to those taken by human athletes caused a high percentage of premature deaths.

Hormonal System: Steroid abuse disrupts the normal production of hormones in the body, causing both reversible and irreversible changes. Changes that can be reversed include reduced sperm production and shrinking of the testicles (testicular atrophy). Irreversible changes include male-pattern baldness and breast development (gynecomastia). In one study of male bodybuilders, more than half had testicular atrophy, and more than half had gynecomastia. Gynecomastia is thought to occur due to the disruption of normal hormone balance.

In the female body, anabolic steroids cause masculinization. Breast size and body fat decrease, the skin becomes coarse, the clitoris enlarges, and the voice deepens. Women may experience excessive growth of body hair but lose scalp hair. With continued administration of steroids, some of these effects are irreversible.

Musculoskeletal System: Rising levels of testosterone and other sex hormones normally trigger the growth spurt that occurs during puberty and adolescence. Subsequently, when these hormones reach certain levels, they signal the bones to stop growing, locking a person into his or her maximum height. When a child or adolescent takes anabolic steroids, the resulting artificially high sex hormone levels can signal the bones to stop growing sooner than they normally would have done.

Cardiovascular System: Steroid abuse has been associated with cardiovascular diseases (CVD), including heart attacks and strokes, even in athletes younger than 30. Steroids contribute to the development of CVD, partly by changing the levels of lipoproteins that carry cholesterol in the blood. Steroids, particularly the oral types, increase the level of low-density lipoprotein (LDL) and decrease the level of high-density lipoprotein (HDL). High LDL and low HDL levels increase the risk of atherosclerosis, a condition in which fatty substances are deposited inside arteries and disrupt blood flow. If blood is prevented from reaching the heart, the result can be a heart attack. If blood is prevented from reaching the brain, the result can be a stroke.

Steroids also increase the risk that blood clots will form in blood vessels, potentially disrupting blood flow and damaging the heart muscle so that it does not pump blood effectively.

Liver: Steroid abuse has been associated with liver tumors and a rare condition called peliosis hepatis, in which blood-filled cysts form in the liver. Both the tumors and the cysts sometimes rupture, causing internal bleeding.

Skin: Steroid abuse can cause acne, cysts, and oily hair and skin.

Infection: Many abusers who inject anabolic steroids use nonsterile injection techniques or share contaminated needles with other abusers. In addition, some steroid preparations are manufactured illegally under nonsterile conditions. These factors put abusers at risk for acquiring life-threatening viral infections, such as HIV and hepatitis B and C. Abusers also can develop infective endocarditis, a bacterial illness that causes a potentially fatal inflammation of the inner lining of the heart. Bacterial infections also can cause pain and abscess formation at injection sites.

What effects do anabolic steroids have on behavior?

Case reports and small studies indicate that anabolic steroids, particularly in high doses, increase irritability and aggression. Some steroid abusers report that they have committed aggressive acts, such as physical fighting, committing armed robbery, or using force to obtain something. Some abusers also report that they have committed property crimes, such as stealing from a store, damaging or destroying others' property, or breaking into a house or a building. Abusers who have committed aggressive acts or property crimes generally report that they engage in these behaviors more often when they take steroids than when they are drug-free.

Some researchers have suggested that steroid abusers may commit aggressive acts and property crimes not because of steroids' direct effects on the brain but because the abusers have been affected by extensive media attention to the link between steroids and aggression. According to this theory, the abusers are using this possible link as an excuse to commit aggressive acts and property crimes.

One way to distinguish between these two possibilities is to administer either high steroid doses or placebo for days or weeks to human

Table 38.2. Possible Health Consequences of Anabolic Steroid Abuse

Hormonal System: Men

- Infertility
- Breast development
- Shrinking of the testicles
- Male-pattern baldness

Hormonal System: Women

- Enlargement of the clitoris
- Excessive growth of body hair
- Male-pattern baldness

Musculoskeletal System

- Short stature
- Tendon rupture

Cardiovascular System

- Heart attacks
- Enlargement of the heart's left ventricle

Liver

- Cancer
- Peliosis hepatis

Skin

- Acne and cysts
- Oily scalp

Infection

- HIV/AIDS
- Hepatitis

Psychiatric Effects

- Homicidal rage
- Mania
- Delusions

volunteers and then ask the people to report on their behavioral symptoms. To date, four such studies have been conducted. In three, high steroid doses did produce greater feelings of irritability and aggression than did placebo; but in one study, the drugs did not have that effect. One possible explanation, according to researchers, is that some but not all anabolic steroids increase irritability and aggression.

Anabolic steroids have been reported also to cause other behavioral effects, including euphoria, increased energy, sexual arousal, mood swings, distractibility, forgetfulness, and confusion. In the studies in which researchers administered high steroid doses to volunteers, a minority of the volunteers developed behavioral symptoms that were so extreme as to disrupt their ability to function in their jobs or in society. In a few cases, the volunteers' behavior presented a threat to themselves and others.

In summary, the extent to which steroid abuse contributes to violence and behavioral disorders is unknown. As with the health complications of steroid abuse, the prevalence of extreme cases of violence and behavioral disorders seems to be low, but it may be under-reported or under-recognized.

Are anabolic steroids addictive?

An undetermined percentage of steroid abusers become addicted to the drugs, as evidenced by their continuing to take steroids in spite of physical problems, negative effects on social relations, or nervousness and irritability. Also, they spend large amounts of time and money obtaining the drugs and experience withdrawal symptoms such as mood swings, fatigue, restlessness, loss of appetite, insomnia, reduced sex drive, and the desire to take more steroids. The most dangerous of the withdrawal symptoms is depression, because it sometimes leads to suicide attempts. Untreated, some depressive symptoms associated with anabolic steroid withdrawal have been known to persist for a year or more after the abuser stops taking the drugs.

What can be done to prevent steroid abuse?

Early attempts to prevent steroid abuse concentrated on drug testing and on educating students about the drugs' adverse effects. A few school districts test for abuse of illicit drugs, including steroids, and studies are currently under way to determine whether such testing reduces drug abuse.

Research on steroid educational programs has shown that simply teaching students about steroids' adverse effects does not convince adolescents that they personally can be adversely affected. Nor does such instruction discourage young people from taking steroids in the future. Presenting both the risks and benefits of anabolic steroid use is more effective in convincing adolescents about steroids' negative effects, apparently because the students find a balanced approach more credible and less biased, according to the researchers. However, the balanced approach still does not discourage adolescents from abusing steroids.

A more sophisticated approach has shown promise for preventing steroid abuse among players on high school sports teams. In the ATLAS program, developed for male football players, coaches and team leaders discuss the potential effects of anabolic steroids and other illicit drugs on immediate sports performance, and they teach how to refuse offers of drugs. They also discuss how strength training and proper nutrition can help adolescents build their bodies without the use of steroids. Later, special trainers teach the players proper weightlifting techniques. An ongoing series of studies has shown that this multicomponent, team-centered approach reduces new steroid abuse by 50%. A program designed for adolescent girls on sports teams, patterned after the program designed for boys, is currently being tested.

What treatments are effective for anabolic steroid abuse?

Few studies of treatments for anabolic steroid abuse have been conducted. Current knowledge is based largely on the experiences of a small number of physicians who have worked with patients undergoing steroid withdrawal. The physicians have found that supportive therapy is sufficient in some cases. Patients are educated about what they may experience during withdrawal and are evaluated for suicidal thoughts. If symptoms are severe or prolonged, medications or hospitalization may be needed.

Some medications that have been used for treating steroid withdrawal restore the hormonal system after its disruption by steroid abuse. Other medications target specific withdrawal symptoms—for example, antidepressants to treat depression, and analgesics for headaches and muscle and joint pains.

Some patients require assistance beyond simple treatment of withdrawal symptoms and are treated with behavioral therapies.

Where can I get further scientific information about steroid abuse?

Fact sheets on anabolic steroids, other illicit drugs, and related topics can be ordered free, in English and Spanish, by calling NIDA Infofax at (888) NIH-NIDA (644-6432) or, for those with hearing impairment, (888) TTY-NIDA (889-6432).

Information on steroid abuse also can be accessed through the NIDA Steroid Abuse website (www.steroidabuse.org). Information on illicit drugs in general can be accessed through NIDA's home page (www.drugabuse.gov) or by contacting the National Clearinghouse for Alcohol and Drug Information (NCADI) website (www.health.org).

Chapter 39

Yaba

What is yaba?

Yaba is a combination of methamphetamine (a powerful and addictive stimulant) and caffeine. Yaba, which means crazy medicine in Thai, is produced in Southeast and East Asia. The drug is popular in Asian communities in the United States and increasingly is available at raves and techno parties.

What does yaba look like?

Yaba is sold as tablets. These tablets are generally no larger than a pencil eraser. They are brightly colored, usually reddish-orange or green. Yaba tablets typically bear one of a variety of logos; R and WY are common logos.

How is yaba used?

Yaba tablets typically are consumed orally. The tablets sometimes are flavored like candy (grape, orange, or vanilla). Another common method is called chasing the dragon. Users place the yaba tablet on aluminum foil and heat it from below. As the tablet melts, vapors rise and are inhaled. The drug also may be administered by crushing the tablets into powder, which is then snorted or mixed with a solvent and injected.

"Yaba Fast Facts: Questions and Answers," National Drug Intelligence Center (NDIC), a component of the U.S. Department of Justice, June 2003.

Who uses yaba?

It is difficult to determine the scope of yaba use in the United States because most data sources do not distinguish yaba from other forms of methamphetamine. Yaba has emerged as a drug of abuse in Asian communities in the United States, specifically in Northern California and in Los Angeles.

Yaba also is becoming increasingly popular at raves, techno parties, and other venues where the drug MDMA (3,4-methylenedioxy-methamphetamine, typically called ecstasy) is used. Drug distributors deliberately market yaba to young people, many of whom have already tried MDMA. The bright colors and candy flavors of yaba tablets are examples of distributors' attempts to appeal to young people.

What are the risks?

Individuals who use yaba face the same risks as users of other forms of methamphetamine: rapid heart rate, increased blood pressure, and damage to the small blood vessels in the brain that can lead to stroke. Chronic use of the drug can result in inflammation of the heart lining. Overdoses can cause hyperthermia (elevated body temperature), convulsions, and death. Individuals who use yaba also may have episodes of violent behavior, paranoia, anxiety, confusion, and insomnia.

Although most users administer yaba orally, those who inject the drug expose themselves to additional risks, including contracting HIV (human immunodeficiency virus), hepatitis B and C, and other blood-borne viruses.

What is it called?

The most common names for yaba are crazy medicine and Nazi speed.

Is yaba illegal?

Yes, yaba is illegal because it contains methamphetamine, a Schedule II substance under the Controlled Substances Act. Schedule II drugs, which include cocaine and PCP, have a high potential for abuse. Abuse of these drugs may lead to severe psychological or physical dependence.

Part Four

Treating Drug Abuse

Chapter 40

Recognizing Drug Paraphernalia

What are drug paraphernalia?

The term drug paraphernalia refers to any equipment that is used to produce, conceal, and consume illicit drugs. It includes but is not limited to items such as bongs, roach clips, miniature spoons, and various types of pipes.

Under federal law the term drug paraphernalia means "any equipment, product, or material of any kind which is primarily intended or designed for use in manufacturing, compounding, converting, concealing, producing, processing, preparing, injecting, ingesting, inhaling, or otherwise introducing into the human body a controlled substance."

What do drug paraphernalia look like?

Identifying drug paraphernalia can be challenging because products often are marketed as though they were designed for legitimate purposes. Marijuana pipes and bongs, for example, frequently carry a misleading disclaimer indicating that they are intended to be used only with tobacco products. Recognizing drug paraphernalia often involves considering other factors such as the manner in which items are displayed for sale, descriptive materials or instructions accompanying the items, and the type of business selling the items.

"Drug Paraphernalia Fast Facts: Questions and Answers," National Drug Intelligence Center, a component of the U.S. Department of Justice, September 2003.

The appearance of drug paraphernalia varies depending upon the manufacturer and intended purpose. Increasingly, bongs, pipes, and other paraphernalia are manufactured in bright, trendy colors and bear designs such as skulls, devils, dragons, and wizards. Manufacturers attempt to glamorize drug use and make their products attractive to teenagers and young adults.

Where are drug paraphernalia sold?

Drug paraphernalia can be obtained through various means. Many large manufacturers market their products over the Internet and through mail-order businesses. In addition, drug paraphernalia frequently are sold at tobacco shops, trendy gift and novelty shops, gas stations, and convenience stores.

What are examples of drug paraphernalia?

- Pipes (metal, wooden, acrylic, glass, stone, plastic, or ceramic)
- Water pipes
- Roach clips
- Miniature spoons
- Chillums (cone-shaped marijuana/hash pipes)
- Bongs
- Cigarette papers
- Cocaine freebase kits

Are drug paraphernalia illegal?

Yes, drug paraphernalia are illegal. The drug paraphernalia statute, U.S. Code Title 21 Section 863, makes it "unlawful for any person to sell or offer for sale drug paraphernalia; to use the mails or any other facility of interstate commerce to transport drug paraphernalia; or to import or export drug paraphernalia."

Chapter 41

Frequently Asked Questions about Drug Addiction Treatment

What is drug addiction treatment?

There are many addictive drugs, and treatments for specific drugs can differ. Treatment also varies depending on the characteristics of the patient.

Problems associated with an individual's drug addiction can vary significantly. People who are addicted to drugs come from all walks of life. Many suffer from mental health, occupational, health, or social problems that make their addictive disorders much more difficult to treat. Even if there are few associated problems, the severity of addiction itself ranges widely among people.

A variety of scientifically based approaches to drug addiction treatment exists. Drug addiction treatment can include behavioral therapy (such as counseling, cognitive therapy, or psychotherapy), medications, or their combination. Behavioral therapies offer people strategies for coping with their drug cravings, teach them ways to avoid drugs and prevent relapse, and help them deal with relapse if it occurs. When a person's drug-related behavior places him or her at higher risk for AIDS or other infectious diseases, behavioral therapies can help to reduce the risk of disease transmission. Case management and referral to other medical, psychological, and social services are crucial

"Frequently Asked Questions," excerpted from *Principles of Drug Treatment*, National Institute on Drug Abuse (NIDA), NIH Pub. No. 99-4180, October 1999, reprinted July 2000; this version updated by David A. Cooke, M.D., April 2004.

components of treatment for many patients. The best programs provide a combination of therapies and other services to meet the needs of the individual patient, which are shaped by such issues as age, race, culture, sexual orientation, gender, pregnancy, parenting, housing, and employment, as well as physical and sexual abuse.

Treatment medications, such as methadone, buprenorphine, LAAM, and naltrexone, are available for individuals addicted to opiates. Nicotine preparations (patches, gum, nasal spray) and bupropion are available for individuals addicted to nicotine.

Medications, such as antidepressants, mood stabilizers, or neuroleptics, may be critical for treatment success when patients have co-occurring mental disorders, such as depression, anxiety disorder, bipolar disorder, or psychosis. Treatment can occur in a variety of settings, in many different forms, and for different lengths of time. Because drug addiction is typically a chronic disorder characterized by occasional relapses, a short-term, one-time treatment often is not sufficient. For many, treatment is a long-term process that involves multiple interventions and attempts at abstinence.

Why can't drug addicts quit on their own?

Nearly all addicted individuals believe in the beginning that they can stop using drugs on their own, and most try to stop without treatment. However, most of these attempts result in failure to achieve long-term abstinence. Research has shown that long-term drug use results in significant changes in brain function that persist long after the individual stops using drugs. These drug-induced changes in brain function may have many behavioral consequences, including the compulsion to use drugs despite adverse consequences—the defining characteristic of addiction.

Understanding that addiction has such an important biological component may help explain an individual's difficulty in achieving and maintaining abstinence without treatment. Psychological stress from work or family problems, social cues (such as meeting individuals from one's drug-using past), or the environment (such as encountering streets, objects, or even smells associated with drug use) can interact with biological factors to hinder attainment of sustained abstinence and make relapse more likely. Research studies indicate that even the most severely addicted individuals can participate actively in treatment and that active participation is essential to good outcomes.

How effective is drug addiction treatment?

In addition to stopping drug use, the goal of treatment is to return the individual to productive functioning in the family, workplace, and community. Measures of effectiveness typically include levels of criminal behavior, family functioning, employability, and medical condition. Overall, treatment of addiction is as successful as treatment of other chronic diseases, such as diabetes, hypertension, and asthma.

According to several studies, drug treatment reduces drug use by 40% to 60% and significantly decreases criminal activity during and after treatment. For example, a study of therapeutic community treatment for drug offenders demonstrated that arrests for violent and nonviolent criminal acts were reduced by 40% or more. Methadone treatment has been shown to decrease criminal behavior by as much as 50%. Research shows that drug addiction treatment reduces the risk of HIV infection and that interventions to prevent HIV are much less costly than treating HIV-related illnesses. Treatment can improve the prospects for employment, with gains of up to 40% after treatment.

Although these effectiveness rates hold in general, individual treatment outcomes depend on the extent and nature of the patient's presenting problems, the appropriateness of the treatment components and related services used to address those problems, and the degree of active engagement of the patient in the treatment process.

How long does drug addiction treatment usually last?

Individuals progress through drug addiction treatment at various speeds, so there is no predetermined length of treatment. However, research has shown unequivocally that good outcomes are contingent on adequate lengths of treatment. Generally, for residential or outpatient treatment, participation for less than 90 days is of limited or no effectiveness, and treatments lasting significantly longer often are indicated. For methadone maintenance, 12 months of treatment is the minimum, and some opiate-addicted individuals will continue to benefit from methadone maintenance treatment over a period of years.

Many people who enter treatment drop out before receiving all the benefits that treatment can provide. Successful outcomes may require more than one treatment experience. Many addicted individuals have multiple episodes of treatment, often with a cumulative impact.

What helps people stay in treatment?

Since successful outcomes often depend upon retaining the person long enough to gain the full benefits of treatment, strategies for keeping an individual in the program are critical. Whether a patient stays in treatment depends on factors associated with both the individual and the program. Individual factors related to engagement and retention include motivation to change drug-using behavior, degree of support from family and friends, and whether there is pressure to stay in treatment from the criminal justice system, child protection services, employers, or the family. Within the program, successful counselors are able to establish a positive, therapeutic relationship with the patient. The counselor should ensure that a treatment plan is established and followed so that the individual knows what to expect during treatment. Medical, psychiatric, and social services should be available.

Since some individual problems (such as serious mental illness, severe cocaine or crack use, and criminal involvement) increase the likelihood of a patient dropping out, intensive treatment with a range of components may be required to retain patients who have these problems. The provider then should ensure a transition to continuing care or "aftercare" following the patient's completion of formal treatment.

Is the use of medications like methadone simply replacing one drug addiction with another?

No. As used in maintenance treatment, methadone and LAAM are not heroin substitutes. They are safe and effective medications for opiate addiction that are administered by mouth in regular, fixed doses. Their pharmacological effects are markedly different from those of heroin.

Injected, snorted, or smoked heroin causes an almost immediate "rush" or brief period of euphoria that wears off very quickly terminating in a "crash." The individual then experiences an intense craving to use more heroin to stop the crash and reinstate the euphoria. The cycle of euphoria, crash, and craving—repeated several times a day—leads to a cycle of addiction and behavioral disruption. These characteristics of heroin use result from the drug 's rapid onset of action and its short duration of action in the brain. An individual who uses heroin multiple times per day subjects his or her brain and body to marked, rapid fluctuations as the opiate effects come and go. These fluctuations can disrupt a number of important bodily functions. Because heroin is illegal, addicted persons often become part of a volatile drug-using street culture characterized by hustling and crimes for profit.

Methadone, buprenorphine, and LAAM have far more gradual onsets of action than heroin, and as a result, patients stabilized on these medications do not experience any rush, In addition, both medications wear off much more slowly than heroin, so there is no sudden crash, and the brain and body are not exposed to the marked fluctuations seen with heroin use. Maintenance treatment with methadone or LAAM markedly reduces the desire for heroin. If an individual maintained on adequate, regular doses of methadone or buprenorphine (once a day) or LAAM (several times per week) tries to take heroin, the euphoric effects of heroin will be significantly blocked. According to research, patients undergoing maintenance treatment do not suffer the medical abnormalities and behavioral destabilization that rapid fluctuations in drug levels cause in heroin addicts.

What role can the criminal justices system play in the treatment of drug addiction?

Increasingly, research is demonstrating that treatment for drug-addicted offenders during and after incarceration can have a significant beneficial effect upon future drug use, criminal behavior, and social functioning. The case for integrating drug addiction treatment approaches with the criminal justice system is compelling. Combining prison- and community-based treatment for drug-addicted offenders reduces the risk of both recidivism to drug-related criminal behavior and relapse to drug use. For example, a recent study found that prisoners who participated in a therapeutic treatment program in the Delaware State Prison and continued to receive treatment in a work-release program after prison were 70% less likely than nonparticipants to return to drug use and incur rearrest.

The majority of offenders involved with the criminal justice system are not in prison but are under community supervision. For those with known drug problems, drug addiction treatment may be recommended or mandated as a condition of probation. Research has demonstrated that individuals who enter treatment under legal pressure have outcomes as favorable as those who enter treatment voluntarily.

The criminal justice system refers drug offenders into treatment through a variety of mechanisms, such as diverting nonviolent offenders to treatment, stipulating treatment as a condition of probation or pretrial release, and convening specialized courts that handle cases for offenses involving drugs. Drug courts, another model, are dedicated to drug offender cases. They mandate and arrange for treatment as an alternative to incarceration, actively monitors progress in treatment, and arrange for other services to drug-involved offenders.

The most effective models integrate criminal justice and drug treatment systems and services. Treatment and criminal justice personnel work together on plans and implementation of screening, placement, testing, monitoring, and supervision, as well as on the systematic use of sanctions and rewards for drug abusers in the criminal justice system. Treatment for incarcerated drug abusers must include continuing care, monitoring, and supervision after release and during parole.

How does drug addiction treatment help reduce the spread of HIV/AIDS and other infectious diseases?

Many drug addicts, such as heroin or cocaine addicts and particularly injection drug users, are at increased risk for HIV/AIDS as well as other infectious diseases like hepatitis, tuberculosis, and sexually transmitted infections. For these individuals and the community at large, drug addiction treatment is disease prevention.

Drug injectors who do not enter treatment are up to six times more likely to become infected with HIV than injectors who enter and remain in treatment. Drug users who enter and continue in treatment reduce activities that can spread disease, such as sharing injection equipment and engaging in unprotected sexual activity. Participation in treatment also presents opportunities for screening, counseling, and referral for additional services. The best drug abuse treatment programs provide HIV counseling and offer HIV testing to their patients.

Where do 12-step or self-help programs fit into drug addiction treatment?

Self-help groups can complement and extend the effects of professional treatment. The most prominent self-help groups are those affiliated with Alcoholics Anonymous (AA), Narcotics Anonymous (NA), and Cocaine Anonymous (CA), all of which are based on the 12-step model, and Smart Recovery. Most drug addiction treatment programs encourage patients to participate in a self-help group during and after formal treatment.

How can families and friends make a difference in the life of someone needing treatment?

Family and friends can play critical roles in motivating individuals with drug problems to enter and stay in treatment. Family therapy is important, especially for adolescents. Involvement of a family member in an individual's treatment program can strengthen and extend the benefits of the program.

Is drug addiction treatment worth its cost?

Drug addiction treatment is cost-effective in reducing drug use and its associated health and social costs. Treatment is less expensive than alternatives, such as not treating addicts or simply incarcerating addicts. For example, the average cost for one full year of methadone maintenance treatment is approximately $4,700 per patient, whereas one full year of imprisonment costs approximately $18,400 per person.

According to several conservative estimates, every $1 invested in addiction treatment programs yields a return of between $4 and $7 in reduced drug-related crime, criminal justice costs, and theft alone. When savings related to health care are included, total savings can exceed costs by a ratio of 12 to 1. Major savings to the individual and society also come from significant drops in interpersonal conflicts, improvements in workplace productivity, and reductions in drug-related accidents.

Chapter 42

Major Types of Drug Treatment Approaches

Drug addiction is a complex disorder that can involve virtually every aspect of an individual's functioning—in the family, at work, and in the community. Because of addiction's complexity and pervasive consequences, drug addiction treatment typically must involve many components. Some of those components focus directly on the individual's drug use. Others, like employment training, focus on restoring the addicted individual to productive membership in the family and society.

Treatment for drug abuse and addiction is delivered in many different settings, using a variety of behavioral and pharmacological approaches. In the United States, more than 11,000 specialized drug treatment facilities provide rehabilitation, counseling, behavioral therapy, medication, case management, and other types of services to persons with drug use disorders.

Because drug abuse and addiction are major public health problems, a large portion of drug treatment is funded by local, state, and federal governments. Private and employer-subsidized health plans also may provide coverage for treatment of d rug addiction and its medical consequences.

Drug abuse and addiction are treated in specialized treatment facilities and mental health clinics by a variety of providers, including

"Drug Addiction Treatment in the United States," excerpted from *Principles of Drug Treatment*, National Institute on Drug Abuse (NIDA), NIH Pub. No. 99-4180, October 1999, reprinted July 2000; this version updated by David A. Cooke, M.D., April 2004.

certified drug abuse counselors, physicians, psychologists, nurses, and social workers. Treatment is delivered in outpatient, inpatient, and residential settings. Although specific treatment approaches often are associated with particular treatment settings, a variety of therapeutic interventions or services can be included in any given setting.

General Categories of Treatment Programs

Research studies on drug addiction treatment have typically classified treatment programs into several general types or modalities, which are described in the following text. Treatment approaches and individual programs continue to evolve, and many programs in existence today do not fit neatly into traditional drug addiction treatment classifications.

Agonist Maintenance Treatment

Agonist maintenance treatment for opiate addicts usually is conducted in outpatient settings, often called methadone treatment programs. These programs use a long-acting synthetic opiate medication, usually methadone or LAAM, administered orally for a sustained period at a dosage sufficient to prevent opiate withdrawal, block the effects of illicit opiate use, and decrease opiate craving. Patients stabilized on adequate, sustained dosages of methadone or LAAM can function normally. They can hold jobs, avoid the crime and violence of the street culture, and reduce their exposure to HIV by stopping or decreasing injection drug use and drug-related high-risk sexual behavior.

Patients stabilized on opiate agonists can engage more readily in counseling and other behavioral interventions essential to recovery and rehabilitation. The best, most effective opiate agonist maintenance programs include individual and/or group counseling, as well as provision of, or referral to, other needed medical, psychological, and social services.

Buprenorphine has been recently approved by the Food and Drug Administration for use in opiate addict treatment in outpatient settings. Like methadone and LAAM, buprenorphine is an opiate. However, it has lesser potency, reducing its potential for abuse, and it can also act as an opiate antagonist (see below) if mixed with another opiate. Physicians who prescribe this drug are required to have special training in addiction medicine and approval from the Drug Enforcement Agency. However, they may be community physicians, rather than only at addiction treatment clinics.

336

Narcotic Antagonist Treatment

Narcotic antagonist treatment using naltrexone for opiate addicts usually is conducted in outpatient settings although initiation of the medication often begins after medical detoxification in a residential setting. Naltrexone is a long-acting synthetic opiate antagonist with few side effects that is taken orally either daily or three times a week for a sustained period of time. Individuals must be medically detoxified and opiate-free for several days before naltrexone can be taken to prevent precipitating an opiate abstinence syndrome. When used this way, all the effects of self-administered opiates, including euphoria, are completely blocked. The theory behind this treatment is that the repeated lack of the desired opiate effects, as well as the perceived futility of using the opiate, will gradually over time result in breaking the habit of opiate addiction. Naltrexone itself has no subjective effects or potential for abuse and is not addicting. Patient noncompliance is a common problem. Therefore, a favorable treatment outcome requires that there also be a positive therapeutic relationship, effective counseling or therapy, and careful monitoring of medication compliance.

Many experienced clinicians have found naltrexone most useful for highly motivated, recently detoxified patients who desire total abstinence because of external circumstances, including impaired professionals, parolees, probationers, and prisoners in work-release status. Patients stabilized on naltrexone can function normally. They can hold jobs, avoid the crime and violence of the street culture, and reduce their exposure to HIV by stopping injection drug use and drug-related high-risk sexual behavior.

Outpatient Drug-Free Treatment

Outpatient drug-free treatment varies in the types and intensity of services offered. Such treatment costs less than residential or inpatient treatment and often is more suitable for individuals who are employed or who have extensive social supports. Low-intensity programs may offer little more than drug education and admonition. Other outpatient models, such as intensive day treatment, can be comparable to residential programs in services and effectiveness, depending on the individual patient's characteristics and needs. In many outpatient programs, group counseling is emphasized. Some outpatient programs are designed to treat patients who have medical or mental health problems in addition to their drug disorder.

337

Long-Term Residential Treatment

Long-term residential treatment provides care 24 hours per day, generally in nonhospital settings. The best-known residential treatment model is the therapeutic community (TC), but residential treatment may also employ other models, such as cognitive-behavioral therapy.

TCs are residential programs with planned lengths of stay of 6 to 12 months. TCs focus on the "resocialization" of the individual and use the program's entire "community," including other residents, staff, and the social context, as active components of treatment. Addiction is viewed in the context of an individual's social and psychological deficits, and treatment focuses on developing personal accountability and responsibility and socially productive lives. Treatment is highly structured and can at times be confrontational, with activities designed to help residents examine damaging beliefs, self-concepts, and patterns of behavior and to adopt new, more harmonious and constructive ways to interact with others. Many TCs are quite comprehensive and can include employment training and other support services on site.

Compared with patients in other forms of drug treatment, the typical TC resident has more severe problems, with more co-occurring mental health problems and more criminal involvement. Research shows that TCs can be modified to treat individuals with special needs, including adolescents, women, those with severe mental disorders, and individuals in the criminal justice system.

Short-Term Residential Programs

Short-term residential programs provide intensive but relatively brief residential treatment based on a modified 12-step approach. These programs were originally designed to treat alcohol problems, but during the cocaine epidemic of the mid-1980s, many began to treat illicit drug abuse and addiction. The original residential treatment model consisted of a three- to six-week hospital-based inpatient treatment phase followed by extended outpatient therapy and participation in a self-help group, such as Alcoholics Anonymous. Reduced health care coverage for substance abuse treatment has resulted in a diminished number of these programs, and the average length of stay under managed care review is much shorter than in early programs.

Medical Detoxification

Medical detoxification is a process whereby individuals are systematically withdrawn from addicting drugs in an inpatient or outpatient setting, typically under the care of a physician. Detoxification is sometimes called a distinct treatment modality but is more appropriately considered a precursor of treatment, because it is designed to treat the acute physiological effects of stopping drug use. Medications are available for detoxification from opiates, nicotine, benzodiazepines, alcohol, barbiturates, and other sedatives. In some cases, particularly for the last three types of drugs, detoxification may be a medical necessity, and untreated withdrawal may be medically dangerous or even fatal.

Detoxification is not designed to address the psychological, social, and behavioral problems associated with addiction and therefore does not typically produce lasting behavioral changes necessary for recovery. Detoxification is most useful when it incorporates formal processes of assessment and referral to subsequent drug addiction treatment.

Treating Criminal Justice-Involved Drug Abusers and Addicts

Research has shown that combining criminal justice sanctions with drug treatment can be effective in decreasing drug use and related crime. Individuals under legal coercion tend to stay in treatment for a longer period of time and do as well as or better than others not under legal pressure. Often, drug abusers come into contact with the criminal justice system earlier than other health or social systems, and intervention by the criminal justice system to engage the individual in treatment may help interrupt and shorten a career of drug use. Treatment for the criminal justice-involved drug abuser or drug addict may be delivered prior to, during, after, or in lieu of incarceration.

Prison-Based Treatment Programs

Offenders with drug disorders may encounter a number of treatment options while incarcerated, including didactic drug education classes, self-help programs, and treatment based on therapeutic community or residential milieu therapy models. The TC model has been studied extensively and can be quite effective in reducing drug use and recidivism to criminal behavior. Those in treatment should be segregated from the general prison population, so that the "prison culture" does not overwhelm progress toward recovery. As might be expected, treatment gains can be lost if inmates are returned to the general prison population after treatment. Research shows that relapse to drug use and recidivism to crime are significantly lower if the drug offender continues treatment after returning to the community.

Community-Based Treatment for Criminal Justice Populations

A number of criminal justice alternatives to incarceration have been tried with offenders who have drug disorders, including limited diversion programs, pretrial release conditional on entry into treatment, and conditional probation with sanctions. The drug court is a promising approach. Drug courts mandate and arrange for drug addiction treatment, actively monitor progress in treatment, and arrange for other services to drug-involved offenders. Federal support for planning, implementation, and enhancement of drug courts is provided under the U.S. Department of Justice Drug Courts Program Office.

As a well-studied example, the Treatment Accountability and Safer Communities (TASC) program provides an alternative to incarceration by addressing the multiple needs of drug-addicted offenders in a community-based setting. TASC programs typically include counseling, medical care, parenting instruction, family counseling, school and job training, and legal and employment services. The key features of TASC include (1) coordination of criminal justice and drug treatment; (2) early identification, assessment, and referral of drug-involved offenders; (3) monitoring offenders through drug testing; and (4) use of legal sanctions as inducements to remain in treatment.

Chapter 43

Scientifically Tested Drug Treatment Components

This section presents several examples of treatment approaches and components that have been developed and tested for efficacy through research supported by the National Institute on Drug Abuse (NIDA). Each approach is designed to address certain aspects of drug addiction and its consequences for the individual, family, and society. The approaches are to be used to supplement or enhance—not replace—existing treatment programs.

This section is not a complete list of efficacious, scientifically based treatment approaches. Additional approaches are under development as part of NIDA's continuing support of treatment research.

Relapse Prevention

Relapse prevention, a cognitive-behavioral therapy, was developed for the treatment of problem drinking and adapted later for cocaine addicts. Cognitive-behavioral strategies are based on the theory that learning processes play a critical role in the development of maladaptive behavioral patterns. Individuals learn to identify and correct problematic behaviors. Relapse prevention encompasses several cognitive-behavioral strategies that facilitate abstinence as well as provide help for people who experience relapse.

"Scientifically Based Approaches to Drug Addiction Treatment," excerpted from *Principles of Drug Treatment*, National Institute on Drug Abuse (NIDA), NIH Pub. No. 99-4180, October 1999, reprinted July 2000; this version updated by David A. Cooke, M.D., April 2004.

The relapse prevention approach to the treatment of cocaine addiction consists of a collection of strategies intended to enhance self-control. Specific techniques include exploring the positive and negative consequences of continued use, self-monitoring to recognize drug cravings early on and to identify high-risk situations for use, and developing strategies for coping with and avoiding high-risk situations and the desire to use. A central element of this treatment is anticipating the problems patients are likely to meet and helping them develop effective coping strategies.

Research indicates that the skills individuals learn through relapse prevention therapy remain after the completion of treatment. In one study, most people receiving this cognitive-behavioral approach maintained the gains they made in treatment throughout the year following treatment.

Supportive-Expressive Psychotherapy

Supportive-expressive psychotherapy is a time-limited, focused psychotherapy that has been adapted for heroin- and cocaine-addicted individuals. The therapy has two main components:

- Supportive techniques to help patients feel comfortable in discussing their personal experiences.

- Expressive techniques to help patients identify and work through interpersonal relationship issues.

Special attention is paid to the role of drugs in relation to problem feelings and behaviors, and how problems may be solved without recourse to drugs.

The efficacy of individual supportive-expressive psychotherapy has been tested with patients in methadone maintenance treatment who had psychiatric problems. In a comparison with patients receiving only drug counseling, both groups fared similarly with regard to opiate use, but the supportive-expressive psychotherapy group had lower cocaine use and required less methadone. Also, the patients who received supportive-expressive psychotherapy maintained many of the gains they had made. In an earlier study, supportive-expressive psychotherapy, when added to drug counseling, improved outcomes for opiate addicts in methadone treatment with moderately severe psychiatric problems.

Individualized Drug Counseling

Individualized drug counseling focuses directly on reducing or stopping the addict's illicit drug use. It also addresses related areas of impaired functioning—such as employment status, illegal activity, family/social relations—as well as the content and structure of the patient's recovery program. Through its emphasis on short-term behavioral goals, individualized drug counseling helps the patient develop coping strategies and tools for abstaining from drug use and then maintaining abstinence. The addiction counselor encourages 12-step participation and makes referrals for needed supplemental medical, psychiatric, employment, and other services. Individuals are encouraged to attend sessions one or two times per week.

In a study that compared opiate addicts receiving only methadone to those receiving methadone coupled with counseling, individuals who received only methadone showed minimal improvement in reducing opiate use. The addition of counseling produced significantly more improvement. The addition of onsite medical/psychiatric, employment, and family services further improved outcomes.

In another study with cocaine addicts, individualized drug counseling, together with group drug counseling, was quite effective in reducing cocaine use. Thus, it appears that this approach has great utility with both heroin and cocaine addicts in outpatient treatment.

Motivational Enhancement Therapy

Motivational enhancement therapy is a client-centered counseling approach for initiating behavior change by helping clients to resolve ambivalence about engaging in treatment and stopping drug use. This approach employs strategies to evoke rapid and internally motivated change in the client, rather than guiding the client stepwise through the recovery process. This therapy consists of an initial assessment battery session, followed by two to four individual treatment sessions with a therapist. The first treatment session focuses on providing feedback generated from the initial assessment battery to stimulate discussion regarding personal substance use and to elicit self-motivational statements. Motivational interviewing principles are used to strengthen motivation and build a plan for change. Coping strategies for high-risk situations are suggested and discussed with the client. In subsequent sessions, the therapist monitors change, reviews cessation strategies being used, and continues to encourage commitment to change or sustained abstinence. Clients are sometimes encouraged to bring a significant other to sessions. This approach has been used successfully with alcoholics and with marijuana-dependent individuals.

Behavioral Therapy for Adolescents

Behavioral therapy for adolescents incorporates the principle that unwanted behavior can be changed by clear demonstration of the desired behavior and consistent reward of incremental steps toward achieving it. Therapeutic activities include fulfilling specific assignments, rehearsing desired behaviors, and recording and reviewing progress, with praise and privileges given for meeting assigned goals. Urine samples are collected regularly to monitor drug use. The therapy aims to equip the patient to gain three types of control:

- **Stimulus control** helps patients avoid situations associated with drug use and learn to spend more time in activities incompatible with drug use.

- **Urge control** helps patients recognize and change thoughts, feelings, and plans that lead to drug use.

- **Social control** involves family members and other people important in helping patients avoid drugs. A parent or significant other attends treatment sessions when possible and assists with therapy assignments and reinforcing desired behavior.

According to research studies, this therapy helps adolescents become drug free and increases their ability to remain drug free after treatment ends. Adolescents also show improvement in several other areas—employment/school attendance, family relationships, depression, institutionalization, and alcohol use. Such favorable results are attributed largely to including family members in therapy and rewarding drug abstinence as verified by urinalysis.

Multidimensional Family Therapy (MDFT) for Adolescents

Multidimensional family therapy (MDFT) for adolescents is an outpatient family-based drug abuse treatment for teenagers. MDFT views adolescent drug use in terms of a network of influences (that is, individual, family, peer, community) and suggests that reducing unwanted behavior and increasing desirable behavior occur in multiple ways in different settings. Treatment includes individual and family sessions held in the clinic, in the home, or with family members at the family court, school, or other community locations.

During individual sessions, the therapist and adolescent work on important developmental tasks, such as developing decision-making, negotiation, and problem-solving skills. Teenagers acquire skills in communicating their thoughts and feelings to deal better with life stressors, and vocational skills. Parallel sessions are held with family members. Parents examine their particular parenting style, learning to distinguish influence from control and to have a positive and developmentally appropriate influence on their child.

Multisystemic Therapy (MST)

Multisystemic therapy (MST) addresses the factors associated with serious antisocial behavior in children and adolescents who abuse drugs. These factors include characteristics of the adolescent (for example, favorable attitudes toward drug use), the family (poor discipline, family conflict, pa rental drug abuse), peers (positive attitudes toward drug use), school (dropout, poor performance), and neighborhood (criminal subculture). By participating in intense treatment in natural environments (homes, schools, and neighborhood settings) most youths and families complete a full course of treatment. MST significantly reduces adolescent drug use during treatment and for at least 6 months after treatment. Reduced numbers of incarcerations and out-of-home placements of juveniles offset the cost of providing this intensive service and maintaining the clinicians' low caseloads.

Combined Behavioral and Nicotine Replacement Therapy for Nicotine Addiction

Combined behavioral and nicotine replacement therapy for nicotine addiction consists of two main components:

- The transdermal nicotine patch or nicotine gum reduces symptoms of withdrawal, producing better initial abstinence.

- The behavioral component concurrently provides support and reinforcement of coping skills, yielding better long-term outcomes.

Through behavioral skills training, patients learn to avoid high-risk situations for smoking relapse early on and later to plan strategies to cope with such situations. Patients practice skills in treatment, social, and work settings. They learn other coping techniques, such as cigarette refusal skills, assertiveness, and time management. The combined treatment is based on the rationale that behavioral and pharmacological treatments operate by different yet complementary mechanisms that produce potentially additive effects.

Community Reinforcement Approach (CRA) Plus Vouchers

Community reinforcement approach (CRA) plus vouchers is an intensive 24-week outpatient therapy for treatment of cocaine addiction. The treatment goals are twofold:

- To achieve cocaine abstinence long enough for patients to learn new life skills that will help sustain abstinence.

- To reduce alcohol consumption for patients whose drinking is associated with cocaine use.

Patients attend one or two individual counseling sessions per week, where they focus on improving family relations, learning a variety of skills to minimize drug use, receiving vocational counseling, and developing new recreational activities and social networks. Those who also abuse alcohol receive clinic-monitored disulfiram (Antabuse) therapy. Patients submit urine samples two or three times each week and receive vouchers for cocaine-negative samples. The value of the vouchers increases with consecutive clean samples. Patients may exchange vouchers for retail goods that are consistent with a cocaine-free lifestyle.

This approach facilitates patient' engagement in treatment and systematically aids them in gaining substantial periods of cocaine abstinence. The approach has been tested in urban and rural areas and used successfully in outpatient detoxification of opiate-addicted adults and with inner-city methadone maintenance patients who have high rates of intravenous cocaine abuse.

Voucher-Based Reinforcement Therapy in Methadone Maintenance Treatment

Voucher-based reinforcement therapy in methadone maintenance treatment helps patients achieve and maintain abstinence from illegal drugs by providing them with a voucher each time they provide a drug-free urine sample. The voucher has monetary value and can be exchanged for goods and services consistent with the goals of treatment. Initially, the voucher values are low, but their value increases with the number of consecutive drug-free urine specimens the individual provides. Cocaine- or heroin-positive urine specimens reset the value of the vouchers to the initial low value. The contingency of escalating incentives is designed specifically to reinforce periods of sustained drug abstinence.

Studies show that patients receiving vouchers for drug-free urine samples achieved significantly more weeks of abstinence and significantly more weeks of sustained abstinence than patients who we re given vouchers independent of urinalysis results. In another study, urinalyses positive for heroin decreased significantly when the voucher program was started and increased significantly when the program was stopped.

Day Treatment with Abstinence Contingencies and Vouchers

Day treatment with abstinence contingencies and vouchers was developed to treat homeless crack addicts. For the first 2 months, participants must spend 5.5 hours daily in the program, which provides lunch and transportation to and from shelters. Interventions include individual assessment and goal setting, individual and group counseling, multiple psychoeducational groups (for example, didactic groups on community resources, housing, cocaine, and HIV/AIDS prevention; establishing and reviewing personal rehabilitation goals; relapse prevention; weekend planning), and patient-governed community meetings during which patients review contract goals and provide support and encouragement to each other. Individual counseling occurs once a week, and group therapy sessions are held three times a week. After 2 months of day treatment and at least 2 weeks of abstinence, participants graduate to a 4-month work component that pays wages that can be used to rent inexpensive, drug-free housing. A voucher system also rewards drug-free related social and recreational activities.

This innovative day treatment was compared with treatment consisting of twice-weekly individual counseling and 12-step groups, medical examinations and treatment, and referral to community resources for housing and vocational services. Innovative day treatment followed by work and housing dependent upon drug abstinence had a more positive effect on alcohol use, cocaine use, and days homeless.

The Matrix Model

The Matrix model provides a framework for engaging stimulant abusers in treatment and helping them achieve abstinence. Patients learn about issues critical to addiction and relapse, receive direction and support from a trained therapist, become familiar with self-help programs, and are monitored for drug use by urine testing. The program includes education for family members affected by the addiction.

The therapist functions simultaneously as teacher and coach, fostering a positive, encouraging relationship with the patient and using that relationship to reinforce positive behavior change. The interaction between the therapist and the patient is realistic and direct but not confrontational or parental. Therapists are trained to conduct treatment sessions in a way that promotes the patient's self-esteem, dignity, and self-worth. A positive relationship between patient and therapist is a critical element for patient retention.

Treatment materials draw heavily on other tested treatment approaches. Thus, this approach includes elements pertaining to the areas of relapse prevention, family and group therapies, drug education, and self-help participation. Detailed treatment manuals contain work sheets for individual sessions; other components include family educational groups, early recovery skills groups, relapse prevention groups, conjoint sessions, urine tests, 12-step programs, relapse analysis, and social support groups.

A number of projects have demonstrated that participants treated with the Matrix model demonstrate statistically significant reductions in drug and alcohol use, improvements in psychological indicators, and reduced risky sexual behaviors associated with HIV transmission. These reports, along with evidence suggesting comparable treatment response for methamphetamine users and cocaine users and demonstrated efficacy in enhancing naltrexone treatment of opiate addicts, provide a body of empirical support for the use of the model.

Chapter 44

Drug Addiction Treatment Medications

Treatment for people who abuse drugs but are not yet addicted to them most often consists of behavioral therapies, such as psychotherapy, counseling, support groups, or family therapy. But treatment for drug-addicted people often involves a combination of behavioral therapies and medications. Medications, such as methadone or LAAM (levo-alpha-acetyl-methadol), are effective in suppressing the withdrawal symptoms and drug craving associated with narcotic addiction, thus reducing illicit drug use and improving the chances of the individual remaining in treatment.

The primary medically assisted withdrawal method for narcotic addiction is to switch the patient to a comparable drug that produces milder withdrawal symptoms, and then gradually taper off the substitute medication. The medication used most often is methadone, taken by mouth once a day. Patients are started on the lowest dose that prevents the more severe signs of withdrawal and then the dose is gradually reduced. Substitutes can be used also for withdrawal from sedatives. Patients can be switched to long-acting sedatives, such as diazepam or phenobarbital, which are then gradually reduced.

Once a patient goes through withdrawal, there is still considerable risk of relapse. Patients may return to taking drugs even though they no longer have physical withdrawal symptoms. A great deal of research is being done to find medications that can block drug craving and treat other factors that cause a return to drugs.

NIDA InfoFacts, National Institute on Drug Abuse (NIDA), June 2003.

Patients who cannot continue abstaining from opiates are given maintenance therapy, usually with methadone. The maintenance dose of methadone, usually higher than that used for medically assisted withdrawal, prevents both withdrawal symptoms and heroin craving. It also prevents addicts from getting a high from heroin and, as a result, they stop using it. Research has shown that maintenance therapy reduces the spread of AIDS in the treated population. The overall death rate is also significantly reduced.

Within various methadone programs, those that provide higher doses of methadone (usually a minimum of 60 mg.) have better retention rates. Also, those that provide other services, such as counseling, therapy, and medical care, along with methadone generally get better results than the programs that provide minimal services.

Another drug recently approved for use in maintenance treatment is LAAM, which is administered three times a week rather than daily, as is the case with methadone. The drug naltrexone is also used to prevent relapse. Like methadone, LAAM and naltrexone prevent addicts from getting high from heroin. However, naltrexone does not eliminate the drug craving, so it has not been popular among addicts. Naltrexone works best with highly motivated patients.

There are currently no medications approved by the Food and Drug Administration (FDA) for treating addiction to cocaine, LSD, PCP, marijuana, methamphetamine and other stimulants, inhalants, or anabolic steroids. There are medications, however, for treating the adverse health effects of these drugs, such as seizures or psychotic reactions, and for overdoses from opiates.

Currently, the National Institute on Drug Abuse (NIDA)'s top research priority is the development of a medication useful in treating cocaine addiction.

For information on hotlines or counseling services, please call the Center for Substance Abuse Treatment (CSAT) National Drug and Alcohol Treatment Routing Service at (800) 662-4357.

Chapter 45

Dual Diagnosis and Integrated Treatment of Mental Illness and Substance Abuse Disorder

What are dual diagnosis services?

Dual diagnosis services are treatments for people who suffer from co-occurring disorders—mental illness and substance abuse. Research has strongly indicated that to recover fully, a consumer with co-occurring disorder needs treatment for both problems—focusing on one does not ensure the other will go away. Dual diagnosis services integrate assistance for each condition, helping people recover from both in one setting, at the same time.

Dual diagnosis services include a different types of assistance that go beyond standard therapy or medication: assertive outreach, job and housing assistance, family counseling, even money and relationship management. The personalized treatment is viewed as long-term and can be begun at whatever stage of recovery the consumer is in. Positivity, hope, and optimism are at the foundation of integrated treatment.

How often do people with severe mental illnesses also experience a co-occurring substance abuse problem?

There is a lack of information on the numbers of people with co-occurring disorders, but research has shown the disorders are very common. According to reports published in the *Journal of the American Medical Association* (*JAMA*):

- Roughly 50% of individuals with severe mental disorders are affected by substance abuse.

- Thirty-seven percent of alcohol abusers and 53% of drug abusers also have at least one serious mental illness.

- Of all people diagnosed as mentally ill, 29% abuse either alcohol or drugs.

The best data available on the prevalence of co-occurring disorders are derived from two major surveys: the Epidemiologic Catchment Area (ECA) Survey (administered 1980–1984), and the National Comorbidity Survey (NCS), administered between 1990 and 1992.

Results of the NCS and the ECA Survey indicate high prevalence rates for co-occurring substance abuse disorders and mental disorders, as well as the increased risk for people with either a substance abuse disorder or mental disorder for developing a co-occurring disorder. For example, the NCS found that:

- 42.7% of individuals with a 12-month addictive disorder had at least one 12-month mental disorder.

- 14.7% of individuals with a 12-month mental disorder had at least one 12-month addictive disorder.

The ECA Survey found that individuals with severe mental disorders were at significant risk for developing a substance use disorder during their lifetime. Specifically:

- 47% of individuals with schizophrenia also had a substance abuse disorder (more than four times as likely as the general population).

- 61% of individuals with bipolar disorder also had a substance abuse disorder (more than five times as likely as the general population).

Continuing studies support these findings, that these disorders do appear to occur much more frequently the previously realized, and that appropriate integrated treatments must be developed.

What are the consequences of co-occurring severe mental illness and substance abuse?

For the consumer, the consequences are numerous and harsh. Persons with a co-occurring disorder have a statistically greater propensity for violence, medication noncompliance, and failure to respond to treatment than consumers with just substance abuse or a mental illness. These problems also extend out to these consumers' families, friends, and co-workers.

Purely healthwise, having a simultaneous mental illness and a substance abuse disorder frequently leads to overall poorer functioning and a greater chance of relapse. These consumers are in and out of hospitals and treatment programs without lasting success. People with dual diagnoses also tend to have tardive dyskinesia (TD) and physical illnesses more often than those with a single disorder, and they experience more episodes of psychosis. In addition, physicians often don't recognize the presence of substance abuse disorders and mental disorders, especially in older adults.

Socially, people with mental illnesses often are susceptible to co-occurring disorders due to "downward drift." In other words, as a consequence of their mental illness they may find themselves living in marginal neighborhoods where drug use prevails. Having great difficulty developing social relationships, some people find themselves more easily accepted by groups whose social activity is based on drug use. Some may believe that an identity based on drug addiction is more acceptable than one based on mental illness.

Consumers with co-occurring disorders are also much more likely to be homeless or jailed. An estimated 50% of homeless adults with serious mental illnesses have a co-occurring substance abuse disorder. Meanwhile, 16% of jail and prison inmates are estimated to have severe mental and substance abuse disorders. Among detainees with mental disorders, 72% also have a co-occurring substance abuse disorder.

Consequences for society directly stem from the above. Just the back-and-forth treatment alone currently given to non-violent persons with dual diagnosis is costly. Moreover, violent or criminal consumers, no matter how unfairly afflicted, are dangerous and also costly. Those with co-occurring disorders are at high risk to contract AIDS, a disease that can affect society at large. Costs rise even higher when these persons, as those with co-occurring disorders have been shown to do, recycle through health care and criminal justice systems again and again. Without the establishment of more integrated treatment programs, the cycle will continue.

Why is an integrated approach to treating severe mental illnesses and substance abuse problems so important?

Despite much research that supports its success, integrated treatment is still not made widely available to consumers. Those who struggle both with serious mental illness and substance abuse face problems of enormous proportions. Mental health services tend not to be well prepared to deal with patients having both afflictions. Often only one of the two problems is identified. If both are recognized, the individual may bounce back and forth between services for mental illness and those for substance abuse, or they may be refused treatment by each of them. Fragmented and uncoordinated services create a service gap for persons with co-occurring disorders.

Providing appropriate, integrated services for these consumers will not only allow for their recovery and improved overall health, but can ameliorate the effects their disorders have on their family, friends, and society at large. By helping these consumers stay in treatment, find housing and jobs, and develop better social skills and judgment, we can potentially begin to substantially diminish some of the most sinister and costly societal problems: crime, HIV/AIDS, domestic violence, and more.

There is much evidence that integrated treatment can be effective. For example:

- Individuals with a substance abuse disorder are more likely to receive treatment if they have a co-occurring mental disorder.

- Research shows that when consumers with dual diagnosis successfully overcome alcohol abuse, their response to treatment improves remarkably.

With continued education on co-occurring disorders, hopefully, more treatments and better understanding are on the way.

What does effective integrated treatment entail?

Effective integrated treatment consists of the same health professionals, working in one setting, providing appropriate treatment for both mental health and substance abuse in a coordinated fashion. The caregivers see to it that interventions are bundled together; the consumers, therefore, receive consistent treatment, with no division between mental health or substance abuse assistance. The approach, philosophy, and recommendations are seamless, and the need to consult with separate teams and programs is eliminated.

Integrated treatment also requires the recognition that substance abuse counseling and traditional mental health counseling are different approaches that must be reconciled to treat co-occurring disorders. It is not enough merely to teach relationship skills to a person with bipolar disorder. They must also learn to explore how to avoid the relationships that are intertwined with their substance abuse.

Providers should recognize that denial is an inherent part of the problem. Patients often do not have insight as to the seriousness and scope of the problem. Abstinence may be a goal of the program but should not be a precondition for entering treatment. If dually diagnosed clients do not fit into local Alcoholics Anonymous (AA) and Narcotics Anonymous (NA) groups, special peer groups based on AA principles might be developed.

Clients with a dual diagnosis have to proceed at their own pace in treatment. An illness model of the problem should be used rather than a moralistic one. Providers need to convey understanding of how hard it is to end an addiction problem and give credit for any accomplishments. Attention should be given to social networks that can serve as important reinforcers. Clients should be given opportunities to socialize, have access to recreational activities, and develop peer relationships. Their families should be offered support and education, while learning not to react with guilt or blame but to learn to cope with two interacting illnesses.

What are the key factors in effective integrated treatment?

There are a number of key factors in an integrated treatment program.

Treatment must be approached in stages. First, a trust is established between the consumer and the caregiver. This helps motivate the consumer to learn the skills for actively controlling their illnesses and focus on goals. This helps keep the consumer on track, preventing relapse. Treatment can begin at any one of these stages; the program is tailored to the individual.

Assertive outreach has been shown to engage and retain clients at a high rate, while those that fail to include outreach lose clients. Therefore, effective programs, through intensive case management, meeting at the consumer's residence, and other methods of developing a dependable relationship with the client, ensure that more consumers are consistently monitored and counseled.

Effective treatment includes motivational interventions, which, through education, support, and counseling, help empower deeply demoralized clients to recognize the importance of their goals and illness self-management.

Of course, counseling is a fundamental component of dual diagnosis services. Counseling helps develop positive coping patterns, as well as promotes cognitive and behavioral skills. Counseling can be in the form of individual, group, or family therapy or a combination of these.

A consumer's social support is critical. Their immediate environment has a direct impact on their choices and moods; therefore consumers need help strengthening positive relationships and jettisoning those that encourage negative behavior.

Effective integrated treatment programs view recovery as a long-term, community-based process, one that can take months or, more likely, years to undergo. Improvement is slow even with a consistent treatment program. However, such an approach prevents relapses and enhances a consumer's gains.

To be effective, a dual diagnosis program must be comprehensive, taking into account a number of life's aspects: stress management, social networks, jobs, housing, and activities. These programs view substance abuse as intertwined with mental illness, not a separate issue, and therefore provide solutions to both illnesses together at the same time.

Finally, effective integrated treatment programs must contain elements of cultural sensitivity and competence to even lure consumers, much less retain them. Various groups such as African-Americans, homeless, women with children, Hispanics and others can benefit from services tailored to their particular racial and cultural needs.

Chapter 46

Frequently Asked Questions about Intervention

What is an intervention? What is its objective?

An intervention is a deliberate process by which change is introduced into peoples' thoughts, feelings and behaviors.

A formal intervention, like we are discussing here, usually involves several people preparing themselves, approaching a person involved in some self-destructive behavior, and talking to the person in a clear and respectful way about the behavior in question with the immediate objectives being for the person to listen and to accept help.

Although the intervention process has been formalized, the idea is not new. Thinking back, most of us can remember a time when someone or something—a teacher, friend, or set of circumstances impressed us in a seminal way which altered how we understood ourselves and changed our perspective. Moments like these constitute turning points where new vistas open allowing us to see things differently and to recognize opportunities we did not know existed before.

The overall objective of an intervention is to begin to relieve the suffering caused by a self-destructive behavior—the suffering of the person engaged in it and the suffering of family and friends.

What self-destructive behaviors are appropriate for intervention?

Any self-destructive behavior can be addressed in an intervention.

Generally people think of substance abuse as being most applicable to intervention. In fact, that will be the example used throughout this discussion. However, eating disorders, gambling, and other compulsive behaviors are appropriate as well. Even an elderly person, no longer able to live alone safely yet resisting assisted-living arrangements, can be helped through the intervention process.

Why is it necessary or desirable to conduct an intervention?

Because nothing else has worked.

Most people attempt to change a person or situation through reason and discussion, usually one-on-one. When this fails, frustration may lead to anger. This can go on for years.

Appeals to reason and one-on-one discussions rarely produce change in someone engaged in self-destructive behaviors.

On the other hand, an intervention that includes several people meaningful to the person, that is executed in a controlled and logical way, that focuses on changing everyone's behavior at least for the moment, is highly effective.

What can my family expect to happen during an intervention?

In order to prepare for an intervention, family members and friends gather to discuss the details with the interventionist. They jointly decide what form the intervention will take, identify who should be included in the intervention, develop education and treatment plans, develop an intervention plan and schedule, and then execute the plans.

Family and friends often enter this process with apprehension and frequently with a high level of frustration and anger. They often feel betrayed, confused, guilty, and defensive. They sometimes blame each other as well as themselves and the addicted person for their difficulties.

All can expect these feelings tempered or resolved during an intervention.

Sharing and expressing feelings gives purpose to the rehashing of old pains, and allows the family and friends to receive comfort and to begin to resolve the built up rage and hurt that has influenced many of their relationships and interactions.

These intervention meetings transform the family in ways necessary for lasting change to occur.

And this cohesive group approaching the addict offers something much better than a confrontation. The group creates a different world for everybody to live in.

How did the idea of intervention develop?

Family intervention, where family and friends band together and encourage a drinker to accept help for his drinking, has been used successfully for over thirty years, ever since Vernon Johnson first began experimenting with the technique in the early 1960's. This intervention technique was and continues to be the standard against which all further developments are compared and measured. And rightfully so. Johnson's classic volume *I'll Quit Tomorrow*, published in 1973, includes the basic rationale and approach to interventions still used today. This approach was published later as a separate book, *Intervention*, in 1986. Both books remain excellent primers on the subject for the professional and layperson alike.

However, there have been many developments over the last few decades. And even though these developments are but variations on Johnson's basic themes, some of them are significant. First of all, people recognized that the intervention technique was applicable to a broader range of environments and issues than just alcoholism in the family as most people originally thought. For example, intervention is now used not only in domestic situations with family and friends, but also in many other environments, among them businesses and corporate boardrooms (often called "Executive" interventions), the military, professional sports, and various professional associations including impaired professional groups in the mental health field. And in addition to addressing alcohol, interventions are also done for people with other drug addictions. Recently they are even being performed around issues not related to chemical dependency at all: eating disorders and violent rages for example.

Thus intervention activity has increased both by serving a wider and more varied population and by addressing a broader range of issues. And concomitant with this increase has been an increase in several other areas including the numbers of people conducting interventions and in refinements and variations on the intervention technique itself.

As the applications of interventions has grown, and as more people with a broader range of backgrounds have become involved in conducting interventions, many refinements on Johnson's original techniques emerged. Some of these refinements are due to the population served. For example, the approach to interventions can vary considerably from one conducted in a safe corporate boardroom to one conducted in a potentially violent poor inner city apartment. Also the mechanics of the intervention often vary depending on the style, training and history of the interventionist: some interventionists are assertive, some relaxed and laid back; some interventions are done by one practitioner, others have more than one: some interventions are done in the drinker's home, others in the interventionist's office; some interventions focus on getting help for the drinker, others on promoting recovery for the whole family.

In short, the acceptance by the general public, the refinements in intervention approaches and techniques, and the range of self-destructive behaviors for which interventions are now appropriate, have all increased substantially since Vernon Johnson first expressed his ideas on the subject over 20 years ago.

Why haven't I heard about interventions before?

Because people don't do them very much. "Intervention" is not a common household word. Interventions are not being used nearly as much as they could be for two major reasons. First of all, people cannot do what they don't know about, and even after the remarkable advances of the last decades, the public still remains generally unaware that the intervention process exists.

Of equal concern, the little that is "known" about interventions is too often simplistic, distorted, incorrect, overstated, understated, or misconceived. For example, the public generally believes an intervention to be an aggressive, intrusive, attack of some kind, rather than being, as it truly should be, the kindest and most loving thing family and friends can do. Unfortunately some are intrusive attacks. Increasingly, however, interventions emphasize love and concern rather than blaming or name calling.

What are the forms or variations an intervention can take?

There is no absolute right way to intervene in someone else's life. In fact, there is a school of thought that argues that any form of intervention is abhorrent, a violation of free speech and of an individual's right to choose. Nevertheless, as individuals and as a society we are always influencing others whether or not we want to, and sometimes we decide to intervene purposefully.

In addition to family interventions there are workplace interventions involving Employee Assistance Programs, executive interventions for senior personnel in professions or corporations, court involved interventions and diversion programs, interventions by Impaired Professional Programs conducted by professional membership organizations, and many others.

When thinking about family interventions, however, there are generally four basic orientations: Simple, Crisis, Classical, and Systems.

- **A. Simple Intervention:** Sometimes just a simple request from someone who matters can turn the tide. Simply ask the person to not drink. Believe it or not, this sometimes works.

  It is extraordinary how many times this has not been done because of a belief that nothing was ever going to change. And if this has not been done, it should always be the first step before any more complicated or involved form of intervention is embarked upon.

- **B. Crisis Intervention:** This is the polar opposite of the Simple Intervention. Crisis Interventions occur in dangerous situations involving reckless driving, weapons, hospital emergency rooms, or violence or threats of violence. It is obvious in these situations that a person is in immediate danger to himself or others. The immediate objective in these cases is to calm the crisis and to create safety for all.

  Remember, a crisis often creates golden opportunities for family members to help someone accept help.

- **C. Classical Intervention:** The most common form of family intervention remains the Johnson's approach or some variation thereof. It has been used for over thirty years for thousands of interventions with great success.

  The focus is on the drinker. The immediate goal is for the drinker to enter treatment, hopefully soon.

  Family involvement varies, but at the very least there is enough involvement to plan the intervention prior to the intervention day. Family involvement is often extensive after intervention day to address problems that arise either for themselves or for the drinker.

Family education is primarily aimed at preparing for the intervention day. There is frequently some additional education after intervention day to help the family adjust to the changing circumstances. Many treatment programs have fine family programs designed to educate the family in addictions and how to take care of themselves when living with a recovering person.

- **D. Family System Intervention:** A family systems intervention focuses on the family. The goal is for everyone in the family to change their ways, at least in regards to the self-destructive behavior, knowing that this changed behavior will have a tremendous influence on the drinker.

  In this view the whole process is considered to be the intervention. Intervention day itself is not nearly as significant as in a more classical approach since the whole family, including the drinker, is considered the subject of the intervention. The drinker is sometimes invited to participate in the process from the beginning.

  Family involvement begins very high and continues to be high whether or not the drinker goes to treatment. The educational process is viewed as integral and emphasizes the basics of addiction, the roles of guilt and shame in the family system, the recognition of enabling and provoking behaviors, and the development of a recovery plan for each family member. The goal is for each family member to change behavior and consequently change the situation or system in which the drinker has thrived.

Note that although these forms of intervention were discussed separately, they are rarely so distinct in practice. Many of the characteristics of one can be found in the others depending on the situation. For example, system considerations are always a factor even in the more classical approaches, but are usually not so openly addressed. Because of the many differences among families and situations, an actual intervention often becomes a blend of several of these forms.

How do you determine which intervention approach to use?

Of the several things that need to be considered, the first is always the issue of urgency and safety. If you are responding to a crisis, the intervention approach you choose will reflect that urgency. Immediately address the crisis and ensure everyone safety. Family education and future plans can come later.

However, if you are dealing with a chronic problem the classic, the family systems, or a blend of these approaches are available to you. Your decision on how to proceed will depend on several factors including what your family members are prepared to do, on their geographic dispersion and to a great extent on the orientation of the interventionist you find to help you.

Discuss with the interventionist the most realistic and practical approach to take given the thoughts, feelings and location of the family members.

Remember, an intervention is often a highly charged emotional experience and the family needs to be working with someone they trust. In theory all of the intervention orientations work. However, most interventionists have developed a personalized approach that leans to one form or the other. Look for someone whose approach makes sense to you. Choose someone you can trust and then let them help you.

What can my family expect in the long run from doing an intervention?

A new dance.

Think of a family's interactions as a well choreographed dance. Everything they do and say to each other has been perfected by hours of rehearsal. Each member recognizes their cues and executes their steps without thinking—day after day after day.

Imagine the dancers circling around one member's drinking problem. Everyone knows the moves by heart, even the drinker. And although everyone hates the dance, no one can imagine how to stop doing what they are doing. In fact wanting to stop has become a part of the dance. Guilt and suffering are also written in. The family could go on like this forever.

An intervention is a controlled or choreographed crisis. The dance, business-as-usual behavior of the drinker and family, is stopped for a long enough time to get everyone's attention.

One day a group of the dancers stand still when they would normally being turning somersaults. At that moment everything changes in the family.

Although the transition is not always smooth and some dancers may bump into each other at first, the important thing is that the dance is brought to a stop; the drinker has no one left to do the old steps with. And at long last the family has the drinker's complete attention.

It now becomes possible for a different dance to begin.

An intervention changes the dance.

Chapter 47

What to Do If Your Child Is Using Drugs

Children are exposed to drugs every day. They see adults taking medicine for headaches, classmates using inhalers for asthma, commercials for medications on TV and in magazines, and even people on the news being arrested for drug use. The subject of drugs can be very confusing—and dangerous—for kids.

The younger a child is when he begins to use drugs, the more likely he is to develop problems associated with drug use, such as acts of violence, unplanned or unprotected sex, school failure, or driving accidents.

The average age that a child first experiments with marijuana is 14. And many kids become curious about drugs even sooner. Even children as young as five can become involved with drugs. Inhalants, in particular, are abused more often by younger children than older ones. According to the National Institute on Drug Abuse, about 6% of U.S. children have tried inhalants by the time they reach the fourth grade.

If you're concerned that your child may be using drugs, keep reading to find out how you can tell and what you can do about it.

"What to Do if Your Kid Is Using Drugs" was provided by KidsHealth, one of the largest resources online for medically reviewed health information written for parents, kids, and teens. For more articles like this one, visit www.KidsHealth.org or www.TeensHealth.org. © 2001 The Nemours Center for Children's Health Media, a division of The Nemours Foundation.

Risk Factors

Young people may use drugs for many reasons that are related to factors such as their self-esteem, how they get along with others, and their environment. No single reason determines who will use drugs and who won't, but there are common risk factors to be aware of:

- Low grades or poor school achievement
- Hostile, defiant behavior
- Tendency to be influenced excessively by peers
- Lack of adequate support or supervision
- History of behavior problems
- History of drug use by siblings or friends

Warning Signs

It can be hard to know the difference between normal childhood behavior and behavior caused by drug use. Changes in hairstyle or dress may alarm parents but may be normal behaviors. On the other hand, changes that are extreme or sudden may signal drug use.

It may help to ask yourself the following questions:

- Does my child seem withdrawn, depressed, or tired?
- Has my child become hostile or uncooperative?
- Have my child's relationships with other family members changed?
- Has my child dropped his old friends?
- Has my child lost interest in or drastically changed his appearance?
- Has my child lost interest in hobbies, sports, or other favorite activities?
- Have my child's eating or sleeping patterns changed?
- Does my child suffer from headaches, nosebleeds, or other physical problems for no apparent reason?
- Have I noticed the odor of chemicals or drugs around my child?
- Do aerosol products at home seem to be used much too quickly?

Positive answers to such questions may indicate drug use. However, these signs may also apply to a child who is not using drugs but who may have other problems, such as depression or an eating disorder.

Be aware of common drug paraphernalia. Possession of items such as pipes, rolling papers, small medicine bottles, cans of whipped cream or other aerosol products, or syringes may signal that your child is using drugs.

What Can a Parent Do?

If you think your child may be using drugs, ask other adults in your child's life if they have noticed changes in your child's behavior. The best place to start is at school—talk with your child's teachers, guidance counselor, school nurse, or coach. Many schools now have prevention specialists on the counseling staff who can help you if you think your child is using drugs.

Communicating with your child at this time is very important. If he is reluctant to talk, enlist the aid of his guidance counselor, doctor, or a local drug treatment referral and assessment center.

Also explore what could be going on in your child's emotional or social life that might prompt drug use. Is there anything going on at home or school that could be responsible for his shift in behavior?

Even when the signs are obvious, parents sometimes have difficulty admitting that their child could have a problem. Anger, guilt, and a sense of failure as a parent are common reactions. If your child is using drugs, it is important to avoid blaming yourself for the problem and to get whatever help is needed as soon as possible.

Be consistent in enforcing whatever punishment your family has chosen for this type of rule violation, such as revoking driving privileges. Do not relent because your child promises never to do it again.

Many young people lie about their drug use. If the evidence suggests that your child is not being truthful, you may wish to have your child evaluated by a health professional, such as an adolescent medicine specialist, experienced in diagnosing children with drug-related problems.

Depending upon the severity of your child's drug use, you will probably need help to intervene. Call your doctor, local hospital, state or local substance abuse agencies, or county mental health society for a referral to a drug treatment program in your area. Your school district should have a substance abuse counselor who can refer you to treatment programs. Parents whose children have been through treatment programs can also provide information and support to help you deal with your feelings.

Tips for Parents

- **Spend time with your child.** Stay involved in your child's life, even as he gets older and seems to need you less and less. Know your child's friends and keep up with his recreational activities, his schoolwork, and his social life. Research shows that parents who take an active interest in their child's life can exert a positive influence and reduce the likelihood that their child will turn to drugs.

- **Be a good listener.** Student surveys reveal that when parents listen to their children's concerns and feelings, kids feel more comfortable talking to them, and are more likely to seek help or stay drug-free. If your child has become involved with drugs, he needs your support now more than ever so that he can begin the recovery process.

- **Provide age-appropriate information.** Make sure that the information you offer fits your child's age. A typical six-year-old can understand that he should keep his body healthy and that there are some things that he should not do because they can hurt his body, like taking any medicines when he is not sick. An eight-year-old can understand a simple lesson about specific drugs, like marijuana or cocaine. If you're watching TV and marijuana is mentioned, take advantage of the opportunity to say something like "Do you know what marijuana is? It's a drug that can hurt you." If your child has more questions, answer them. You can teach older children the same message, while adding more specific information about particular drugs and their effects.

- **Establish a clear family position on drugs.** It's OK simply to say, "We don't allow any drug use, and children in this family are not allowed to take drugs. The only time you can take any drugs is when the doctor or Mom or Dad gives you medicine because you are sick. Drugs can hurt your body and make you very sick; some may even kill you. Does anyone have any questions?"

- **Set a good example.** If your kids see you drinking or taking drugs irresponsibly, it undermines your credibility. Be careful not to pop pills—even over-the-counter medications—casually. Your behavior needs to reflect your belief that drugs must be used responsibly.

- **Stress critical thinking skills.** Movies, music, and TV barrage kids with distorted messages about drugs, making it seem that using drugs is cool. You can help counteract these messages by helping your children to think critically about what they hear and view.

- **Repeat the message.** Teach your child the facts about drugs—and keep repeating this important information. Be sure to answer your child's questions as often as he asks them.

Chapter 48

Access to Recovery: Taking Action to Heal America's Substance Users

What Is Access to Recovery?

In his State of the Union Address, President Bush announced a new three-year, $600 million federal treatment initiative, Access to Recovery to help Americans suffering from substance abuse and addiction find needed treatment by providing vouchers to individuals needing assistance. This new investment in our nation's communities will broaden the base of recovery support and make treatment services available to help 300,000 more Americans combat their addiction over the next three years.

Last year, approximately 100,000 men and women seeking treatment for drug addiction did not receive the help they needed. The president's plan is designed to ensure that Americans without private treatment coverage and struggling with addiction have access to a comprehensive continuum of effective treatment services and recovery support options, including faith- and community-based programs, and ensure that these options are more readily available.

Access to Recovery will ensure access and accountability for alcohol and drug abuse services by allowing individuals greater choices among appropriate programs. It would enable eligible individuals to use federal alcohol and drug abuse vouchers to obtain

This chapter begins with "Access to Recovery—Taking Action to Heal America's Substance Users," Office of National Drug Control Policy (ONDCP), July 2003. It also includes "Access to Recovery," and "Access to Recovery: How It Will Work," ONDCP news releases dated June 2003.

help at all effective treatment organizations, including faith-based and community-based organizations. This would expand treatment utilization and accountability, thereby broadening and strengthening the current system.

Access to Recovery will provide a way for the federal government to monitor state implementation of the program to prevent fraud and abuse; ensure quality of care; and evaluate the effectiveness of the program. It would also enable nonprofit and proprietary organizations to have a greater opportunity to participate through full and open competition.

Under the president's plan, people who are seeking drug and alcohol treatment and support services will be assessed, presented with a voucher to pay for a range of appropriate care and services, and then referred to a variety of providers who offer that care.

States will work with a consortium of public and private entities to jointly administer the program, including health care providers, faith-based and community-based organizations, workplaces, and schools to help alcohol and drug abusers receive vouchers for the treatment and support services that are best suited to their individual needs. States would be required to monitor the outcomes and costs of the voucher program and to make adjustments based on the extent to which improved client outcomes are or are not achieved in a cost-effective manner.

For many Americans seeking treatment, the transforming power of faith will now be available to heal those suffering from alcohol and drug abuse. Access to Recovery will serve as a model for states in administering other Department of Health and Human Services alcohol and drug abuse grant funding permissible under proposed Charitable Choice regulations. Access to Recovery will:

- Help 100,000 individuals per year who need and want drug and alcohol treatment services, but lack the financial resources to access them.

- Ensure that a comprehensive continuum of effective drug and alcohol treatment and support service options, including faith- and community-based programs, become more readily available. This includes any Medicaid beneficiary who has been excluded from receiving treatment in residential treatment settings.

- Allow health care providers, faith-based groups, and other community service organizations, workplaces, and schools to assist drug users in receiving the treatment and recovery support services best suited to their individual needs.

- Require state leadership, treatment delivery improvements, and encourage full and open competition among public and private providers, in order to better reach and serve those in need.

- Require states to create a system to monitor program costs and outcomes and establish accountability for delivery of effective treatment.

- Serve as a model for administering other Department of Health and Human Services alcohol and drug abuse grant funding.

How Access to Recovery Will Work

- Those individuals seeking drug and alcohol treatment and recovery support will be assessed and receive a voucher to pay for a range of appropriate services.

- The states will work with a consortium of public and private entities to jointly administer the program, distribute vouchers and deliver alcohol and drug treatment and other services.

- States will be required to monitor client outcomes and to make adjustments based on the cost effectiveness of services received.

- The key to accountability of this new treatment initiative will be in the linking of reimbursement for services to demonstrated abstinence from drug and alcohol use by clients following discharge.

Facts about Access to Recovery

Background: President Bush announced in his State of the Union Address a new substance abuse treatment initiative, Access to Recovery. This new initiative will provide people seeking drug and alcohol treatment with vouchers to pay for a range of appropriate community-based services. The president proposed $600 million in new funds over the next three years for Access to Recovery. The first $200 million installment is included in the 2004 budget for the Substance Abuse and Mental Health Services Administration (SAMHSA).

Too Many Americans Do Not Receive Help. The economic costs associated with drug abuse are estimated at around $110 billion. The human costs are measured in lost jobs, lost families, and lost lives. In 2001, 5 million of the 6.1 million people needing treatment for an illicit drug problem never got help. Of the 5 million, only 377,000 reported that they felt they needed treatment for their drug problem, including 101,000 people who knew they needed treatment, sought help, but were unable to find care.

Addiction Treatment Works; Recovery Is Real. With treatment, even hard-to-reach populations reduce their illegal drug use by nearly half. Further, addiction treatment reduces criminal activity by 80%. It markedly increases employment and decreases homelessness, results in substantially improved physical and mental health, and reduces risky sexual behaviors. When tailored to the needs of the individual, addiction treatment is as effective as treatments for other illnesses, such as diabetes, hypertension, and asthma.

The president's proposal concerning Access to Recovery will establish a state-run voucher program for substance abuse treatment built on three principles:

- **Consumer Choice.** The process of recovery is a personal one. Achieving recovery can take many pathways: physical, mental, emotional, or spiritual. With a voucher, people in need of addiction treatment and recovery support will have the choice to select the programs and providers that will help them most. Increased choice protects individuals and encourages quality.

- **Results Oriented.** Payment to providers will be linked to demonstration of treatment effectiveness and recovery, measured by outcomes such as: abstinence from drugs and alcohol, no involvement with the criminal justice system, attainment of employment or enrollment in school, and stable housing.

- **Increased Capacity.** The initial phase of Access to Recovery will support treatment for approximately 100,000 people per year and expand the array of services available including medical detoxification, inpatient and outpatient treatment modalities, residential services, peer support, relapse prevention, case management, and other recovery-promoting services.

How It Will Work: Governors are key to assuring a coordinated approach among various state departments that come into contact with people with addictive disorders: state drug and alcohol authorities; mental health authorities; departments of education, child welfare, Medicaid, and criminal justice agencies. Therefore, SAMHSA is asking governors' offices to apply for Access to Recovery funds. Funds will be awarded through a competitive grant process.

States will have considerable flexibility in designing their approach and may target efforts to areas of greatest need, to areas with a high degree of readiness or to specific populations including adolescents. Specific requirements, including eligibility criteria, will be spelled out in a Request For Applications that will be developed in partnership with states and treatment providers.

Critically, states must use the new funds to supplement, not supplant, current funding and build on existing programs, including SAMHSA's Substance Abuse Prevention and Treatment (SAPT) Block Grant. The president has requested $1.785 billion for the SAPT Block Grant in Fiscal Year (FY) 2004, an increase of $63 million over the FY03 amount. The Block Grant, with its required state maintenance of effort, provides the basic national addiction treatment infrastructure.

Access to Recovery: How It Will Work

Background: The Nation's substance abuse treatment system is shaped, supported, and maintained by the states. These services are funded primarily through state revenues and federal programs, including SAMHSA's Substance Abuse Prevention and Treatment (SAPT) Block Grant and Targeted Capacity Expansion (TCE) grants, and Medicaid dollars.

While these resources continue to help millions of Americans obtain and sustain recovery from addiction, too many people who seek help are unable to find care. By providing those individuals with vouchers to pay for the care they need, Access to Recovery will foster consumer choice, improve service quality, and increase treatment capacity. Vouchers, along with other state-operated programs, provide an unparalleled opportunity to create profound change in substance abuse treatment financing and service delivery in America, change that both will reduce human suffering and save countless dollars in lost productivity.

Competitive Grant Program: An Access to Recovery workgroup is developing a Request for Applications (RFA) with input from a broad array of stakeholders in the field, among them service providers, states, and technical experts. The workgroup is examining potential standards for participating states, performance measures, service cost ranges, and assessment and placement instruments.

An Executive Steering Committee with White House and Department of Health and Human Services (HHS) leadership is providing overall policy guidance. The RFA will be issued after funds are appropriated by Congress.

Governors' offices will be eligible to apply because Governors are key to assuring a coordinated approach among various state departments that come into contact with people with addictive disorders: state drug and alcohol authorities; mental health authorities; departments of education, child welfare, Medicaid, and criminal justice agencies.

States Will Have Flexibility. Governors applying for Access to Recovery funds will have considerable discretion in the design and focus of the model they select. They may choose to implement the program through a state or sub-state agency, or may implement some or all of the program in partnership with a private entity. States may target the program to areas of greatest need, to areas with a high degree of readiness to implement such an effort, or to specific populations, including adolescents.

Grant applications must delineate a process for screening, assessment, referral, and placement for treatment appropriate for the individual client. Clients will be assessed wherever they present, will be given a voucher for identified services, and will be referred to appropriate service providers.

Grant applications will be expected to detail how the provider base will be expanded and how a broad array of provider organizations will become eligible for voucher reimbursement. Critically, Access to Recovery funds will be required to supplement, not supplant, current funding, thus expanding both capacity and available services.

Applications Must Be Results-Oriented. In both program design and implementation, state grant applications must delineate a process to monitor outcomes, among them: drug or alcohol use, involvement with the criminal justice system, employment, social support, living situation, access to care, and program retention. These performance data will be used to measure not only treatment success but also the ultimate success of the voucher program itself. Successful state applicants will establish:

- Need based on data on rates of abuse and dependence

- Documentation of the most feasible approaches consistent with the voucher program's guiding principles

- Eligibility criteria for providers

- Eligibility criteria for clients

- Criteria for matching clients with appropriate treatment and support services

- Standard costs/reimbursement for treatment modalities

- Effective approaches to address those with special needs (e.g., homeless populations, co-occurring populations, persons living in rural areas)

Chapter 49

Barriers to Drug Abuse Treatment

In Brief

- In 2002, about 6 million persons with illicit drug dependence or abuse did not receive specialty treatment for their illicit drug problem. Among these untreated illicit drug abusers, only 6% perceived an unmet need for treatment.

- In 2002, an estimated 17 million persons with alcohol dependence or abuse did not receive specialty treatment for their alcohol problem. Among these untreated alcohol abusers, only 4.5% perceived an unmet need for treatment.

- Among those who perceived an unmet need for treatment, the most common reasons reported for not receiving treatment were not being ready to stop using the substance and the cost of treatment.

Studies show that many individuals who have substance use problems do not receive treatment for those problems.[1,2] The National Survey on Drug Use and Health (NSDUH) asks persons aged 12 or older to report on their symptoms of dependence on or abuse of alcohol or

"Reasons for Not Receiving Substance Abuse Treatment," *The NSDUH Report*, November 7, 2003, based on: Office of Applied Studies. (2003). *Results from the 2002 National Survey on Drug Use and Health: National findings* (DHHS Publication No. SMA 03-3836, NHSDA Series H-22). Rockville, MD: Substance Abuse and Mental Health Services Administration.

illicit drugs. "Any illicit drug" includes marijuana/hashish, cocaine (including crack), inhalants, hallucinogens, heroin, or prescription-type drugs used nonmedically. NSDUH defines dependence or abuse using criteria in the American Psychiatric Association's Diagnostic and Statistical Manual of Mental Disorders (DSM-IV), which includes such symptoms as withdrawal, tolerance, use in dangerous situations, trouble with the law, and interference in major obligations at work, school or home during the past year (Table 49.1).[3]

Table 49.1. DSM-IV Diagnosis of Substance Abuse or Dependence.

A person is defined with abuse of a substance if he or she is not dependent on that substance and reports one or more of the following symptoms in the past year.

1. Recurrent use resulting in failure to fulfill major role obligations at work, school, or home
2. Recurrent substance use in situations in which it is physically hazardous (e.g., driving an automobile)
3. Recurrent substance-related legal problems
4. Continued use despite having persistent or recurrent social or interpersonal problems

A person is defined as being dependent on a substance if he or she reports three or more of the following symptoms in the past year.

1. Tolerance—discovering less effect with same amount (needing more to become intoxicated)
2. Withdrawal (characteristic withdrawal associated with type of drug)
3. Using more or for longer periods than intended
4. Desire to or unsuccessful efforts to cut down or control substance use
5. Considerable time spent in obtaining or using the substance or recovering from its effects
6. Important social, work, or recreational activities given up or reduced because of use
7. Continued use despite knowledge of problems caused by or aggravated by use

Source: Reprinted with permission from the *Diagnostic and Statistical Manual of Mental Disorders*, Text Revision, Copyright 2000. American Psychiatric Association.

Respondents were also asked whether they had received treatment for a substance use problem. In these analyses, an individual was defined as receiving treatment only if he or she reported receiving specialty treatment for alcohol or illicit drugs in the past year.[4] Specialty treatment is delivered at alcohol or drug rehabilitation facilities (inpatient or outpatient), hospitals (inpatient only), and mental health centers. It excludes treatment at an emergency room, private doctor's office, self-help group, prison or jail, or hospital as an outpatient. Persons are classified as needing treatment for a substance problem if they were dependent on or abused a substance or received specialty substance treatment in the past 12 months.[5]

Respondents who had not received specialty treatment were asked whether there was any time during the past 12 months when they felt they needed treatment or counseling for their alcohol or drug use but did not receive it. Those who answered that they felt they needed treatment ("perceived unmet treatment need") were then asked to identify the reasons they did not receive treatment.[6]

In this report, estimates of treatment need, treatment, perceived unmet treatment need and reasons for not receiving treatment are presented separately for illicit drugs and for alcohol. Because many people have problems with both alcohol and illicit drugs, there is considerable overlap in these estimates.[7] For simplicity, the analyses in this report do not separate this population with multiple substance problems.

Illicit Drug Treatment Need

In 2002, about 7.7 million persons aged 12 or older were classified as needing treatment for an illicit drug problem. Of these, 1.4 million (about 18%) received specialty treatment in the past year. The rate of treatment need for an illicit drug problem was approximately twice as high for males as for females. The rate was highest among young adults aged 18 to 25. Among racial/ethnic groups, American Indians or Alaska Natives and blacks had the highest rate of treatment need. Among the approximately 6 million persons with untreated illicit drug dependence or abuse, only 6% (362,000) reported perceived unmet treatment need.

Alcohol Treatment Need

In 2002, almost 18.6 million persons aged 12 or older were classified as needing treatment for an alcohol problem. Of these, 1.5 million (about 8%) received specialty treatment in the past year. The rate of treatment need for alcohol problems was approximately twice as high for males as for females, and the rate of treatment need for young adults aged 18 to 25 was approximately three times higher than in other age groups. Among racial/ethnic groups, American Indians or

Table 49.2. Percentage of Persons Aged 12 or Older Who Needed Treatment for an Illicit Drug Problem or an Alcohol Problem* in the Past Year, by Demographic Characteristics: 2002.

	Percent Needed Treatment for Illicit Drug Problem	Percent Needed Treatment for Alcohol Problem
Total	3.3	7.9
Gender		
Male	4.3	11.2
Female	2.4	4.9
Age Group		
12 to 17	5.7	6.0
18 to 25	8.6	18.0
26 or older	2.0	6.4
Race/Ethnicity**		
American Indian or Alaska Native	4.8	12.6
Black	4.7	7.4
White	3.0	8.0
Asian	1.2	3.6
Hispanic	4.0	8.6
Native Hawaiian or Other Pacific Islander	3.5	7.1

* Respondents were classified as needing treatment for an illicit drug or alcohol problem if they met at least one of three criteria during the past year: (1) dependent on any illicit drug or alcohol; (2) abuse of any illicit drug or alcohol; or (3) received treatment for an illicit drug or alcohol problem at a specialty facility (i.e., drug and alcohol rehabilitation facilities [inpatient or outpatient], hospitals [inpatient only], and mental health centers). Illicit drugs include marjuana/hashish, cocaine (including crack), inhalants, hallucinogens, heroin, or prescription-type psychotherapeutic (nonmedical use).

** Individuals reporting two or more races were not included in this analysis.

Source: Substance Abuse and Mental Health Services Administration (SAMHSA) 2002 National Survey on Drug Use and Health (NSDUH).

Alaska Natives had the highest rate of treatment need. Among the 17 million persons with untreated alcohol dependence or abuse, only 4.5% (761,000) reported perceived unmet treatment need.

Reasons for Not Receiving Specialty Treatment

Among the 362,000 persons who perceived an unmet treatment need for an illicit drug use problem in the past year, the most common reasons given for not receiving treatment were not being ready to stop using illicit drugs (39%) and thinking the cost of treatment would be too high (37%). Twenty-six percent reported that the stigma associated with receiving treatment was a reason for not receiving treatment, and 20% reported that they did not know where to get treatment.

Among the 761,000 persons who perceived an unmet need for alcohol treatment in the past year, nearly half (49%) reported that they were not ready to stop using alcohol. Approximately 40% reported that the cost of treatment contributed to their not receiving treatment. Twenty-four percent reported concerns regarding stigma associated with seeking treatment, and 12% reported they did not know where to receive treatment.

Notes

1. Office of Applied Studies. (2003). *Results from the 2002 National Survey on Drug Use and Health: National findings* (DHHS Publication No. SMA 03-3836, NHSDA Series H-22). Rockville, MD: Substance Abuse and Mental Health Services Administration.

2. Office of Applied Studies. (2002). *National and State Estimates of the Drug Abuse Treatment Gap: 2000 National Household Survey on Drug Abuse* (NHSDA Series H-14, DHHS Publication No. SMA 02-3640). Rockville, MD: Substance Abuse and Mental Health Services Administration.

3. American Psychiatric Association. (1994). *Diagnostic and statistical manual of mental disorders (4th ed.)*. Washington, D.C.: Author.

4. An individual who was dependent on or had abused illicit drugs was counted as receiving treatment only if they received specialty treatment in the past year for illicit drugs. An

individual who was dependent on or had abused alcohol was counted as receiving treatment only if they received specialty treatment in the past year for alcohol. Individuals who reported receiving specialty substance abuse treatment but were missing information on whether the treatment was specifically for alcohol or illicit drugs were not counted in estimates of specialty illicit drug treatment or in estimates of specialty alcohol treatment.

5. An estimated 632,000 persons who were not classified with dependence or abuse of illicit drugs received specialty treatment for an illicit drug problem in the past year, and an estimated 538,000 persons who were not classified with dependence or abuse of alcohol received specialty treatment for an alcohol problem in the past year.

6. Response options were (1) you had no health care coverage, and you couldn't afford the cost; (2) you did have health care coverage, but it didn't cover treatment for [alcohol or drugs], or didn't cover the full cost; (3) you had no transportation to a program, or the programs were too far away, or the hours were not convenient; (4) you didn't find a program that offered the type of treatment or counseling you wanted; (5) you were not ready to stop using [alcohol or drugs]; (6) there were no openings in the programs; (7) you did not know where to go to get treatment; (8) you were concerned that getting treatment or counseling might cause your neighbors or community to have a negative opinion of you; (9) you were concerned that getting treatment or counseling might have a negative effect on your job; and (10) some other reason or reasons. Respondents who had other reasons were asked to indicate the specific reason(s) they did not receive treatment. The responses then were grouped into broader categories. Response options #3, #4, and #6 above were not included in the analyses for this report.

7. An estimated 3 million persons were classified with dependence on or abuse of both illicit drugs and alcohol.

Chapter 50

New Insights into Relapse

Drug addiction is a chronic relapsing disorder. As when patients in treatment for hypertension or asthma temporarily lose control, relapse to drug abuse does not mean treatment does not work, or the patient is not making an effort, or he or she will never have a productive life with long-term freedom from disease. Nevertheless, relapse is perhaps the most frustrating and demoralizing feature of drug addiction, for those who have it and those who would help them.

Clinical observation and research tell us that three types of stimulus can trigger intense drug craving, leading to renewed abuse:

- Priming: "Just one" exposure to the formerly abused substance— be it a cigarette, a drink, or an illegal drug—can precipitate rapid resumption of abuse at previously established levels or greater.

- Environmental cues (people, places, or things associated with past drug use): One vivid illustration of the power of such cues is a negative one: A small percentage of American service personnel became addicted to heroin while overseas during the Vietnam War. When they were removed from that environment, the great majority, after detoxification, reported no further problems with opiates.

By Glen R. Hanson, Ph.D., D.D.S., NIDA Acting Director, National Institute on Drug Abuse (NIDA), *NIDA Notes*, Volume 17, Number 3, October 2002.

- Stress: Both acute and chronic stress can contribute to the establishment, maintenance, and resumption of drug abuse. Patients and treatment providers alike point to stress as the most common cause of relapse. The impact of stress recently was highlighted when researchers documented increased rates of smoking and alcohol consumption by New Yorkers after the September 11, 2001, attacks.

Our knowledge of relapse is incorporated in science-based drug treatments. In cognitive-behavioral therapy, for example, patients learn to confront the consequences of their drug use, recognize the environmental cues and potentially stressful situations that trigger strong drug cravings, and develop strategies to steer clear or respond without relapsing. Recent research has shown that patients who benefit from cognitive-behavioral therapy may even show further improvement after treatment has ended and with passing time.

Science-based medical treatments buffer patients against the craving that leads to relapse. Methadone and other opioid agonist agents block the euphoric effects of opioids and stabilize brain processes whose disruption is linked to craving. Naltrexone, an opioid antagonist, blocks opioid-induced euphoria and counters opioid craving with an aversive effect. Disulfiram (Antabuse) is used to treat alcohol abuse, and it is currently being tested to determine whether it also can offset cocaine craving. Anti-anxiety agents are prescribed to moderate stress.

New research findings appear to shed light on one of the deepest mysteries involving drug relapse: We know that former abusers of addictive drugs remain vulnerable to powerful drug cravings for months or years after establishing abstinence. What accounts for the extraordinary persistence of drug cravings?

Scientists have known for some time that addictive drugs hyperactivate key brain circuits that provide pleasure and are closely linked to motivation and memory. Research also has shown that drugs change brain cells in these circuits in numerous ways, some of which might be linked to craving. However, these changes generally last only as long as a drug is actually present, or a little longer. To explain how craving can recur after long abstinence, researchers need to show that the drugs change the cells in ways that change back slowly or not at all.

The natural place to look for long-lasting drug-induced alterations is in the same circuits that produce short-term effects. Key cells in these circuits are located in an area called the midbrain; they manufacture a chemical called dopamine and release it in a nearby area called the nucleus accumbens, where it produces powerful mood effects.

During the past three years, research teams at Yale and Texas Southwestern Universities demonstrated that repeated exposure to cocaine produces alterations in gene activity in the nucleus accumbens that can persist for weeks. Last year, researchers at the University of Michigan showed that cocaine self-administration changes the actual shape of these neurons—a change that is long lasting or even permanent. Moreover, its specific nature—a proliferation of signal receptors—might be expected to contribute to craving by heightening the cells' general reactivity.

Further research will tell whether these changes are critically important to long-term vulnerability to drug craving, or whether they play a relatively minor role. The studies were conducted with laboratory animals and cocaine, and we need to find out whether they also apply in humans and with other drugs. Although uncertainties remain, these new results provide powerful confirmation of the neurobiological and chronic nature of drug addiction, evidenced at still more fundamental levels of brain cell operation. The studies also demonstrate the power of new neuroscience tools to elucidate the underlying causes of drug abuse. Ultimately, we need approaches this powerful to gain the understanding necessary to solve the mysteries of craving and generate treatments that help all patients move beyond the reach of relapse.

Part Five

Health Risks Related to Drug Abuse

Chapter 51

Hepatitis C and Drug Abuse

What is hepatitis C?

Hepatitis C, a viral disease that destroys liver cells, is the most common blood-borne infection in the United States. Approximately 36,000 new cases of acute hepatitis C infection occur each year in the United States, according to the Centers for Disease Control and Prevention (CDC) in Atlanta. People with acute hepatitis C virus (HCV) infection may exhibit such symptoms as jaundice, abdominal pain, loss of appetite, nausea, and diarrhea. However, most infected people exhibit mild or no symptoms.

About 85% of people with acute hepatitis C develop a chronic infection. Chronic hepatitis is an insidious disease whose barely discernible symptoms can mask progressive injury to liver cells over two to four decades. An estimated 4 million Americans are infected with chronic hepatitis C, according to CDC.

Chronic hepatitis C often leads to cirrhosis of the liver and liver cancer and causes between 8,000 and 10,000 deaths a year in the United States. It is now the leading cause of liver cancer in this country and results in more liver transplants than any other disease.

"Facts about Drug Abuse and Hepatitis C," *NIDA Notes*, Volume 15, Number 1, March 2000, National Institute on Drug Abuse (NIDA); updated by David A. Cooke, M.D., April 2004.

How is HCV transmitted?

People become infected with the hepatitis C virus (HCV) through direct contact with an infected person's blood. Although this contact can occur in a number of ways, injection drug use now accounts for at least 60% of HCV transmission in the United States, according to CDC. This estimate may be conservative because about 10% of people newly diagnosed with HCV do not report an identifiable risk factor. Some of these cases may represent people who are reluctant to identify injection drug use as a risk factor. Because HCV is highly transmissible through the blood, anyone who has ever injected drugs is at risk for liver disease and should be tested for the virus.

Injecting drug users (IDUs) contract hepatitis C by sharing contaminated needles and other drug injection paraphernalia. One recent study found that 64.7% of IDUs who had been injecting for one year or less were already infected with the virus. Overall prevalence of HCV was 76.5% among IDUs who had been injecting drugs for six years or less.

Additional research indicates that rates of hepatitis C among past or current IDUs are extremely high in a number of cities in the United States. For example, last year a NIDA- and CDC-funded study detected HCV infection in approximately 85% of 3,000 IDUs in Seattle. Researchers in Texas reported similar percentages in several Texas cities and noted that many recovering IDUs who tested positive for HCV reportedly had not injected for 5 to 15 years.

Hepatitis C, HIV/AIDS [human immunodeficiency virus/acquired immune deficiency syndrome], and hepatitis B share common risk factors for infection. IDUs have a high prevalence of co-infection with the viruses that cause these diseases. It is important to test IDUs for all three viruses.

Prior to the development of sophisticated HCV blood screening tests in the early 1990s, blood transfusions accounted for a substantial proportion of HCV infections. Now, there is only 1 chance in 100,000 that someone will get HCV from transfused blood or blood products. However, people who received blood transfusions prior to July 1992 should be tested for HCV.

The risk of perinatal transmission of hepatitis C is relatively low. About 5 of every 100 infants born to HCV-infected women become infected. However, about 17 out of every 100 infants born to HCV-infected women who are also infected with HIV become infected with HCV. HCV infection among women with HIV also is associated with increased maternal-infant transmission of HIV.

Can HCV infection be prevented?

Although there are vaccines for other forms of hepatitis, none exists to protect against HCV. However, prevention of illegal drug injection would eliminate the greatest risk factor for HCV infection in the United States, according to CDC. Therefore, drug addiction treatment can play a major role in reducing HCV transmission. Research shows that drug users who enter and remain in treatment reduce high-risk activities, such as sharing needles and other drug injection paraphernalia, that are responsible for spreading HCV. AIDS outreach and HIV prevention programs for out-of-treatment drug users that reduce HIV risk also reduce the risk of HCV transmission.

How can HCV infection be treated?

Available antiviral drugs to eliminate the virus and reduce liver injury are not highly effective for patients with chronic hepatitis C. Side effects can be severe and the treatment is costly, lengthy, and effective for only 30% to 50% of those with the disease.

Chapter 52

AIDS and Drug Abuse

Behavior associated with drug abuse is now the single largest factor in the spread of HIV infection in the United States. HIV is the human immunodeficiency virus, which causes acquired immunodeficiency syndrome, or AIDS. AIDS is a condition characterized by a defect in the body's natural immunity to diseases, and individuals who suffer from it are at risk for severe illnesses that are usually not a threat to anyone whose immune system is working properly. Although many individuals who have AIDS or carry HIV may live for many years with treatment, there is no known cure or vaccine.

Using or sharing unsterile needles, cotton swabs, rinse water, and cookers, such as when injecting heroin, cocaine, or other drugs, leaves a drug abuser vulnerable to contracting or transmitting HIV. Another way people may be at risk for contracting HIV is simply by using drugs of abuse, regardless of whether a needle and syringe are involved. Research sponsored by the National Institute on Drug Abuse (NIDA) and the National Institute on Alcohol Abuse and Alcoholism has shown that drug and alcohol use interfere with judgment about sexual (and other) behavior, making it more likely that users have unplanned and unprotected sex. This places them at increased risk for contracting HIV from infected sex partners.

"Drug Abuse and AIDS," NIDA InfoFacts, National Institute on Drug Abuse (NIDA), June 2003.

Infection Rates

Half of all new infections with HIV now occur among injecting drug users (IDUs), according to a review of 1996 data from the Centers for Disease Control and Prevention (CDC).[1] This review used data gathered from the nation's 96 largest cities, where HIV infection rates are the highest. Most newly HIV-infected IDUs live in northeastern cities from Boston to Washington, D.C., as well as in Miami and San Juan, Puerto Rico. In these cities, where injection drug use rates are the highest among the 96 cities surveyed, an average of 27% of all IDUs are HIV-infected.

The 96 metropolitan areas surveyed have an estimated 1.5 million IDUs, 1.7 million gay and bisexual men, and 2.1 million at-risk heterosexuals (men and women who have sex with IDUs or gay and bisexual men). Among these three risk groups, there are currently an estimated 565,000 HIV infections, with 38,000 new infections occurring each year. Using these data to make nationwide projections, the review concludes that there are about 700,000 current HIV infections, with 41,000 new HIV infections occurring each year in the United States.

An estimated 19,000 IDUs are infected each year in these areas, indicating an HIV incidence rate of about 1.5 infections per 100 IDUs per year. Infection rates are lower for the other two high-risk groups. Although gay and bisexual men still represent the group with the greatest number of current HIV infections, the rate of infection—except in

Table 52.1. HIV Infections Among At-Risk Populations in America's 96 Largest Cities.

Risk Group	Estimated Number in Risk Group	Estimated Percent HIV Positive	Estimated New HIV Infections Each Year per 100 Group Members
Injecting drug users	1.5 million	14.0%	1.5
Men who have sex with men	1.7 million	18.3	0.7
At-risk heterosexuals*	2.1 million	2.3	0.5

* Men and women who are at risk because they have sex with injecting drug users and/or bisexual or gay men.

young and ethnic/ minority gay men—is much lower now than it was a decade ago. For gay and bisexual men, the HIV infection rate per 100 persons per year is 0.7; for at-risk heterosexuals, the rate is 0.5 infections per 100 persons per year. At-risk heterosexual women out-number at-risk heterosexual men about 4 to 1.

Prevention of HIV among IDUs

It is clear from research that drug abuse treatment is a proven means of preventing the spread of HIV and AIDS, especially when combined with prevention and community-based outreach programs for at-risk people. These efforts can reduce or eliminate drug use and drug-related HIV risk behaviors such as needle sharing and unsafe sex practices. One study comparing HIV infection rates among drug abusers enrolled in methadone treatment programs to rates among those not in treatment found that those not in treatment were nearly seven times more likely to have become infected with HIV during the first 18 months. The study also found that the longer drug abusers remained in treatment, the less likely they were to become infected.

In addition, drug treatment programs help reduce the spread of other blood-borne infections, including hepatitis B and C viruses. Adequate medical care for HIV or AIDS and any related illnesses is also critical to reducing spread.

For More Information

To learn more about resources for HIV/AIDS information or HIV testing in your area, call the National AIDS Hotline at (800) 342-2437 (in Spanish, 800-344-7432; deaf, 800-243-7889), or the National AIDS Clearinghouse at (800) 458-5231, or write P.O. Box 6003, Rockville, MD 20849-6003.

Note

1. Holmberg, S.D. The estimated prevalence and incidence of HIV in 96 large U.S. metropolitan areas. *American Journal of Public Health* 86(5):642-654, 1996.

Chapter 53

Drug Use and Infectious Diseases

The use of illicit drugs is associated with the transmission of HIV/ AIDS (human immunodeficiency virus/acquired immune deficiency syndrome) and other infectious diseases, such as hepatitis B and C and tuberculosis. Furthermore, drug use can result in many other health problems. With the establishment of National Institute on Drug Abuse (NIDA)'s new Center for AIDS and Other Medical Consequences of Drug Abuse, NIDA has the unique opportunity to assess both short- and long-term medical consequences associated with drug use. It has long been known that injection drug use is related to a significant percentage of new AIDS cases each year. More recently, research has indicated that hepatitis C is spreading rapidly among injection drug users, with current estimates indicating infection rates of 65% to 90% among this population.

Since AIDS was first identified in 1981, more than 1 million Americans have become infected with HIV. According to the Centers for Disease Control and Prevention (CDC), drug use remains the second most common mode of exposure among AIDS cases nationwide. Through June 1997, injection-related AIDS cases accounted for 32% of total diagnoses.

Overall and in each age group surveyed, respondents who had used illicit drugs in the past year were more likely than those who had not to have had a blood test for HIV. In addition, illicit drug users were

Excerpted from *Sixth Triennial Report to Congress: Research on the Nature and Extent of Drug Use in the United States*, National Institute on Drug Abuse (NIDA), October 1999. Reviewed by David A. Cooke, M.D., April 2004.

more likely than nonusers to be sexually active and to have had two or more sexual partners within the past year. At the same time, those illicit drug users who reported having two or more sexual partners within the past year were less likely to say that they always used a condom.

Approximately 170,000 new acute hepatitis C virus (HCV) infections occur annually, of which approximately 36% are estimated to be related to intravenous drug use. In 1992, the last year for which data are available, the estimated cost of drug use associated with HCV treatment was $429.8 million. HCV is most commonly transmitted through intravenous drug use and blood transfusions and is rarely acquired through sexual contact. In contrast to the epidemiological trends of hepatitis B virus (HBV), the proportion of reported HCV cases acquired through intravenous drug use remains high (12% versus 36%, respectively). The risk of acquiring HCV through intravenous drug use also increases as the duration and frequency of drug use increases. According to an Australian study, approximately 66% of intravenous drug users acquire HBV within two years of regular intravenous drug use, and virtually 100% of intravenous drug users acquire HCV within eight years of regular use. However, the results of this study should be used with caution because characteristics of intravenous-drug-user populations (such as needle-sharing) have been shown to vary across and within countries.

Intravenous drug users contract both HBV and HCV by sharing contaminated needles. Studies have shown that intravenous drug users are at high risk to acquire HBV and HCV, as seroprevalence rates range from 65% to 90%. During 1993, 12% of HBV infections and 36% of HCV infections were attributed to persons who used intravenous drugs. These estimates may be conservative because at least 30% of adults who reported HBV and HCV cases did not specify a risk factor. It is possible that some persons with unidentifiable risk factors were reluctant to identify intravenous drug use as a risk factor.

As in HIV infection, intravenous drug users can infect not only other intravenous drug users but also their sexual partners. Transmission of HBV through heterosexual activity has been increasing each year, and perinatal transmission of HBV by mothers who use intravenous drugs or have sexual intercourse with an intravenous drug user is common, with transmission rates reaching 90%. However, sexual and perinatal transmission of HCV is rare.

Chapter 54

Fetal and Childhood Development

The impact of drug abuse and addiction on our nation's children is particularly onerous. Today, National Institute on Drug Abuse (NIDA) estimates that 5.5% of women use some illicit drug during pregnancy, translating into approximately 221,000 babies who have the potential to be born drug exposed. The full extent of the effects of prenatal drug exposure on a child is still not known completely, but science has shown that babies born to mothers who use drugs during pregnancy are often delivered prematurely, have low birth weights and smaller head circumferences, and are often shorter in length than infants not exposed in utero to drugs. Estimating the full extent of the consequences of maternal drug use is difficult, and determining the specific hazard of a particular drug to the unborn child is even more problematic given that typically more than one substance is used.

Although it is difficult, researchers are making progress in resolving these questions. For example, one group of investigators has demonstrated that there are cocaine receptors in the brains of fetal rats and that cocaine will bind to these brain sites. Such binding could be a mechanism by which cocaine could modify brain development and later behavior through modification of brain activity during fetal development. With this new information, researchers may be able to pinpoint

Excerpted from *Sixth Triennial Report to Congress: Research on the Nature and Extent of Drug Use in the United States*, National Institute on Drug Abuse (NIDA), October 1999. Reviewed by David A. Cooke, M.D., June 2004.

the specific sites in the developing brain that are most vulnerable to cocaine and to develop better treatment strategies for prenatal cocaine exposure.

Drug use can also have a significant negative impact on the health of children who are exposed to nicotine or illegal drugs by growing up in a household where drugs and tobacco are abused. In addition, the use of drugs during childhood and adolescence can be particularly damaging to the child's developing body and psyche.

Participants at a NIDA-sponsored conference recently concluded that many childhood psychiatric disorders are strongly associated with subsequent substance use, although a causal role remains to be established. Furthermore, the meeting participants stressed that because other biological and environmental influences can increase or reduce the risk of drug use, the mere existence of a specific psychiatric disorder does not predestine a child to later drug use. However, research has shown that conduct disorder and anxiety disorders are more clearly associated than other disorders with later drug use. Bipolar (manic-depressive) disorder may constitute a risk factor, depression in the presence of another disorder may increase risk, and some subtypes of ADHD may also increase risk. The coexistence of more than one childhood psychiatric disorder has been found to greatly increase the risk for later drug use.

Effects of Maternal Drug Use

Recent results from a longitudinal study add to the growing body of evidence for the importance of studying the amount of exposure when examining developmental outcomes associated with use of drugs during pregnancy. Although there were no overall differences between mothers who used drugs and those who did not on gestational age, birth weight, or birth length, there was a significant relationship between the amount of cocaine used in the third trimester and newborn length and head circumference. Similarly, the reported amount of cocaine use in the third trimester was negatively associated with measures of state regulation, alertness, and the ability of the infant to orient to the environment. These findings raise concerns about later developmental abilities of these infants.[1]

Another study examined the effects of maternal substance use on the costs to neonatal care. The findings from this investigation suggest that exposure to drugs in newborns resulted in total hospital charges almost double those of nonexposed newborns. The results demonstrated a consistent pattern of effects on charges, mortality, and resource use in the hospital of drug-exposed newborns due, in part, to longer lengths of stay and higher intensity care per day. The investigators suggest that their results confirm the policy concern that maternal substance use has severe consequences for the baby's health and that these costs are often borne by others.[2]

What might be the effect of prenatal drug exposure on the child's development? Children with histories of prenatal polydrug exposure that included cocaine scored significantly lower on standardized test measures of language development than nonexposed children, according to one group of investigators. Nearly half of the children in the drug-exposed group qualified for early intervention services. Significant differences between groups were also noted on measures of infant development. All the children studied were living in stable, drug-free environments at the time of the study. Nevertheless, the results indicate that, due to the cumulative effects of prenatal history, children with histories of prenatal drug exposure should be considered at risk for language delay.[3]

Cocaine's Effects on the Developing Brain

In September 1997, the New York Academy of Sciences, with support from NIDA, held a landmark conference titled "Cocaine: Effects on the Developing Brain." This was the first time that basic and clinical investigators had come together to discuss what is and is not known about the developmental consequences of prenatal cocaine exposure. Much of the research reported at this meeting came from longitudinal studies that NIDA has been supporting. For example, since 1991 NIDA has been a cosponsor, with the National Institute on Child Health and Human Development, Center for Substance Abuse Treatment, and Administration for Children and Families, of the Maternal Lifestyles Study (MLS), which has been examining the health and developmental consequences of illicit drug exposure during pregnancy in 1,400 children, who will be followed into their school years, when problems of learning disabilities, hyperactivity, and emotional disorders tend to emerge.

So far, analysis of the data from the MLS has shown that exposure to cocaine during fetal development may lead to subtle but significant deficits later on, especially with behaviors that are crucial to success in the classroom, such as blocking out distractions and concentrating for long periods. Other studies are also showing subtle cognitive and learning problems in some middle school children who were exposed to cocaine before birth.

Childhood and Adolescent Development

NIDA has spent, and continues to spend, significant effort study-ing the factors that put children at risk for later drug use to develop new interventions. One recent study, for example, attempted to iden-tify developmental correlates of alcohol and tobacco use among el-ementary school children. Children's current alcohol and tobacco use was strongly related to low scores of several measures of child com-petence, both self-report and teacher rated. Use of these substances was also associated with less effective parenting behaviors and with parental use of alcohol and tobacco. The researchers conclude that children's early experiences with tobacco and alcohol are associated with weak competence development and exposure to socializing fac-tors that promote risk taking.[4]

Another group of investigators examined the childhood, early ado-lescent, and late adolescent predictors of young adult drug use and delinquency to explore the effects of drug use on delinquent behav-ior. Data on childhood aggression, early and late adolescent drug use and delinquency, and young adult drug use and delinquency were gathered during the course of a 20-year longitudinal study of children. Overall, the results were consistent, with drug use and delinquency during early and late adolescence serving as the mediator between childhood aggression and young adult drug use. Adolescent drug use was associated with later delinquency. The findings indicated that childhood aggression was related to both young adult drug use and delinquency. In addition, there was stability of drug use and delin-quency between early adolescence and young adulthood, and drug use during early adolescence had an impact on delinquency not only in early adolescence but also in late adolescence and young adulthood. The findings suggest that a decrease in drug use during adolescence should decrease delinquency in early and late adolescence and in young adulthood.[5]

Previous research has noted that schools vary in substance use prevalence rates, but explanations for school differences have received little empirical attention. To examine this issue, investigators assessed variability across 36 elementary schools in rates of early adolescent alcohol, cigarette, and marijuana use. Characteristics of neighbor-hoods and schools were measured using student, parent, and archi-val data. The findings of this study show substantial variation across schools in substance use. Contrary to expectations, lifetime alcohol and cigarette use rates were higher in schools located in neighborhoods having greater social advantages as indicated by the perceptions of residents and archival data.[6] Perhaps not surprisingly, a recent study examining factors mediating the effects of parental emotional and instrumental support on adolescents' use of tobacco, alcohol, and marijuana found that parental support was inversely related to substance use. Further analysis of the data from this study indicated that the effect of parental support was mediated through multiple pathways, although in general, the major mediators were higher levels of behavioral coping and academic competence and less tolerance for deviance and behavioral undercontrol. Multiple-group analysis suggested buffering effects occurred because high support reduced the effect of risk factors and increased the effect of protective factors. Results of this study support the position that enhanced coping ability is an important mechanism through which social support contributes to adjustment.[7]

A child's level of cognitive skills may also be a factor in early drug use. A longitudinal study of the relationships between several cognitive skills and drug use over time found a small but significant association between drug use and weak cognitive and affective self-management strategies in early adolescence; this relationship became stronger over time. The exacerbation of these cognitive weaknesses with increased drug use may contribute to impaired social, emotional, and psychological growth in late adolescence. The investigators note that deficits in cognitive efficacy may actually precede and perhaps predispose to problematic drug use. Weaknesses in cognitive skills and learning disabilities may be undetected factors that underlie recognized risk factors such as low self-esteem, academic failure, and school dropout.[8]

Of course, not all children who try drugs continue to use them. To assess risk factors for escalation of substance use once it begins, researchers grouped adolescents according to substance use patterns over three assessments and then examined variables differentiating the groups. The four groups—nonusers, minimal experimenters, late starters, and escalators—were identified through analysis of changes in cigarette, alcohol, and marijuana use among a cohort of eighth and ninth graders enrolled in public schools. By modeling group differences based on variables from stress-coping theory, problem behavior theory, and peer-association theory, the researchers identified measures predictive of subsequent escalation in substance use. Compared with nonusers and minimal experimenters, late starters and escalators had higher life stress, lower parental support, lower academic competence, more deviant attitudes, and more nonadaptive modes of coping; they also were higher in measures of parental and peer substance use. This study also found, in contrast with earlier work, that substance use experimenters, compared with nonusers, had higher stress, more maladaptive coping, more deviance-prone attitudes, lower levels of parental support, and lower levels of self-control. The findings support the idea that some people enter adolescence with less parental support and more life stress, have less adaptive patterns of coping and competence, and tend to gravitate to groups of peer substance users. To the extent that these factors prevail and are not offset, these adolescents become involved in a network of active users. The experience-regulating function of substance use becomes more salient, and they are primed to continue substance use at increasing rates.[9]

The effect of a parent's drug use on the child is well documented. However, a recent study suggests that the sensitive period for the influence of a father's substance use disorder on a son's behavioral problems starts when the son is about six years old. These results suggest the importance of early intervention to reduce paternal substance use to prevent intergenerational transmission of behavioral problems and of substance use, given that externalizing behavioral problems in male children and adolescents are among the best predictors of subsequent substance use in early and late adolescence.[10]

Notes

1. Eyler, F.D.; Behnke, M.; Conlon, M.; et al. Birth outcome from a prospective, matched study of prenatal crack/cocaine use: I. Interactive and dose effects on health and growth. *Pediatrics* 101:229-237, 1998; and Eyler, F.D.; Behnke, M.; Conlon, M.; et al. Birth outcome from a prospective, matched study of prenatal crack/cocaine use: II. Interactive and dose effects on neurobehavioral assessment. *Pediatrics* 101:237-241, 1998.

2. Norton, E.C.; Zarkin, G.A.; Calingaert, B.; and Bradley, C.J. The effect of maternal substance abuse on the cost of neonatal care. *Inquiry* 33:247-257, 1996.

3. Johnson, J.M.; Seikel, J.A.; Madison, C.M.; et al. Standardized test performance of children with a history of prenatal exposure to multiple drugs/cocaine. *Journal of Communication Disorders* 30:45-72, 1997.

4. Jackson, C.; Henriksen, L.; Dickinson, D.; and Levine, D.W. Early use of alcohol and tobacco: Relation to child competence

and parental behavior. *American Journal of Public Health* 87:359-364, 1997.

5. Brook, J.S.; Whiteman, M.; Finch, S.J.; and Cohen, P. Young adult drug use and delinquency: Childhood antecedents and adolescent mediators. *Journal of the American Academy of Child Adolescent Psychiatry* 35(12):1584-1592, 1996.

6. Ennett, S.T.; Flewelling, R.L.; Lindrooth, R.C.; and Norton, E.C. School and neighborhood characteristics associated with school rates of alcohol, cigarette, and marijuana use. *Journal of Health and Social Behavior* 38:55-71, 1997.

7. Wills, T.A., and Cleary, S.D. How are social support effects mediated? A test with parental support and adolescent substance use. *Journal of Personality and Social Psychology* 71:937-952, 1996.

8. Scheier, L.M., and Botvin, G.J. Effects of early adolescent drug use on cognitive efficacy in early-late adolescence: A developmental structural model. *Journal of Substance Abuse* 7(4): 379-40, 1995; and Scheier, L.M., and Botvin, G.J. Cognitive effects of marijuana. (Letter.) *Journal of the American Medical Association* 275(20):1547, 1996.

9. Wills, T.A.; McNamara, G.; Vaccaro, D.; and Hirky, A.E. Escalated substance use: A longitudinal grouping analysis from early to middle adolescence. *Journal of Abnormal Psychology* 105(2):166-180, 1996.

10. Moss, H.B.; Clark, D.B.; and Kirisci, L. Timing of paternal substance use disorder cessation and effects of problem behaviors in sons. *American Journal on the Addictions* 6(1):30-37, 1997.

Chapter 55

Significant Deficits in Mental Skills Observed in Toddlers Exposed to Cocaine before Birth

A study conducted by researchers from Case Western Reserve University in Cleveland found that children exposed to cocaine before birth were twice as likely to have significant delays in mental skills by age two, compared to other toddlers with similar backgrounds but whose mothers had not used cocaine during pregnancy. It is probable, according to the researchers, that these cocaine-exposed children will continue to have learning difficulties and an increased need for special educational services when they reach school age.

The study, which was funded by the National Institute on Drug Abuse (NIDA), is published in the April 17, 2002 issue of the *Journal of the American Medical Association.*

Dr. Glen R. Hanson, acting NIDA director, said, "This study adds important new evidence to a growing body of knowledge. It is the first report of a clear-cut relationship between prenatal cocaine and mental test performance at age two. These findings remind us of the importance of continued efforts to determine which children and families are at risk because of exposure to cocaine, so we can prevent or ameliorate negative consequences of using this drug." He added, "It is important that in this research process, we avoid inadvertently labeling or stigmatizing large numbers of toddlers because of drug use by their mothers during pregnancy. We want to use this type of research to help us be more effective in how we work with these children."

NIDA News Release, National Institute on Drug Abuse (NIDA), April 19, 2002.

The investigators followed the developmental course of 415 infants, whose pregnant mothers were recruited into the study at a large urban county teaching hospital between the years 1994 and 1996. All of the pregnant women recruited into the study were from high-risk and low-socioeconomic status backgrounds. Urine samples were collected from the women and meconium samples were collected from each baby. These samples were screened for maternal drug use. Two hundred and eighteen infants were found to be cocaine-exposed and 197 to be cocaine-free.

Each infant was tested for developmental progress at 6.5, 12, and 24 months of age. The infants were administered the Bayley Scales of Infant Mental and Motor Development, a widely used assessment of infant development. Scores on this assessment measure memory, language, and problem-solving abilities, as well as gross and fine motor control and coordination.

While no effects on the Bayley Motor Scale were detected, the cocaine-exposed children performed more poorly on the Bayley Mental Scale than unexposed children, after adjusting for other variables (such as use of alcohol, tobacco, or other drugs; maternal age; prenatal care, and home environment quality). Although mental development index scores decreased over time for both groups of infants, children prenatally exposed to cocaine had scores that decreased faster. From 6.5 to 24 months, the average score for infants exposed to cocaine declined by 14 points compared to nine points for unexposed children.

Almost 14% of the cocaine-exposed infants had scores in the mental retardation range, 4.89 times higher than expected in the general population. The percentage of children with mild or greater delays was 38%, almost double the rate of the non-cocaine-exposed group. Infants of mothers with evidence of higher and more frequent cocaine use during pregnancy fared the worst.

Lead investigator Dr. Lynn T. Singer said that there are several possible mechanisms by which cocaine exposure during pregnancy may affect infant outcome. Developing neural systems of the fetal brain may be directly and adversely affected by cocaine exposure. Another possible explanation is that cocaine use during pregnancy may constrict the vascular system, subsequently decreasing blood flow through the placenta and resulting in low oxygen levels (hypoxemia) in the fetus.

Differences in the cocaine-exposed infants were noted at birth. These infants had lower gestational age, lower birth weight, and smaller head circumference and length than unexposed babies. There were more preterm, low birth weight and small-for-gestational age infants in the exposed group. There were 11 deaths by the time the infants were two years old, eight in cocaine-positive children and three in cocaine-negative children. Sudden infant death syndrome (SIDS) was the leading cause of death in both groups.

An estimated 1 million children have been born after fetal cocaine exposure since the mid-1980s, when the so-called crack epidemic emerged with the availability of a cheap, potent, smokable form of cocaine.

Chapter 56

Methamphetamine Abuse Linked to Brain Damage

A new magnetic resonance imaging (MRI) technology that measures blood flow in the brain corroborates earlier positron emission tomography (PET) scan studies that showed evidence of brain abnormalities caused by methamphetamine abuse. Perfusion MRI, or pMRI, measures blood flow into key brain regions by producing images based on hundreds of electronic cross-sections showing brain structure and blood flow.

Dr. Linda Chang and colleagues at Brookhaven National Laboratory in Upton, NY, used pMRI scans to document blood-flow abnormalities in test subjects in brain regions that control response times and immediate, short-term memory. Their research correlated these abnormalities with response times during cognitive testing, where methamphetamine abusers consistently reacted more slowly on computerized tasks than did closely matched nonusers. The slower reaction times, evident in abusers even after months of abstinence, are seen as evidence of brain injury.

In earlier research, Dr. Chang, together with Dr. Nora Volkow and others at Brookhaven, used PET scans to measure brain metabolism, or glucose consumption levels. Scientists know that the more active brain areas use more glucose, which is fuel for cells, and that this indicates higher localized metabolism. The National Institute on Drug Abuse

"New Imaging Technology Confirms Earlier PET Scan Evidence: Methamphetamine Abuse Linked to Human Brain Damage," by Neil Swan, *NIDA Notes*, Volume 18, Number 2, August 2003, National Institute on Drug Abuse (NIDA).

(NIDA)-supported PET studies revealed that methamphetamine abusers showed regional increases and decreases in glucose metabolism that were consistent with mounting evidence that methamphetamine abuse injures brain cells.

Explaining the significance of her latest study, Dr. Chang said, "We used pMRI to show that methamphetamine abuse is related to changes in blood flow in the same critical regions of the human brain in which PET scans have shown increases in glucose usage in methamphetamine abusers. Finding similar patterns of drug-related changes or abnormalities in the brain using two different scanning technologies makes the evidence of methamphetamine-induced damage to brain cells more credible."

In the pMRI study, increased brain blood flow was detected in the parietal regions of methamphetamine abusers' brains. These regions are involved in receiving and processing information from the sensory receptors in the skin, muscles, and joints and in the integration of auditory, visual, and somatic information. Dr. Chang's study also found that methamphetamine users had decreased blood flow in other areas of the brain's parietal regions and in the frontal and basal ganglia regions. These regions are involved in controlling response speed and attention span and in coordinating motor functions and psychomotor speed.

Dr. Chang theorizes that increased blood flow in parietal regions indicates an increase in activity by glial cells, or supporting cells, rather than neurons, or nerve cells, since glia have a higher metabolic rate than neurons. Glia are a cell type that gears up to try to shield and repair nerve cells that are damaged or exposed to toxins, such as drugs. Animal experiments have demonstrated similar glial responses to repair drug-induced injury. On the other hand, Dr. Chang reports, decreased blood flow observed in the parietal and other brain regions might indicate that nerve cells there are already damaged beyond glial cells' power to repair them.

Forty subjects participated in Dr. Chang's study—20 abstinent methamphetamine abusers and 20 nonusers. Each control group member was selected to match one of the methamphetamine abusers by age and gender, an unusually precise matching. Those in the abusers' group had abused an average of 2.8 g or more of methamphetamine a day, an average of 6.5 days a week, for approximately eight years, but had been abstinent for an average of eight months.

The researchers administered standard neuropsychological tests, on which the methamphetamine abusers performed within normal ranges, and a battery of more sensitive computerized tests designed to detect subtle or early signs of cognitive decline. The battery, called the CalCAP, assesses a range of cognitive functions, including brief, sustained, and divided attention; immediate memory; rapid visual scanning; discrimination between various forms or shapes; and language skills.

Three of the CalCAP tests showed the most dramatic results. In the simple reaction time test, subjects are asked to press a keyboard key as soon as they see anything appear on the computer screen. Average reaction time for the methamphetamine users was 21% slower than that of the nonusers, as measured in milliseconds.

The single-digit recognition test involves immediate memory and requires subjects to press a key when they see a specific letter, but only when the letter appears immediately after another specific letter ("X" only after "A"). Methamphetamine abusers' average response time was 30% slower than that of the nonusers.

The sequential reaction time tests also involves immediate memory. Numbers are flashed one at a time on the computer screen and the participant is asked to press a key whenever the currently flashing number matches the one just before (one-back target) or when the current number matches the one two flashes before (two-back target). On the one-back test, methamphetamine abusers' average response time was 21.5% slower than that of the nonusers; on the two-back test, their response time was 18% slower.

Altogether, the nine CalCAP tests revealed consistently slower response times for methamphetamine abusers, particularly on tasks that required working memory, the immediate storage of information, and mental concentration. Dr. Chang interprets these results as evidence of subclinical Parkinsonism—brain damage that is not yet noticeable in routine activities but which in more severe form could produce the symptoms associated with Parkinson's disease, a chronic neurological condition marked by physical slowness, tremors, unstable posture, and a peculiar gait.

"The computer response tasks measure response times very precisely, in ways not noticeable in everyday activities but consistent with subclinical Parkinsonism," says Dr. Chang. "This possibility is further supported by numerous studies with animals that have indicated that methamphetamine may injure the brain's dopamine system, which is involved with working, or immediate, memory."

"The important advance here is not that we have confirmed earlier PET scan evidence of brain injury in methamphetamine abusers, but that we have done so with a new imaging technology that is simpler and relatively inexpensive to administer," comments Dr. Chang.

PET scans involve injection of radioactive materials into the blood of test subjects, a procedure that can be extremely sensitive in detecting small quantities of specific molecules in the brain, but that is expensive, technically difficult, and more invasive to test subjects.

"Because of the need to limit excess radiation exposure, PET scans can be repeated on a subject only once or twice in a given year, but these pMRI scanning procedures can be performed relatively often on the same person, even daily if required," she says. "If blood-flow scans continue to prove viable for viewing and measuring evidence of drug-induced brain damage, they could hold potential for development as clinical tools to measure the effectiveness, over time, of a variety of pharmacological and behavioral therapies for drug addiction.

"These MRI techniques might also prove valuable in studying the long-term brain damage attributed to drug use and whether the damage can be reversed," concludes Dr. Chang.

Chapter 57

Drugged Driving

In Brief

- In 2001, over 8 million persons aged 12 or older reported driving under the influence of illegal drugs during the past year.

- Rates of drugged driving increased from 2000 to 2001 for young adults aged 18 to 34.

- Among adults aged 18 or older, those who were unemployed were more likely than full- or part-time workers to report driving under the influence of illegal drugs during the past year.

The *National Household Survey on Drug Abuse* (NHSDA) asks respondents aged 12 or older to report whether they had driven a vehicle during the past 12 months while under the influence of illegal drugs alone or in combination with alcohol. Respondents aged 15 or older were asked about their current employment status.

Office of Applied Studies. (2002). Results from the *2001 National Household Survey on Drug Abuse: Volume I. Summary of national findings* (NHSDA Series H-17, DHHS Publication No. SMA 02-3758). Rockville, MD: Substance Abuse and Mental Health Services Administration.

Prevalence of Driving under the Influence of Illegal Drugs

In 2001, over 8 million persons aged 12 or older, or 3.6% of the U.S. population, reported driving under the influence of illegal drugs during the past year. This was an increase from the rate of 3.1% in 2000.

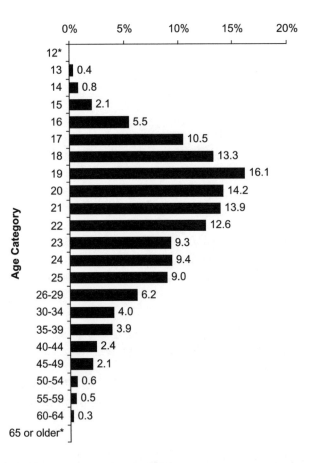

Figure 57.1. *Percentages of Persons Aged 12 or Older Reporting Driving under the Influence of Illegal Drugs During the Past Year, by Detailed Age Categories: 2001.*

Demographic Variations in Drugged Driving

In 2001, rates of drugged driving generally followed the same patterns as rates of overall current illicit drug use. The rate of drugged driving increased with each year of age to 16% among 19 year olds and generally decreased with increasing age among those aged 20 or older (Figure 57.1).[1] Rates of drugged driving increased from 2000 to 2001 for most ages from 18 years to 34 years of age (Figure 57.2).

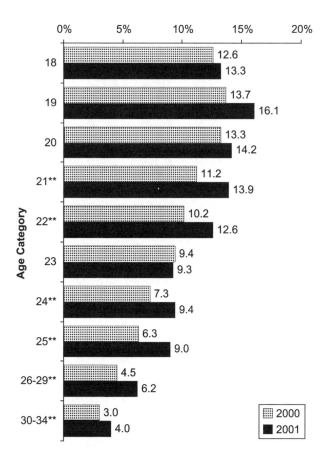

Figure 57.2. *Percentages of Persons Aged 18 to 34 Reporting Driving under the Influence of Illegal Drugs, by Detailed Age Categories: 2000 and 2001.*

In 2001, males (5%) were more than twice as likely as females (2%) to report driving under the influence of illegal drugs.[1] The 2001 rate of drugged driving among males was an increase from 4% in 2000.

In 2001, the rate of drugged driving was higher among white persons than among Hispanic, black, or Asian persons (Figure 57.3). The 2001 rate of drugged driving among white persons (4%) increased from 3% in 2000.

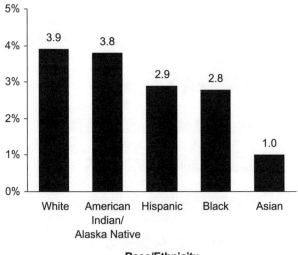

Figure 57.3. *Percentages of Persons Aged 12 or Older Reporting Driving under the Influence of Illegal Drugs During the Past Year, by Race/ Ethnicity: 2001.*

Employment Status and Drugged Driving

Among adults aged 18 or older, those who were unemployed or classified as full- or part-time students were the most likely to report driving under the influence of illegal drugs in the past year, followed by part-time workers and full-time workers (Figure 57.4). Drugged driving rates were lowest among persons not in the labor force, such as retired or disabled persons, and homemakers.

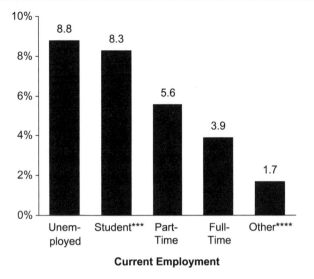

Figure 57.4. Percentages of Adults Aged 18 or Older Reporting Driving under the Influence of Illegal Drugs During the Past Year, by Current Employment Status: 2001.

Note

1. This pattern of drugged driving parallels the pattern of abuse of or dependence on alcohol or illicit drugs. For more information about abuse and dependence in the NHSDA, see: J. Epstein (2002). *Substance abuse, dependence, abuse, and treatment: Data from the 2000 National Household Survey on Drug Abuse* (NHSDA Series: DHHS Report No. SMA 02-3642). Rockville, MD: Substance Abuse and Mental Health Services Administration.

Chapter 58

Risky Sexual Activity and Drug Abuse

In recent years, researchers have begun to explore the intersection of alcohol or drug use and sexual "risk behaviors"—activities that put people at increased risk for STDs [sexually transmitted diseases], unintended pregnancy, and sexual violence. Risky sexual activities include using condoms inconsistently, having multiple sexual partners over one's lifetime, or having intercourse with a casual partner. Studies conducted to date indicate that drinking and illicit drug use often occur in association with risky sexual activity. Still, a direct link between substance use and these sexual behaviors can be difficult to document.

Public health experts hope that creating a greater awareness of the potential relationship between substance use and risky sexual activity can influence individuals who rely on drinking or drugs to help reduce inhibitions, increase sociability, or enhance sexual arousal. Some people may drink or use drugs to gain courage, relieve pressure, or justify behavior they might otherwise feel is uncomfortable or unwise—without considering the potential consequences. In addition, determining how the use of alcohol or other substances influence sexual risk-taking can help to inform efforts by health care providers,

"Substance Use and Risky Sexual Activity," (#3214), The Henry J. Kaiser Family Foundation, February 2002. This information was reprinted with permission from the Henry J. Kaiser Family Foundation. The Kaiser Family Foundation, based in Menlo Park, California, is a nonprofit, independent national health care philanthropy and is not associated with Kaiser Permanente or Kaiser Industries.

educators, social workers, and policymakers to create effective programs for substance abuse prevention and treatment, STD and HIV [human immunodeficiency virus] prevention, and sexual health education.

This issue update examines the current available data concerning drinking, drug use, and risky sexual activity—including the degree to which these behaviors may be related. It also outlines the ways in which these behaviors can lead to potentially harmful health consequences.

Sex, Drinking, and Drug Use: How Common?

A national survey of Americans aged 18 to 59 found that 90 percent of men and 86 percent of women had sex in the year prior to the survey.[1] More than 80 percent of adults have ever used alcohol and more than half have had a drink in the past month.[2] Illicit drug use is less common, particularly among adults aged 35 and older. About half of adults aged 18–35 say they have ever tried an illicit drug, as have about a third of those 35 and older.[2]

Fifty-two percent of boys and 48 percent of girls in 9th–12th grades report having ever had sex and 36 percent of high school students say they have had sex recently.[3] Seventy-nine percent of high school students say they have tried alcohol and more than half of all high school students in 1997 reported having used at least one illicit drug and a quarter reported frequent drug use.[4,5]

Researching the Links: Substance Use and Risky Sexual Activity

Drinking and Sex

Increased alcohol use seems to be associated with an increased likelihood of sexual activity. When men aged 18 to 30 were asked to report their episode of heaviest drinking in the last year, 35 percent said that they had sex after consuming five to eight drinks and 45 percent had sex after consuming eight or more drinks, compared with 17 percent of those who had one or two drinks. Among women aged 18 to 30, 39 percent had sex while consuming five to eight drinks and 57 percent had sex when consuming eight or more drinks, compared with 14 percent of women who had one or two drinks.[6]

There is some evidence that heavy alcohol use[7] is associated with having multiple sex partners, which is a primary risk factor for transmission of STDs, including HIV. Seven percent of adults who report never drinking or drinking less than once a month say that they have had two or more sex partners in the last year, compared with fifteen percent of those who say they drink monthly, and 24 percent of those who drink weekly.[8]

Among adults aged 18 to 30, binge drinkers[9] are twice as likely as those who do not binge drink to have had two or more sex partners in the previous year. (That is, seven percent of those who never binge drink compared with 40 percent of those who report monthly binge drinking.)[8] This is true even after controlling for other factors—including age, sex, marital status, and drug use—that can affect a person's likelihood of having multiple sex partners.[2,8] Heavy drinkers[7] are five times as likely as non-heavy drinkers to have at least ten sex partners in a year.

Drugs and Sex

About two million adults—one man in 100 and one woman in 200—admit to using drugs before having sex in the past year.[4,10] Illicit drug users are also more likely than non-users to have multiple sex partners. One study found that 52 percent of those who used marijuana in the previous year had two or more sex partners during the same period, compared with sixteen percent of those who had not smoked pot.[6] There is even more extensive research documenting the relationship between the use of crack or injection drugs and an increased number of sexual partners.[4,11] And, people who are receiving treatment for alcohol and drug use or who use multiple drugs are more likely than others to engage in risky sexual activity. A study of alcoholics found that those who also have drug problems are more likely than those who do not to have multiple sex partners.[4,12]

Alcohol, Drugs, and Condom Use

Results from research about how drinking might influence condom use have been contradictory.[4] An analysis of thirty studies on the interplay between alcohol use and failure to use condoms found that ten showed an association between the two behaviors, fifteen demonstrated no such association, and five had mixed results.[4] At the same time, studies of "high-risk" groups—such as users of crack cocaine[4] and injection drug users[4]—have tended to more consistently suggest links between illicit drug use and reduced use of condoms.[4]

As researchers gather more data, they may be able to refine their understanding of the relationship between substance abuse and condom use. It is possible that drinking or drug use by themselves, for instance, may not sufficiently explain inconsistent condom use. However, studying people who use multiple substances over the course of their lifetimes—or who use of multiple substances within a given time period—may yield more useful information. One recent analysis of data about young adults aged 18 to 30 found that the more different substances a person had ever used, the less likely he or she is to have used a condom at last sex.[13] Similarly, people who use multiple substances—such as alcoholics who also use drugs—do appear to be less likely to use condoms.[4,12]

Unintended Consequences

Sexually Transmitted Diseases (STDs)

Approximately fifteen million new cases of sexually transmitted diseases (STDs) occur annually in the United States.[14] By age 24, one in three sexually active people will have contracted an STD—and many may not realize when they become infected.[14] Of the 900,000 people currently living with HIV in the U.S., up to a third remain unaware of their HIV status.[15] STDs and substance use are associated in several ways.

To the extent that alcohol and drug users are more likely than others to have sex with multiple partners, their risk of being exposed to STDs—and thus becoming infected—increases. For HIV, in particular, the current profile of someone considered at "high risk" for infection involves multiple and simultaneous risk-taking behaviors, including having multiple sex partners as well as using illicit drugs and trading sex for drugs or money.[16]

In addition to the potential for increased STD exposure, substance use may make a person biologically more susceptible to infection. Alcohol, for instance, can have a substantial impact on the immune system of a heavy drinker, interfering with the body's mechanisms for destroying viruses. This process, in turn, enhances a person's vulnerability to HIV infection or the development of AIDS-related illnesses.[4] Drug use can indirectly result in other types of physical vulnerability. For example, it has been theorized that because drugs like crack cocaine, amphetamines, and nitrates can delay ejaculation, they may be associated with longer or particularly vigorous sexual activity—thus increasing the potential for physical trauma during sex that makes it easier to transmit HIV.[4] The spread of other blood-borne and sexually transmitted infections, such as hepatitis, have previously been associated with both decreased immunity and genital trauma.

STDs among Risk Takers

There is significant research on STDs among alcoholics and crack cocaine users. Rates of STDs are high in geographic areas where rates of substance use are high.[17] STD prevalence rates in these communities range from 30 to 87 percent, compared with about 1.6 percent of all adults.[4] Adults who report having gotten drunk in the last year are almost twice as likely as those who did not to have ever had an STD.[18] Problem drinkers[19] are three times more likely than nondrinkers to have ever contracted an STD.[18] Heterosexual men and women who abuse alcohol (and not injection drugs) are six and twenty times more likely, respectively, to be HIV positive than individuals in the general population.[20] Alcohol use has also been found to be associated with risky sexual behaviors in vulnerable populations, including the mentally ill, runaway youth, and the HIV-negative female partners of men with HIV.[17]

Adults who use illicit drugs have almost three times the risk of nonusers of contracting an STD.[18] Non-injection drug use, particularly of crack cocaine, has proven to be a significant risk factor for HIV and other STDs, with drug-for-sex exchanges and unprotected sex with multiple partners among crack users accounting for the rapid spread of HIV through drug and sex networks.[18] Use of multiple substances—such as having alcohol and drug problems at the same time—is also associated with a higher likelihood of having had an STD and being HIV positive.[4,12]

Injection Drugs and HIV/AIDS

Because of the AIDS epidemic, researchers have extensively studied the connections between injection drug abuse and HIV transmission. Sharing drug needles is known to be a primary route of HIV transmission. Drug use also contributes to the spread of HIV to people who have sex with a drug user and to children born to HIV-infected mothers who acquired the infection from sharing needles or having sex with an infected drug user.

Injection drug use or sex with partners who inject drugs account for a larger proportion of female than male AIDS cases in the U.S. (59 percent and 31 percent of all cases, respectively, since the epidemic began). Today, more than 48,000 women in the U.S. have been diagnosed with AIDS attributed to injection drug use, and more than a third of AIDS cases in adult and adolescent women diagnosed from July 1998 through June 1999 reported injection drug use as their risk exposure.[22]

Unintended Pregnancy

More than 3 million unintended pregnancies occur every year in the U.S., nearly half—47 percent—among women who were not using a regular method of birth control. [23] While there is no explicit data linking unintended pregnancy and substance use, the two may be related to the extent that drinking or drug use is associated with a lesser likelihood of using condoms and/or a greater likelihood of having "casual" sexual encounters—intercourse taking place outside the context of an ongoing relationship, during which contraceptives of any kind are less likely to be used.[24]

The ability to conduct research in this area is complicated by the fact that the use of contraceptives, including condoms, is inconsistent in the general population. Of the 9.8 million women using barrier contraceptives such as the male condom, the female condom, and the diaphragm, one-third report not using their method every time they have intercourse.[25] And, whether a woman uses contraception—and which method she chooses—is known to change over time, influenced by a host of personal and lifestyle factors. For example, while more than one-third (37%) of teenage women using contraceptives choose condoms as their primary method, these numbers decline as women grow older and marry.[26]

Sexual Assault and Violence

Substance use, particularly drinking alcohol, appears to play a role in a significant number of crimes of sexual violence—whether it is the victim or the perpetrator who uses. Substance use during instances of sexual violence and rape is estimated to range from 30 to 90 percent for alcohol use, and from 13 to 42 percent for the use of illicit substances.[4] These statistics, however, are difficult to gather and track. A study of arrested sex offenders found that 42 percent of them tested positive for drugs at the time of their arrest.[4]

When it comes to date rapes among college students, alcohol use by the victim, perpetrator, or both, has been implicated in 46 to 75 percent of the incidents.[4] Other drugs that disable a potential sexual assault victim, particularly Rohypnol and GHB [gamma hydroxy-butyrate], have been anecdotally implicated in date rape scenarios.[4] In addition to the immediate physical and emotional damage caused by sexual assault, women and girls who experience sexual violence may be unable to implement practices to protect themselves against unintended pregnancy or STDs.

Trading Sex for Money or Drugs

Research examining rates of substance abuse among prostitutes finds that from 40 to 86 percent of prostitutes use drugs and that some also drink while working.[4] Meanwhile, 43 percent of women and 10 percent of men in alcohol treatment programs say they have traded sex for money or drugs.[4] Risk behaviors other than substance abuse are also implicated among people who engage in prostitution or sex trade. Studies have shown that condom use is highly inconsistent in cases of sex for drug or money exchanges: One of the many small studies of non-injecting, crack-using women who traded sex for money found that only 38 percent said that they always used a condom with their paying partners.[4] Prostitutes tend to have higher rates of infection with HIV and other STDs than the general population, and are more likely to report having been sexually victimized.[4]

Making the Connections: Implications for the Future

Researchers believe that the association between substance use and risky sexual activities could stem from a host of personal factors, including a reduction in sexual inhibitions because of the actual pharmacological effect of alcohol or drugs and cognitive impairment caused by drinking or drug use. A particular individual's personality or risk-taking tendencies may also influence which, if any, risk behaviors they engage in. And assumptions that alcohol or drugs will enhance a person's sexual attraction, behavior, or performance can also have an impact. For example, adolescents who expect alcohol to lead them to be less inhibited sexually are more likely to participate in risky sexual behavior when they drink.[27]

Similarly, the social context of drinking or alcohol use may be an important factor. Social environments that support the use of alcohol and other drugs may also support the meeting of new sexual partners,[28] which may help to explain the relationship between recent substance use and the likelihood of having multiple partners.[13]

The ability of researchers to determine how substance abuse and sexual risk-taking are connected also has important implications for education and treatment efforts. If sexual risk-taking is caused by lessened inhibitions due to substance use, then education might warn about the impact of alcohol and drugs on one's judgment and the potential consequences of such situations, such as the increased risk of STD and HIV transmission. On the other hand, if personality or other unique factors of individuals influence sexual-risk taking and substance use, then prevention efforts might be better focused on particular groups of people with more specific messages to help them channel potentially destructive risk-taking impulses into healthier activities.[29]

For additional free copies of this publication (#3214), please contact our Publication Request Line at 1-800-656-4533.

References

1. Laumann EO et al., *The Social Organization of Sexuality: Sexual Practices in the United States*, Chicago, IL: The University of Chicago Press, 1994.

2. Department of Health and Human Services, SAMHSA, Office of Applied Studies, *Summary of Findings from the 1998 National Household Survey on Drug Abuse*, Rockville, MD: Department of Health and Human Services, 1999.

3. Centers for Disease Control and Prevention, *Youth Risk Behavior Surveillance*, 1999. "Recently" was defined as having intercourse in the three months prior to being surveyed.

4. The National Center of Addiction and Substance Abuse (CASA) at Columbia University. (1999). *Dangerous liaisons: Substance abuse and sex*. New York, The National Center on Addiction and Substance Abuse (CASA) at Columbia University.

5. "Heavy drug use" was defined as using any drug at least 20 times in one's lifetime.

6. Graves KL, Risky sexual behavior and alcohol use among young adults: Results from a national survey, *American Journal of Health Promotion*, 1995, vol. 10.

7. "Heavy drinkers" were defined as those who have ever had twenty or more drinks in one day; or who reported drinking at

least seven drinks each day for two weeks; or who reported drinking seven or more drinks at least once a week for two months.

8. Leigh BC et al., The relationship of alcohol use to sexual activity in a U.S. national sample, *Social Science and Medicine*, 1994, vol. 39.

9. "Binge drinkers" were defined as those who consume five or more drinks at one sitting.

10. Michael RT et al., *Sex in America: A Definitive Survey*, Boston: Little Brown, 1994.

11. National Institute on Drug Abuse and National Institutes of Health, *A Collection of NIDA Notes: Articles on Drugs and AIDS*, 1996.

12. Scheidt DM and M Windle, A comparison of alcohol typologies using HIV risk behaviors among alcoholic inpatients, *Psychology of Addictive Behaviors*, 1997, vol. 11.

13. Santelli JS et al., Timing of alcohol and other drug use and sexual risk behaviors among unmarried adolescents and young adults, *Family Planning Perspectives*, 2001, vol. 33.

14. American Social Health Association/Kaiser Family Foundation, *Sexually Transmitted Diseases in America: How Many Cases and At What Cost?* Menlo Park, CA: The Henry J Kaiser Family Foundation, 1998, and the Centers for Disease Control and Prevention (CDC), *Tracking the Hidden Epidemics: Trends in STDs in the United States 2000*, Atlanta, GA: CDC, 2001.

15. Kaiser Family Foundation, *Critical Policy Brief: Challenges in the Third Decade of the AIDS Epidemic*, Menlo Park, CA: The Henry J Kaiser Family Foundation, 2001.

16. http://grants.nih.gov/grants/guide/pa-files/PA-01-023.html.

17. Eng TR and WT Butler, eds., The Hidden Epidemic: Confronting Sexually Transmitted Diseases, Washington D.C.: *National Academy Press*, 1997.

18. Eriksen KP and KF Trocki, Sex, alcohol, and sexually transmitted diseases: a national survey, *Family Planning Perspectives*, 1994, vol. 26.

19. "Problem drinkers" were defined as ever having had three of eight major symptoms indicating an increased tolerance or desire for alcohol; impaired control over drinking; symptoms of withdrawal; or increased social disruption.

20. Avins AL et al., HIV infection and risk behaviors among heterosexuals in alcohol treatment, *JAMA*, 1994, vol. 271.

21. Scheidt DM and M Windle, A comparison of alcohol typologies using HIV risk behaviors among alcoholic inpatients, *Psychology of Addictive Behaviors*, 1997, vol. 11.

22. Centers for Disease Control and Prevention (CDC), HIV/AIDS Surveillance in Women, L264 Slide Series, 1999, which draws on information from various HIV/AIDS Surveillance Reports. See also http://grants.nih.gov/grants/guide/pa-files/PA-01 -023.html.

23. The Alan Guttmacher Institutes, *Facts in Brief: Induced Abortion*, New York, NY: AGI, 2000.

24. Anderson JE et al., Condom use and HIV risk behaviors among U.S. adults: Data from a national survey, *Family Planning Perspectives*, 1999, vol. 31. (*National Household Survey of Drug Abuse*).

25. Piccinino LJ and Mosher WD, Trends in contraceptive use in the US: 1982–1995, *Family Planning Perspectives*, 1998, vol. 30.

26. National Center for Health Statistics, Fertility, family planning, and women's health: New data from the 1995 NSFG, *Vital and Health Statistics*, 1997, series 23.

27. Dermen KH et al., Sex-related alcohol expectancies as moderators of the relationship between alcohol use and risky sex in adolescents, *Journal of Studies on Alcohol*, 1998, vol. 59.

28. Fergusson DM and Lynskey MT, Alcohol misuse and adolescent sexual behaviors and risk taking, *Pediatrics*, 1996, vol. 98.

29. Kim N et al., Effectiveness of the 40 adolescent AIDS-risk re-education interventions; quantitative review, *Journal of Adolescent Health*, 1997, vol. 20.

Chapter 59

Drug Use and
the Risk of Suicide
among Youths

In Brief

- In 2000, approximately 3 million youths were at risk for suicide during the past year.

- Youths who reported past year alcohol or illicit drug use were more likely than youths who did not use these substances to be at risk for suicide.

- Only 36% of youths at risk for suicide during the past year received mental health treatment or counseling.

The National Household Survey on Drug Abuse (NHSDA) asks youths aged 12 to 17 whether they had thought seriously about killing themselves or tried to kill themselves during the 12 months before the survey interview.[1] For the purpose of this report, youths who thought about or tried to kill themselves during the past year were considered to be at risk for suicide. Responses were analyzed by geographic regions for comparative purposes.[2]

Respondents were also queried about their use of alcohol and illicit drugs during the 12 months before the survey interview. "Any illicit

"Substance Use and the Risk of Suicide among Youths," *The NHSDA Report*, July 12, 2002, based on: Substance Abuse and Mental Health Services Administration. (2001). *Summary of findings from the 2000 National Household Survey on Drug Abuse* (NHSDA Series: H-13, DHHS Publication No. SMA 01-3549). Rockville, MD.

433

drug" refers to marijuana/hashish, cocaine (including crack), inhalants, hallucinogens, heroin, or prescription-type drugs used nonmedically. Youths were also asked whether they had received treatment or counseling services during the past year for emotional or behavioral problems that were not caused by alcohol or drugs.[3] Respondents who received treatment or counseling were asked to identify reasons for the last time they received these services.[4]

Suicide Risk among Youths

Suicide is an important cause of mortality among youths in the United States.[5] The 2000 NHSDA estimated that almost 3 million youths were at risk for suicide during the past year. Of youths at risk for suicide, 37% actually tried to kill themselves during the past year.

Females (16%) were almost twice as likely as males (8%) to be at risk for suicide during the past year. The likelihood of suicide risk was also greater among youths aged 14 to 17 than it was among those aged 12 or 13 (Figure 59.1). The likelihood of suicide risk was similar among white, black, Hispanic, and Asian youths.

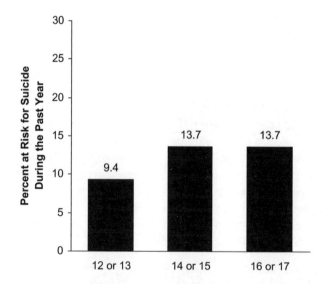

Figure 59.1. *Percentages of Youths Aged 12 to 17 at Risk for Suicide During the Past Year, by Age: 2000. (Source: Substance Abuse and Mental Health Services Administration [SAMHSA] 2000 NHSDA)*

Substance Use and Suicide Risk

Prior research has associated substance use with an increased risk of suicide among youths.[6] The 2000 NHSDA found that youths who reported alcohol or illicit drug use during the past year were more likely than those who did not use these substances to be at risk for suicide during this same time period. For instance, youths who reported past year use of any illicit drug other than marijuana (29%) were almost three times more likely than youths who did not (10%) to be at risk for suicide during this time period (Figure 59.2).

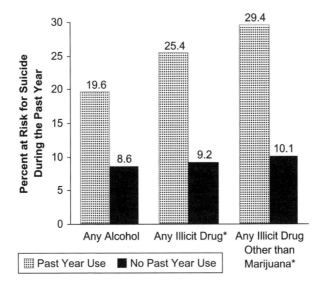

Figure 59.2. *Percentages of Youths Aged 12 to 17 at Risk for Suicide During the Past Year, by Past Year Alcohol or Illicit Drug Use: 2000. (Source: SAMHSA 2000 NHSDA)*

Regional Differences of Suicide Risk

Regionally, youths from the West (14%) were more likely to be at risk for suicide during the past year than those who lived in the Midwest (12%) or Northeast (11%) (Figure 59.3). The risk of suicide was

435

similar among youths from large metropolitan, small metropolitan, and non-metropolitan counties.

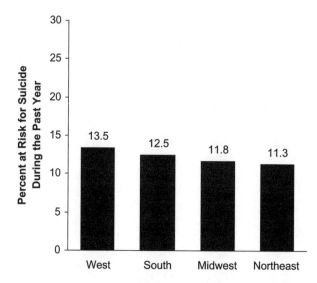

Figure 59.3. *Percentages of Youths Aged 12 to 17 at Risk for Suicide During the Past Year, by Geographic Region: 2000. (Source: SAMHSA 2000 NHSDA)*

Mental Health Treatment Utilization among Suicidal Youths

Research has demonstrated that the most effective way to prevent suicide is through the early identification and treatment of those at risk.[6] Yet, according to the 2000 NHSDA, only 36% of youths at risk for suicide during the past year received mental health treatment during this same time period. Fewer than one-fifth of youths at risk for suicide received help from a private therapist, psychologist, psychiatrist, social worker, or counselor (Table 59.1). More than 15% received treatment from school counselors, school psychologists, or having regular meetings with teachers. Among youths at risk for suicide who received mental health treatment, 38% reported suicidal thoughts or attempts as the reason for the last time they received these services.[7]

Table 59.1. Percentages of Youths Aged 12 to 17 at Risk for Suicide During the Past Year Reporting that They Received Mental Health Services During this Same Time Period, by Location of Treatment: 2000.

Location of treatment	Percent reporting that they received mental health services during the past year
Any treatment	35.5
Private therapist, psychologist, psychiatrist, social worker, or counselor	19.4
School counselor, school psychologist, or having regular meetings with teachers	15.1
Mental health clinic or center	6.5
In-home therapist, counselor, or family preservation worker	6.3
Pediatrician or other family doctor	5.3
Overnight or longer stay in any type of hospital	5.2
Special education classes while in a regular classroom or in a special classroom, a special program, or in a special school	4.6
Partial day hospital or day treatment program	3.8
Overnight or longer stay in a residential treatment center	3.5
Overnight or longer stay in foster care or in a therapeutic foster care home	2.0

Source: SAMHSA 2000 NHSDA.

Notes

1. Respondents were asked whether they tried to kill themselves during the past year if they reported thinking seriously about killing themselves during the same time period and/or they answered affirmatively to at least one of the following questions: (a) "During the past 12 months, has there been a time when nothing was fun for you and you just weren't interested in anything?" (b) "During the past 12 months, has there been a time when you had less energy than you usually do?" or (c) "During the past 12 months, has there been a time when you felt you couldn't do anything well or that you weren't as good-looking or as smart as other people?"

2. Regions include the following groups of States: Northeast Region: Maine, New Hampshire, Vermont, Massachusetts, Rhode Island, Connecticut, New York, New Jersey, Pennsylvania. Midwest Region: Wisconsin, Illinois, Michigan, Indiana, Ohio, North Dakota, South Dakota, Nebraska, Kansas, Minnesota, Iowa, Missouri. South Region: Alabama, Kentucky, Mississippi, Tennessee, West Virginia, Virginia, Maryland, Delaware, District of Columbia, North Carolina, South Carolina, Georgia, Florida, Texas, Oklahoma, Arkansas, Louisiana. West Region: Idaho, Nevada, Arizona, New Mexico, Utah, Colorado, Wyoming, Montana, California, Oregon, Washington, Hawaii, Alaska.

3. Respondents were asked about treatment or counseling services provided by any of the following: Overnight or longer stay in any type of hospital; overnight or longer stay in a residential treatment center; overnight or longer stay in foster care or in a therapeutic foster care home; treatment or counseling at a partial day hospital or day treatment program; visiting a mental health clinic or center; visiting a private therapist, psychologist, psychiatrist, social worker, or counselor; treatment or counseling from an in-home therapist, counselor, or family preservation worker; visiting a pediatrician or other family doctor; receiving special education services while in a regular classroom or in a special classroom, a special program, or in a special school; or talking to school counselors, school psychologists, or having regular meetings with teachers.

4. Respondents were asked to select reasons from a list of options, which included: 1) Thought about killing self or tried to kill self, 2) felt depressed, 3) felt very afraid or anxious, 4) were breaking rules or "acting out," 5) had eating problems, and 6) some other reason.

5. Catallozzi, M., Pletcher, J.R., & Schwarz, D.F. (2001). Prevention of suicide in adolescents. *Current Opinions in Pediatrics*, 13, 417-422.

6. National Institute of Mental Health. (1999, November 26). "Suicide Facts." Retrieved April 2, 2002 from http://www.nimh.nih.gov/publicat/suicidefacts.cfm

7. Youths who reported they received mental health services through special education services while in a regular classroom or in a special classroom, a special program, or in a special school were not asked the reason for the last time they received these services and were totally excluded from this analysis.

Part Six

Drug Abuse Prevention

Chapter 60

Lessons from Prevention Research

In more than 20 years of drug abuse research, the National Institute on Drug Abuse (NIDA) has identified important principles for prevention programs in the family, school, and community. NIDA-supported researchers have tested these principles in long-term drug abuse prevention programs and have found them to be effective.

- Prevention programs should be designed to enhance "protective factors" and move toward reversing or reducing known "risk factors." Protective factors are those associated with reduced potential for drug use. Risk factors are those that make the potential for drug use more likely:

  - Protective factors include strong and positive bonds within a prosocial family; parental monitoring; clear rules of conduct that are consistently enforced within the family; involvement of parents in the lives of their children; success in school performance; strong bonds with other prosocial institutions, such as school and religious organizations; and adoption of conventional norms about drug use.

  - Risk factors include chaotic home environments, particularly in which parents abuse substances or suffer from mental illnesses; ineffective parenting, especially with children with difficult temperaments or conduct disorders; lack of

NIDA InfoFacts, National Institute on Drug Abuse (NIDA), February 2004.

mutual attachments and nurturing; inappropriately shy or aggressive behavior in the classroom; failure in school performance; poor social coping skills; affiliations with deviant peers or peers displaying deviant behaviors; and perceptions of approval of drug-using behaviors in family, work, school, peer, and community environments.

- Prevention programs may target a variety of drugs of abuse, such as tobacco, alcohol, inhalants, and marijuana or may target a single area of drug abuse such as the misuse of prescription drugs.

- Prevention programs should include general life skills training and training in skills to resist drugs when offered, strengthen personal attitudes and commitments against drug use, and increase social competency (e.g., in communications, peer relationships, self-efficacy, and assertiveness).

- Prevention programs for children and adolescents should include developmentally appropriate interactive methods, such as peer discussion groups and group problem solving and decision making, rather than didactic teaching techniques alone.

- Prevention programs should include parents' or caregivers' components that train them to use appropriate parenting strategies, reinforce what the children are learning about drugs and their harmful effects, and that open opportunities for family discussions about the use of legal and illegal substances and family policies about their use.

- Prevention programs should be long-term (throughout the school career), with repeat interventions to reinforce the original prevention goals. For example, school-based efforts directed at elementary and middle school students should include booster sessions to help with the critical transitions such as from middle to high school.

- Family-focused prevention efforts have a greater impact than strategies that focus on parents only or children only.

- Community programs that include media campaigns and policy changes, such as new regulations that restrict access to alcohol, tobacco, or other drugs, are more effective when they are accompanied by school and family interventions.

- Community programs need to strengthen norms against drug use in all drug abuse prevention settings, including the family, the school, the workplace and the community.

- Schools offer opportunities to reach all populations and also serve as important settings for specific subpopulations at risk for drug abuse, such as children with behavior problems or learning disabilities and those who are potential dropouts.

- Prevention programming should be adapted to address the specific nature of the drug abuse problem in the local community.

- The higher the level of risk of the target population, the more intensive the prevention effort must be and the earlier it must begin.

- Prevention programs should be age-specific, developmentally appropriate, and culturally sensitive.

- Effective prevention programs are cost-effective. For every $1 spent on drug use prevention, communities can save $4 to $5 in costs for drug abuse treatment and counseling.[1]

The following are critical areas for prevention planners to consider when designing a program:

- **Family Relationships:** Prevention programs can teach skills for better family communication, discipline, and firm and consistent rulemaking to parents of young children. Research also has shown that parents need to take a more active role in their children's lives, including talking with them about drugs, monitoring their activities, getting to know their friends, and understanding their problems and personal concerns.

- **Peer Relationships:** Prevention programs focus on an individual's relationship to peers by developing social-competency skills, which involve improved communications, enhancement of positive peer relationships and social behaviors, and resistance skills to refuse drug offers.

- **The School Environment:** Prevention programs also focus on enhancing academic performance and strengthening students' bonding to school, by giving them a sense of identity and achievement and reducing the likelihood of their dropping out of school. Most curriculums include the support for positive peer relationships (described above) and a normative education component designed to correct the misperception that most students are using drugs. Research has also found that when children understand the negative effects of drugs (physical, psychological, and social), and when they perceive their friends' and families' social disapproval of drug use, they tend to avoid initiating drug use.

- **The Community Environment:** Prevention programs work at the community level with civic, religious, law enforcement, and governmental organizations and enhance antidrug norms and prosocial behavior through changes in policy or regulation, mass media efforts, and community-wide awareness programs. Community-based programs might include new laws and enforcement, advertising restrictions, and drug-free school zones— all designed to provide a cleaner, safer, drug-free environment.

Note

1. Pentz, M.A. "Costs, benefits, and cost effectiveness of comprehensive drug abuse prevention." In W. J. Bukoski, ed. *Cost Effectiveness and Cost Benefit Research of Drug Abuse Prevention: Implications for Programming and Policy*. NIDA Research Monograph. In Press.

Chapter 61

Talking to Your Child about Drugs

If you think you don't need to discuss drug use with your kids, you're not alone: According to a recent survey from the National Center on Addiction and Substance Abuse at Columbia University, many parents have a "don't ask, don't tell" approach when it comes to drugs. Nearly half the middle- and high-school kids surveyed said their parents had never talked to them about the dangers of drug use.

Read on to find out why and how you should talk to your kids about drugs, even if they haven't started school yet.

Why Do I Need to Talk to My Kid about Drugs?

Why should you talk to your kids about drugs even before they're likely to be exposed to them? Just as you inoculate your children against life-threatening illnesses like measles when they are small, you can "immunize" your children against drug use by giving them the facts before they are presented with the substance.

"If we as parents do not take the responsibility to educate our children about drugs, they are going to get the information from other people, and that information may not be right," explains Lisa Elliott, PhD, a children's behavioral health specialist. "Often, without that informa-

This information was provided by KidsHealth, one of the largest resources online for medically reviewed health information written for parents, kids, and teens. For more articles like this one, visit www.KidsHealth.org or www.TeensHealth.org. © 2001 The Nemours Center for Children's Health Media, a division of The Nemours Foundation.

tion, because of peer influence and the desire to fit in, kids will just go ahead and experiment, and they have no idea what they're doing."

What Should I Say to My Kid?

Preschool to Age 7

Before you get anxious about talking to your young children, take heart. You've probably already laid the groundwork for a discussion. When you tell your preschooler, "This medicine is for Tommy's earache, but too much will make Tommy sick," or "We only take the medicine when the doctor tells us to," you've already planted the idea that some substances can harm the body.

At this age, some children may also be ready for the message that drinking coffee or a lot of soda that contains caffeine isn't good for kids.

"These types of discussions are laying the foundations for healthy behaviors in the home," says Scott Basinger, PhD.

For slightly older children, between ages four and seven, the talks can be more extensive. Dr. Elliott suggests telling kids this age to say no if a stranger offers them candy and to then tell an adult they trust. She advises role-playing those scenarios with kids who are at the upper end of this age scale, so they can practice self-control saying no.

Anthony Acquavella, MD, MPH, an adolescent medicine specialist, suggests watching for teachable moments. For example, when you're watching television with your children and you see someone smoking, use this opportunity to talk about cigarettes.

"Smoking is a good lead-in, because it's so in the media," Dr. Acquavella says. "You can start out along the lines of, 'think about this, you're putting all this junk in your body,' and then continue on from there to other drugs. That's a way to start bringing up the topic that there are chemicals out there that could harm you, whether they're legal or illegal."

The tone of these discussions should be calm; take the time to listen to what your kids have to say. Be specific about the effects of the drugs you're discussing: how they make a person feel physically, the risk of overdose, and the other long-term damage they might cause. To give your kids the facts, you might have to do a little research.

Ages 8 to 12

As your kids grow older, you can open up conversations about drugs with them by asking them what they think. "Ask open-ended questions,"

Dr. Basinger says. "Kids don't want preaching—they're looking for Dad to sit back and say, 'I saw a program on drugs when I was on my job, and I'm wondering, what do you guys learn at school? Are there drugs at your school? What do you know about them?'"

Even if this doesn't immediately result in a discussion, you've made your kids aware and gotten them thinking about it. If you show your kids that you're willing to talk to them openly and hear what they have to say, they might be more willing to come to you for help in the future.

News items, such as steroids in professional sports, can be springboards for casual conversations about current events. These discussions can provide your children with information about the risks of drugs, Dr. Acquavella adds.

"We had five girls die in a car accident not too long ago, and the autopsy showed they were 'huffing,'" he says of the practice of sniffing toxic fumes from aerosol cans. "And one of the physicians on TV said, as tragic as this is, this is the perfect moment for parents to bring up the discussion."

Talk openly about how to safely use products such as nail polish or permanent markers in a well-ventilated area because the fumes can hurt the body. This is a worthwhile lesson to bring up when you're painting or doing similar projects.

Although inhalants like the computer keyboard cleaner used by the girls in the accident are a problem—some surveys suggest one in five children have tried them by eighth grade—two other perfectly legal substances more commonly lead children to try illegal drugs.

"You have to have clear standards on smoking and alcohol use with your kids, because those are generally known as the gateway drugs," Dr. Elliott says. Dr. Basinger adds that two or three times as many kids who end up in drug treatment centers smoke, compared to those without drug problems.

Your own behaviors will influence whether your kids try tobacco and alcohol. "It's hard to tell a kid, you shouldn't smoke and you shouldn't drink, when you're sitting there with a cigarette in one hand, and a Jim Beam in the other," Dr. Acquavella says.

Ages 13 to 17

At this age, your kids are likely to know other kids who abuse alcohol or drugs and to have friends who drive. It's important to impress the dangers of driving under the influence on your kids. "When kids are driving, or they're in cars with older kids who are driving, I think you have to sit down and say, 'people use drugs, people drink, and I don't want you in a car where anybody's under the influence,'" Dr. Acquavella advises. Talk about the legal issues—convictions for driving under the influence—and the possibility that they or someone else might be killed or seriously injured.

It's a good idea to set up a written or unwritten contract on the conditions of going out or using the car. You can promise to pick your kid up at any time (even 2 AM!) without asking questions if she promises to call you when the person who gave her a ride has been drinking or using drugs.

"Say, 'you can call me anytime, day or night, if you're worried about getting in the car with somebody, and I will come and get you,'" says Dr. Acquavella. "'I won't yell, I won't scream. The next day, we'll talk about why you were in that situation, but I won't be crazy about it.'"

The contract can also detail other situations: for example, if you find out someone has been drinking or using drugs in your car while your kid is using it, driving privileges will be suspended for 6 months.

"As long as you put it up front, and don't surprise them, I think it works out better," says Acquavella. "They know the rules to begin with; they can't argue with them. But you have to be consistent."

Risk Factors and Tips for Parents

"No one is immune to drugs," says Dr. Acquavella. "You can be the best parent, your kid can be the best kid, you can have a wonderful relationship, and he can just be in the wrong place at the wrong time and start something."

However, certain groups of kids seem more prone to using drugs than others use. One powerful predictor for drug use is having friends who use drugs. The best way to combat this is to know your child's friends—and their parents.

"Get involved in the schools, and know what's going on," suggests Dr. Acquavella. "Know your neighborhood, because different places have different trends in drug use." If your child's school runs an anti-drug program, get involved. You might learn something!

Kids who are isolated from the mainstream for example, lesbian and gay teens or kids who are depressed or have been abused, are also more likely to use drugs. Pay attention to how your kids are feeling and get them medical treatment promptly if they need it.

A warm, open family environment, where kids are encouraged to talk about their feelings, where their achievements are praised and their self-esteem bolstered will encourage kids to come forward with their questions and concerns.

"It sounds schmaltzy, but it's true," says Dr. Acquavella. "You have to know your kids, and what they're doing. Tell them and reiterate that there's always an open avenue of discussion. If they hear it often enough, then maybe they'll come forth. But if you say, 'we don't discuss that in this house,' then they'll go elsewhere."

Chapter 62

A Parent's Guide to Preventing Inhalant Abuse

Inhalant Abuse Can Kill

It can kill suddenly, and it can kill those who sniff for the first time.

Every year, young people in this country die of inhalant abuse. Hundreds suffer severe consequences, including permanent brain damage, loss of muscle control, and destruction of the heart, blood, kidney, liver, and bone marrow.

Today more than 1,000 different products are commonly abused. The National Institute on Drug Abuse reported in 1996 that one in five American teenagers have used inhalants to get high.

Many youngsters say they begin sniffing when they're in grade school. They start because they feel these substances can't hurt them, because of peer pressure, or because of low self-esteem. Once hooked, these victims find it a tough habit to break.

These questions and answers will help you identify inhalant abuse and understand what you can do to prevent or stop this problem.

What is inhalant abuse?

Inhalant abuse is the deliberate inhalant or sniffing of common products found in homes and schools to obtain a "high."

CPSC Document #389, Consumer Product Safety Commission (CPSC), 1995. Reviewed by David A. Cooke, M.D., April 2004.

What are the effects of inhalant abuse?

Sniffing can cause sickness and death. For example, victims may become nauseated, forgetful, and unable to see things clearly. Victims may lose control of their body, including the use of arms and legs. These effects can last 15 to 45 minutes after sniffing.

In addition, sniffing can severely damage many parts of the body, including the brain, heart, liver, and kidneys.

Even worse, victims can die suddenly—without any warning. "Sudden Sniffing Death" can occur during or right after sniffing. The heart begins to overwork, beating rapidly but unevenly, which can lead to cardiac arrest. Even first-time abusers have been known to die from sniffing inhalants.

What products are abused?

Ordinary household products, which can be safely used for legitimate purposes, can be problematic in the hands of an inhalant abuser. The following categories of products are reportedly abused: glues/adhesives, nail polish remover, marking pens, paint thinner, spray paint, butane lighter fluid, gasoline, propane gas, typewriter correction fluid, household cleaners, cooking sprays, deodorants, fabric protectors, whipping cream aerosols, and air conditioning coolants.

How can you tell if a young person is an inhalant abuser?

If someone is an inhalant abuser, some or all these symptoms may be evident:

- Unusual breath odor or chemical odor on clothing
- Slurred or disoriented speech
- Drunk, dazed, or dizzy appearance
- Signs of paint or other products where they wouldn't normally be, such as on the face or fingers
- Red or runny eyes or nose
- Spots and/or sores around the mouth
- Nausea and/or loss of appetite
- Chronic inhalant abusers may exhibit such symptoms as anxiety, excitability, irritability, or restlessness

What could be other telltale behaviors of inhalant abuse?

Inhalant abusers also may exhibit the following signs:

- Sitting with a pen or marker near nose
- Constantly smelling clothing sleeves
- Showing paint or stain marks on the face, fingers, or clothing
- Hiding rags, clothes, or empty containers of the potentially abused products in closets and other places

What is a typical profile of an inhalant abuser in the United States?

There is no typical profile of an inhalant abuser. Victims are represented by both sexes and all socioeconomic groups throughout the United States. It's not unusual to see elementary and middle-school age youths involved with inhalant abuse.

How does a young person who abuses inhalants die?

There are many scenarios for how young people die of inhalant abuse. Here are some of them:

- A 13-year-old boy was inhaling fumes from cleaning fluid and became ill a few minutes afterwards. Witnesses alerted the parents, and the victim was hospitalized and placed on life support systems. He died 24 hours after the incident.

- An 11-year-old boy collapsed in a public bathroom. A butane cigarette lighter fuel container and a plastic bag were found next to him. He also had bottles of typewriter correction fluid in his pocket. CPR failed to revive him, and he was pronounced dead.

- A 15-year-old boy was found unconscious in a backyard. According to three companions, the four teenagers had taken gas from a family's grill propane tank. They put the gas in a plastic bag and inhaled the gas to get high. The victim collapsed shortly after inhaling the gas. He died on the way to the hospital.

What can you do to prevent inhalant abuse?

One of the most important steps you can take is to talk with your children or other youngsters about not experimenting even a first time with inhalants. In addition, talk with your children's teachers, guidance counselors, and coaches. By discussing this problem openly and stressing the devastating consequences of inhalant abuse, you can help prevent a tragedy.

If you suspect your child or someone you know is an inhalant abuser, what can you do to help?

Be alert for symptoms of inhalant abuse. If you suspect there's a problem, you should consider seeking professional help.

Contact a local drug rehabilitation center or other services available in your community, or:

National Inhalant Prevention Coalition
Toll-Free: (800) 269-4237
Website: www.inhalants.org

National Drug and Alcohol Treatment Referral Service
Toll-Free: (800) 662-HELP

National Clearinghouse for Alcohol and Drug Information
Toll-Free: (800) 729-6686
Website: www.health.org

Other related websites: www.projectknow.org and www.freevibe.com

Chapter 63

Drug Abuse Prevention Programs

Drug use, violence, delinquency, teen pregnancy, and other prob-lem behaviors among young people are causes for grave concern in the United States. Despite a decade of success in reducing drug use in youth, the prevention field is currently losing ground again. Five years of rising adolescent drug use (Johnston, O'Malley, & Bachman, 1996) has increased the urgency to identify successes and improve the dissemination of prevention programs that work. Although skeptics say prevention doesn't work, the research literature contains a num-ber of research-based prevention strategies with sufficient program effectiveness in Phase III Controlled Intervention Trials to warrant dissemination (Falco, 1993; Kumpfer, 1997a; Kumpfer & Alder, 1997; National Institute on Drug Abuse [NIDA], 1997; Tobler & Stratton, 1997).

The recent, highly publicized failure of the popular Drug Abuse Resistance Education (DARE) program (Ennett, Tobler, Ringwalt, & Flewelling, 1994) has highlighted the importance of enhanced dissemi-nation of programs that work. Hence, a major task for the prevention field and funding agencies is to improve the identification and dis-semination of the most effective prevention programs to schools and communities. In the ideal model of the five phases of research proposed

"Identification of Drug Abuse Prevention Programs," Literature review by Karol L. Kumpfer, Ph.D., National Institute on Drug Abuse (NIDA), May 2003. For convenience in identifying sources, parenthetical references in the text have been retained. The complete citations are available online at www.drugabuse.gov/about/organization/hsr/da-pre/KumpferLitReviewPartC.html#ref.

by Jansen, Glynn and Howard (1996), prevention programs implemented at the state and local levels should be based on tested interventions in Phase III controlled intervention trials further tested for generalizability on Phase IV. These Phase III controlled intervention trials likewise should address the most salient precursors of drug use and abuse as suggested by Phase I and II biomedical and etiological research. This logical, smooth flow of research into practice is not happening.

Major gaps are occurring in the linkage between product research and product dissemination. An ideal research-based approach flows smoothly from basic biomedical research through the five phases of research to implementation of models in nationwide prevention and health services programs (Jansen, Glynn, & Howard, 1996). This review of the research and practice literature suggests that the most commonly used programs typically are the most highly commercially marketed programs, which rarely have solid research results. Although some popular prevention programs are based on similar principles, they are generally not of equal intensity, do not control fidelity as well, or do not have well-trained implementers.

The research-based programs with effectiveness results usually are those developed and tested in federally funded Phase III clinical trials, generally by university researchers. Because few university researchers have the time or the knowledge to market their programs commercially, funding sources need to support the dissemination of research-based approaches. Practitioners also have a responsibility to question the effectiveness of the programs they are planning to implement and to select a prevention program by matching the prevention intervention to the risk characteristics of the proposed participants.

Types of Prevention Interventions

A major issue in the prevention field is the degree to which programs should be targeted to specific at-risk groups or spread across all groups with no differentiation. A growing body of research (Thornberry, 1987; Thornberry, Lizotte, Krohn, Farnworth, & Jang, 1994) suggests that there are rather stable developmental trajectories for childhood conduct problems leading to drug use and delinquency in adolescence. This is encouraging some prevention providers to target the highest risk youth through selective or indicated prevention programs.

The research literature suggests that childhood antisocial behaviors or conduct disorders, anger, rebelliousness and anxiety, and shyness are predictive of later adolescent delinquency and substance use/abuse (Elliott, Huizinga, & Ageton, 1985a, 1985b; Kellam, Ensminger, & Simon, 1980; Windel, 1990). Early childhood aggression recently has become a major focus for prevention research, because it is a developmental marker for a variety of negative adolescent outcomes including delinquency and substance use (Hinshaw, Lahey, & Hart, 1993; Loeber, 1990). Aggressive children do not improve without some type of early intervention. If no prevention intervention is provided, their externalizing behaviors deteriorate as they grow older (Coie, Terry, Lenox, Lochman, & Hyman, 1995), leading to increased risk for substance use (Lochman & Wayland, 1994).

To help practitioners better match appropriate interventions to target populations, prevention experts redefined prevention approaches based on the groups for which they were designed (IOM, 1994). They concluded that there are three distinct types of prevention approaches:

1. Universal prevention strategies designed to prevent precursors of drug use or initiation of use in general populations, such as all students in a school

2. Selective prevention strategies designed to target groups or subsets of the general population, such as children of drug users or poor school achievers

3. Indicated prevention strategies created for participants who are already manifesting drug use initiation or precursors of drug abuse, such as conduct disorders, thrill seeking, aggression, and delinquency

Advantages, disadvantages, and examples of effective prevention programs for alcohol and drug abuse are discussed for each of these three categories of prevention.

Universal Prevention Programs

Universal prevention programs include strategies designed to be delivered universally to general populations of youth and families. They can be provided by community groups or governments, churches, schools, and private nonprofit agencies. Media campaigns and public education are used to inform people about the programs. If delivered in schools, programs are provided for all students in the grades for which they are intended. These programs are generally shorter and less intensive than selective or indicated prevention strategies. Staff do not have to be as well trained because these approaches are often supported by video materials and highly structured curriculum materials. In schools, they can be led by the regular teachers or special external staff trained to deliver the program in the classroom.

Advantages and Disadvantages of Universal Prevention Programs

A major advantage of universal prevention strategies is that they are frequently less expensive per participant because of shorter length, do not require special recruitment strategies or incentives for participation, and should include high-risk youth and families. Schools are the primary locus for drug abuse prevention efforts, because they allow universal access to all youth in schools. Hence, all students regardless of risk status can be accessed and served through universal school-based programs. Although some schools would rather "get back to basics" and not overburden teachers with additional tasks, most states mandate school drug prevention programs, health education, and teenage pregnancy and acquired immunodeficiency syndrome (AIDS) education. Many schools recognize that addressing behavioral and emotional risk factors (i.e., anger and lack of emotional control, conduct disorders, aggression, and lack of life and social skills) also helps to improve school achievement and success.

Unfortunately, at-risk youth and families frequently do not participate because of lack of attendance and involvement (e.g., school dropout, truancy, frequent absences, or illness) or beliefs that the content does not meet their individual needs. Universal school-based prevention programs must be targeted at the majority of students, so they frequently do not contain content tailored for ethnic students. The intensity, dosage, content, and method of delivery may be insufficient to change risk factors in higher risk students; hence, their effectiveness may be diminished, producing insufficient or temporary outcomes.

As shown in Table 63.1, a number of traditionally popular drug prevention approaches currently are being implemented in schools and communities. The major types are (a) cognitive and affective prevention approaches, (b) social influence approaches, (c) personal and social skills training, (d) youth-led approaches, (e) school climate change approaches, (f) community partnership approaches, and (g) parent involvement approaches. The earliest approaches implemented in schools and then tested in federal research were drug education and affective education approaches.

Table 63.1. Types of Universal School-Based Prevention Programs

Cognitive and Affective Prevention Approaches

- Public Awareness and Media Campaigns
- Drug Education: Information Dissemination
- Comprehensive School Health Education (Piper et al., 1993)
- Affective Education (Battistich et al., 1996; Schaps et al., 1986)

Social Influence Approaches

- The Social Influence Approach (Evans et al., 1978)
- Psychological Inoculation (Evans et al., 1978)
- Social Resistance Skills (Pentz et al., 1989; Ellickson & Bell, 1990)
- Normative Education, All Stars Program (Hansen, 1996)

Personal and Social Skills Training

- Life Skills Training (Botvin, 1995)
- Violence Prevention Programs (Gainer et al., 1993)

Youth-Led or Involvement Approaches
Center for Substance Abuse Prevention [CSAP], 1996

- Youth Councils
- President's Crime Prevention Council Projects
- CDC's Kids Coalition and Smoking Prevention Projects

School Climate Change Approaches

- Project PATHE (Gottfredson, 1986)
- Project HIPATHE (Kumpfer, Turner, & Alvarado, 1991)
- School Transitional Environment Project (Felner et al., 1993)
- Aban Aya Project (Flay, 1997, in press)
- Child Development Project (Battistich et al., 1996)

County Partnership Approaches

- Robert Wood Johnson's Fighting Back
- PCSAP's Community Partnerships

Family-Focused Approaches (conducted at school)

- Parent Drug Education Homework Involvement (Pentz et al., 1989)
- Parent Education or Training (Hawkins & Catalano, 1994)
- Iowa Strengthening Families Program (Kumpfer, Molgaard, & Spoth, 1996)
- Phased Family Involvement: Adolescent Transition Program (Dishion et al., 1996)

Cognitive and Affective Approaches

Information strategies include media campaigns, films, pamphlets, clearinghouse resource centers, radio-TV public service announcements, health fairs, advertisements, hot lines, and speaking engagements. This approach, which is a major method for providing information for adults, also is being implemented in schools and communities to target youth. Media campaigns provide needed information and affect the community's social norms when combined with other community prevention strategies (Wallack, 1986). In addition, the public demand for information about drugs is increasing and should be satisfied by accurate and scientifically credible messages. Since 1987, the Partnership for a Drug-Free America (1994) has produced more than 400 antidrug ads for their national campaigns worth $1.8 billion in media donations. According to Wartella and Middlestadt (1991), communication campaigns can be effective (a) when there is widespread acceptance of the campaign, (b) when media creates awareness and knowledge of the issues, (c) when information is used to recruit individuals, (d) when interpersonal communication channels such as peer networks are used to reinforce behavior changes (Rogers & Storey, 1987).

Media education is a prevention approach that seeks to educate youth about methods the media use to influence people. Media education was part of the social influence approach developed by Evans and colleagues (1978) at the University of Houston; it has been revised by many other researchers. The basis is McGuire's (1964, 1968) persuasive communication theory. Few studies have tested the efficacy of this approach only, rather than in combination with other strategies.

Drug Education Approaches: Information Dissemination

These programs seek to increase youths' awareness of drugs and of their health and social consequences. Many schools and colleges provide information on tobacco, alcohol, and other drug use as part of their health education classes or drug prevention programs. Drug education is based on the implicit assumption that adolescents behave in a logical manner and will not use drugs if they are given information. Botvin (1995) summarized, however, some of the ways drug education can be counterproductive and actually increase drug use in vulnerable students: (a) stressing the dangers of drug use may attract high-risk thrill seekers, (b) discussing pharmacological effects can arouse curiosity to try drugs firsthand, and (c) providing information on modes of administration tells students how to use drugs. Some studies (Swisher, Crawford, Goldstein, & Yura, 1971) show how information on drugs can increase experimentation. Providing new information to young children on commonly available household products used as inhalants can increase use, and presenting drug use as normative may suggest to some youth that they should use drugs to be normal and accepted. For some teenagers, any perceived short-term social benefit can override concerns with long-term consequences. Although research (Glasgow & McCaul, 1985; Goodstadt, 1980; Schaps, Bartolo, Moskowitz, Palley, & Churgin, 1981; Tobler, 1986) suggests that knowledge alone has not been effective in reducing drug use, it can be important to comprehensive programming and is crucial for lethal drugs or drug combinations. Additionally, education on drug consequences can serve as a basis for supporting peer norms that are unfavorable to drug use.

There is substantial evidence (Johnston et al., 1996) that information on the physical consequences of drug use is highly correlated with reduced use. Hence, providing accurate information, particularly about the most dangerous drugs, through credible sources or interesting group activities should be a part of universal programming. Unfortunately, there has been little research on ways to maximize the effectiveness of this approach. Prior programs that focused on physical consequences were rejected by researchers because it was thought the approach was ineffective when implemented alone (McCaul & Glasgow, 1985; Tobler, 1986). Also, these programs frequently relied on "scare tactics" by noncredible sources who provided inaccurate information, and the approach was rejected by youth. Some research (O'Neil, Glasgow, & McCaul, 1983) suggests that if these programs are creatively implemented with exciting interactive classroom activities, the results are positive, particularly in males.

Comprehensive School Health Education Programs

Comprehensive school health programming, including substance abuse prevention, is rapidly being promoted. The American School Health Association (ASHA) and the Centers for Disease Control (CDC) are recommending that school health programs have one integrated curriculum for AIDS and prevention, substance use, teen pregnancy, violence prevention, gang prevention, and other health risks of youth. An example of an evaluated comprehensive school health curriculum is the NIDA-funded Healthy for Life Curriculum in Wisconsin (Piper et al., 1993). This program includes 56 sessions implemented in school classes over a 3-year period. Such an integrated approach is laudatory if it remains intensive and is imbedded within a total school commitment to reduce risk factors for substance use.

Affective Education Approaches

In the late 1960s, the drug culture flourished, affecting youth culture in music, dress, attitudes about traditional institutions, and drug use. It was hypothesized that youth heavily involved in use of marijuana, psychedelics, and sometimes heroin were lacking in self-esteem. As a logical consequence, affective approaches were developed that sought to improve self-esteem as a mediator of drug use (Kumpfer & Turner, 1990/1991). These approaches used ineffective methods such as "feel good" experiential games and classroom activities, rather than phased behavioral skills training. Affective programs have had no demonstrated impact on drug use itself (Kearney & Hines, 1980; Kim, 1988), but have had some impact on mediators such as school bonding and self-esteem (Battistich, Schaps, Watson, & Solomon, 1996). Despite their weaknesses, as verified in meta-analysis (Tobler, 1986), these approaches are still popular in schools and continue to be evaluated in NIDA research to determine their long-term effectiveness.

Although only a partial focus of the Napa Project, affective education programs aiming to increase youth self-concept or self-esteem were implemented and evaluated (Schaps, Moskowitz, Malvin, & Scheffer, 1986). Although there was no effect on 7th- grade males or 8th-grade males or females, this project produced a 1-year decrease in use of alcohol and marijuana, but not tobacco, in 7th-grade girls (Schaps et al., 1986). These approaches, which did not appear to have negative effects, probably lacked sufficient dosage to single-handedly modify self-esteem or any actual precursors of drug use. Self-esteem has a distal, tangential, and complex relationship to drug use; hence, these prevention intervention studies may have been targeting the wrong risk factors. Studies have found high self-esteem in drug users, particularly when they begin use and before hitting the proverbial "rock bottom."

Social Influence Approaches

This approach was the major school focus from the 1980s to the early 1990s. It has been extremely popular as a basis of many commercially marketed programs, because research suggests it is capable of reducing initiation to tobacco use and sometimes marijuana and alcohol use by 30% to 50%; however, booster sessions are needed or results decrease in 3 years (Pentz et al., 1989). Originally developed by Evans and his colleagues (1978) at the University of Houston, the approach has been revised by many other researchers. The bases are McGuire's (1964, 1968) persuasive communication theory and social and behavioral change theory.

The typical curriculum includes at least three major approaches: (a) social resistance skills training, from three to 12 sessions over two years in junior high taught by teachers or peer leaders (girls respond better to peer leaders), on how to resist peer offers; (b) psychological inoculation by an analysis of advertising appeals; and (c) normative education. Some studies also include a public commitment not to use drugs. The social resistance skills or refusal skills approach involves having students recognize high-risk situations in which they might use drugs and role-play how to resist. The psychological inoculation approach developed by Evans consists of exposure to progressively stronger persuasive messages through films, media, and role-plays. Students recognize advertising appeals and formulate counter arguments to those appeals.

Student Taught Awareness and Resistance Project (STAR and I-STAR)

This approach includes a two-year, middle-school social influence curriculum based on earlier successes with Project SMART developed by this research team in Southern California (Pentz, 1995, 1997; Pentz, et al., 1989; Rohrbach, Graham, Hansen, Flag, & Johnson, 1987). The curriculum is implemented by trained teachers (Smith, McCormick, Steckler, & McLeroy, 1993). Although discussed in this section as an example of a social influence curriculum, Project STAR is more of a multicomponent program combining the classroom curriculum with comprehensive community interventions including mass media campaigns, parent involvement in homework, community coalition development, and health policy changes. A longitudinal follow-up study of participants when they were seniors in high school showed 30% less marijuana use, 25% less cigarette use, and 20% less alcohol use compared to controls.

Normative Education Approaches

These are based on interventions developed by Evans and associates (1978) to correct students' overestimations of the prevalence of drug use. Prior research (Fishbein, 1977) suggested that adolescents tend to believe that more youth are using tobacco, alcohol, and other drugs than actually are. Providing periodic classroom surveys of tobacco use and publishing the results corrected misjudgments that almost all students were smoking and reduced smoking rates by half over the control rate. Perkins and Berkowitz (1992) tested the normative education approach with college students and found it to be effective in reducing drug use rates.

Adolescent Alcohol Prevention Trial (AAPT)

AAPT is an elementary school classroom program for 5th graders with booster sessions in the seventh grade (Donaldson, Graham, & Hansen, 1994). It offers normative education and resistance skills training, which in combination were more effective than resistance skills only. Hansen and Graham (1991) tested the relative contribution of the normative education component versus the peer resistance component in AAPT. The normative education program was more effective and significantly reduced alcohol consumption, marijuana use, and cigarette smoking. The results suggested that previously reported positive effects of peer resistance skills training programs may have been caused primarily by the normative education components in the programs. Ellickson and Bell (1990) similarly concluded that the lack of effectiveness on alcohol reduction after one year of their social influence resistance training program, ALERT Drug Prevention, may have been because more positive peer norms existed for alcohol than for tobacco or marijuana. AAPT served as the basis for the improved All Stars Program (Hansen, 1996), which focuses even more on normative education.

All Stars Program

This program was created by Hansen (1996), who first worked with Evans (1978). The 13-session classroom curriculum focuses on normative education. Trained teachers use highly interactive classroom activities, role-plays, games, debates, art projects, videotaped performances, and active discussion. A symbolic ring and certificates are awarded at graduation. The program targets three of four variables that Hansen's meta-analysis research (Hansen, Rose, & Dryfoos, 1993; Hansen & Rose, in press; Hansen, under review) suggests mediate drug use: (a) personal commitments to avoid drugs; (b) life goals, values, and ideals incongruent with the high-risk behaviors; and (c) conventional beliefs about social norms regarding high-risk behaviors. The fourth mediator, bonding with prosocial institutions, is only indirectly addressed; that is, youth enjoy school more and possibly bond with the teacher or students in the class.

Pilot study results suggest the program was implemented with fidelity. Compared to students who received DARE in the seventh grade, the All Stars students (N = 102) had significantly better outcomes on all four mediators and rated the program more highly. Given the relatively small number of subjects compared to the significance levels (p <.0001 to .0002 and F-values of 34.74 to 14.31), the effect sizes are quite large for a school-based program. There were gender x condition main effects for commitment and ideals, but not for expressed bondedness and normative beliefs. One reason for the very large statistical differences between the two compared programs is that the DARE students significantly decreased on these four variables between the pre- and posttest, whereas the All Stars students significantly increased. The worsening of "key mediators for drug use as students mature is normal and is the primary reason for increases in drug use over time" (Hansen, 1996, p. 1368). Without a no-treatment control group, it is difficult to tell whether the DARE program helped to reduce this decrease in positive mediators or whether these students were totally unaffected by the DARE program and were similar to a no-treatment control.

Personal and Social Skills Training

These approaches are becoming more popular because of the long-term effectiveness of Botvin's Life Skills Training Program. The bases are Bandura's social learning theory (Bandura, 1986) and Jessor's problem behavior theory (Jessor & Jessor, 1977). Other underlying assumptions are that drug use is functional; that it is socially learned through modeling, imitation, and reinforcement; and that it is influenced by an adolescent's cognition, attitudes, and beliefs. The curricula include teaching of generic personal self-management skills and social skills by teachers, health educators, college students, and same-age or older peer leaders. Programs last for seven to 20 sessions with 10 to 15 sessions as the average and are taught in health or drug education classes or in science, social studies, or physical education classes.

The immediate results of these programs are very positive, with 40% to 80% reductions in drug use. However, most studies found erosion of results within three years or by the end of high school (Ellickson & Bell, 1990).

Life Skills Training (LST) Program

The LST program (Botvin, Baker, Dusenbury, Botvin, & Diaz, 1995; Botvin, Baker, Filazzola, & Botvin, 1990; Botvin, Schinka, Epstein, & Diaz, 1995) is one of the programs highlighted in the NIDA (1997) monograph. It is a three-year, middle school personal and social skills program including 30 sessions of drug resistance skills, normative education, and self-management, communication, and other life skills. A 6-year follow-up study with 6,000 students in 56 schools found that weekly use of polydrugs (tobacco, alcohol, and an illegal drug) was 66% lower than control schools. Any use of tobacco, alcohol, or marijuana was 44% lower than control schools. Program fidelity was better in teachers who attended annual training workshops and received on-going support.

Because LST and other programs are conducted in schools, the programs have not been modified to be culturally appropriate, except for some changes in reading level, language, role play scenarios, and examples appropriate for the target population. In a New York State study with 74% Hispanic students and 11% African American students, Botvin found positive effects in knowledge of consequences, smoking prevalence, social acceptability of smoking, decision making, normative expectations of adult smoking, and peer smoking. Similar results were found in two New Jersey studies with 78% to 87% African American students (Botvin, Batson, et al., 1989; Botvin & Cardwell, 1992).

Violence Prevention Programs

Social problem-solving skills training has been combined with education on the relationship between drugs and violence. A 15-session program was implemented daily (50 minutes) in fifth grades for three weeks by experienced trainers (including an attorney, a trauma nurse, and a paraplegic former drug dealer). An evaluation (Gainer, Webster, & Champion, 1993) found positive effects on youth responses to hypothesized social conflict situations and beliefs about aggression and violence.

Summary of Effectiveness of Social Influence and Social Skills Training Programs

Although social skills training approaches employ a wide variety of intervention methods, most of them use behavioral skills training techniques involving demonstrations of effective and ineffective behaviors, trainer demonstrations, participant role plays with feedback, and reinforcement for behavior changes. These programs often address a wide variety of general social skills or competencies, such as assertiveness to avoid negative influences (offers to use drugs), communication skills, decision making, ability to restore self-esteem, anger and stress management, and social skills to make prosocial friends.

The IOM (1994) review of substance abuse prevention concluded that when combined, peer resistance and normative approaches have some effectiveness in "producing modest significant reductions during early adolescence in the onset and prevalence of cigarette smoking, alcohol, and marijuana use across a number of experimental studies conducted by a variety of investigators" (Ellickson & Bell, 1990; Hansen, 1992; Hansen, Johnson, Flay, Graham, & Sobel, 1988; McAlister, Perry, Killen, Slinkard, & Maccoby, 1980). Peer-led classes appear to be more effective than teacher-led classes (Botvin et al., 1990; Goplerud, 1990; McAlister, 1983; Perry, Klepp, Halper, Hawkins, & Murray, 1986; Perry et al., 1989). Bruce and Emshoff (1992) hypothesized that "peers may provide a more credible message in helping to form antidrug norms or may help to create a more realistic context for the acquisition and practice of peer refusal skills."

School-based universal programs are not without potential risk for high-risk or drug-using students. Several studies have found increased use of tobacco and alcohol in students who were already using these substances (Ellickson & Bell, 1990; Gottfredson, 1990; Moskowitz, 1989). The IOM (1994) concluded that school campaigns that show drug use as nonnormative behavior may further isolate students who are already using drugs. Special selective prevention approaches are needed to avoid isolating high-risk students from positive, nonusing friends.

Youth-Led or Youth Involvement Approaches

The youth-led or youth involvement approach seeks to promote protective mediators for drug use, such as self-empowerment, leadership, planning, decision making, opportunities for success, team-building skills, and commitments to remain drug free through school and community advocacy. The interactive, skill-building approach employed in youth-led programs has been supported by the meta-analysis of Tobler and Stratton (1997). However, the leadership training and empowerment aspects have been less researched. Most of these activities are currently being implemented as universal prevention programs in schools and communities; however, such implementers are making major efforts to involve high-risk youth. The underlying assumption appears to be that at-risk youth will respond more favorably to substance abuse prevention programs if other young people from the same community play substantial and meaningful roles in the management and operation of such programs. The primary hypothesis is that youth-led approaches to prevention will be more successful than adult-led activities in reducing substance abuse and other problem behaviors.

Published research supports this hypothesis. A few school-based social influence researchers (Botvin et al., 1990; McAlister, 1983; Perry et al., 1986; Perry et al., 1989) have found that peer-led classes appear to be more effective than teacher-led classes. However, the operationalization of this concept in practice in communities today is much broader than simply training youth to implement a researcher-designed and researcher-controlled curriculum. It is difficult to define youth-led strategies, and much confusion exists. The critical elements or principles of successful youth-led prevention activities have not yet been defined, because researchers have not tested these approaches in Phase III Controlled Intervention Trials. Many of these youth-led approaches have grown out of grassroots ideas within comprehensive community partnership grants funded by CSAP, CDC, and the National Institute of Justice (NIJ). Hence, they have not been tested as independent components.

The major approaches currently being funded are (a) youth councils and youth governments; (b) the President's Crime Prevention Council Projects, including the Office of Juvenile Justice and Delinquency Prevention (OJJDP) 1996 and 1997 Ounce of Prevention grants; and (c) CDC's Kids Coalition and Smoking Prevention youth minigrants.

Youth Councils

Youth councils for crime and substance abuse prevention exist in many of our cities and states as Governor's Youth Councils and Mayor's Youth Councils. Generally, they are staffed by prevention or youth specialists who solicit nominations of youth from their area to serve for a year on a youth council. Youth councils vary in their attempts to recruit high-risk youth as well as high-status peer leaders. Dishion and Andrews' (1995) research on the iatrogenic effects of clustering problem youth suggests that having a mix of youth would produce better effects, but this is an empirical question worth testing in the area of youth-led activities. Sometimes prosocial, high-status voluntary college interns are used as assistants and positive role models.

470

Activities include participating in community service projects, such as neighborhood cleanups, and advising the governor or mayor on youth issues, recreation, and sports.

Youth Governments

Although not new, a more intensive skill-building approach is implementation of youth governments. This approach involves having high-risk youth, who show promise, serve as youth officials for each major part of state, county, or city government. Hence, students would serve as the youth city mayor, the city treasurer, the commissioner of social services or health, and so on. These youth spend time with their mentor, the government official serving in the same public office, after school and on weekends, shadowing their activities and learning professional competencies and aspirations. In addition, the youth government meets and makes recommendations on public services or laws from the perspective of community youth. If implemented as intended, youth governments could provide substantial skills training and increase commitments to traditional values. This promising approach has not been evaluated in the published research literature.

The President's Crime Prevention Council Projects

These constitute a systematic attempt to involve youth more in prevention activities (e.g. OJJDP's 1996 and 1997 Ounce of Prevention grantee projects). A review of these funded projects reveals that these grantees are working primarily within community coalition or partnership models. Although the grantees were asked to focus on youth-led organizations, the funded projects were still adult-led and adult-supported, probably because youth-led organizations are rare. Most of the coalitions or collaboratives are examining existing youth and family services and creating plans to improve those services—hopefully with youth input. Because of the broad definition of youth-led activities, these coalitions are implementing many different types of approaches, including mapping and publishing projects of youth services and resources in the community, needs assessments of youth needs or gap analyses of services compared to needs, peer leadership and mediation projects, cross-age tutoring and mentoring, youth-staffed support lines, and other youth activities within coalitions, including serving as youth representatives on coalition advisory boards or councils. For a summary of youth activities for the nine fiscal year 1996 Ounce of Prevention grantees, see Table 63.2.

Table 63.2. Ounce of Prevention Youth-Led Activities

San Francisco Link:	Cross-training youth workers, functional mapping of services, and monthly neighborhood forums
Boston Coalition Kids First Initiative Against Drugs:	Counseling services for children witnessing violence, education, work readiness, and job opportunities
St. Louis Development Corporation:	Community forum where youth and residents develop action agendas
Youth Violence Prevention Coalition, Louisville, KY:	Community partnership and plan created by youth, service providers, and citizens, including a directory of youth services
DC Forum:	Community collaborative to plan and coordinate youth services with a centralized information system
San Diego YMCA:	Collaborative of three youth and family-focused programs to increase youth and adult involvement and crease database of youth and community services
Akron Mayor's Collaborative:	Collaborative to provide after-school activities, mentors and tutors, conflict resolution, peer mediation, newsletter, and Info-Line
Youth Empowerment Services (YES), Albany, KY:	Collaborative to expand interagency council to provide central services, information, and a referral point
YouUnited Way, Burlington, VT:	Coordination of 18 strategies to create central information and referral services for youth, public health, and safety services, plus review of existing youth programs

CDC's Kids Coalition and Smoking Prevention Activities

Another approach to youth-led activities has been spearheaded by the CDC through their funding to state health departments for IM-PACT (Initiatives to Mobilize for the Prevention and Control of Tobacco Use). One spin-off of these grants has been the development of Kids Coalitions to lobby for passage of clean air acts and for a tax increase on tobacco. In addition, this year CDC funded states to implement youth minigrants ($500). Through IMPACT KIDS (Kids Involved in Discouraging Smoking) minigrants in schools, one adult supervisor works with a group of at least five students to implement specified community environmental change prevention approaches. Funded activities have included (a) measuring the amount of tobacco advertising and placement of tobacco products in stores; (b) developing an antitobacco website and a talk line or referral service; (c) conducting compliance checks for "tobacco stings" with law enforcement, conducting retail education on laws concerning youth access to tobacco, and publishing surveys of tobacco accessibility at businesses; (d) developing peer education or student-led programs to teach other students about tobacco prevention and reduction; (e) encouraging tobacco legislative advocacy including writing and seeking legislators or council members to introduce and support youth-written legislation; (f) developing antitobacco messages that target teenagers and displaying them in schools and businesses; (g) enhancing efforts to reduce tobacco promotion and advertising, and supporting the implementation of teen tobacco reduction and cessation programs.

Evaluations of CDC-funded youth-led activities have been limited and consist primarily of process evaluations demonstrating that the proposed activities were implemented. Outcome evaluations on the hypothesized changes in the youth involved—such as increased commitment to remain tobacco free, increased involvement with non-tobacco-using peers, increased school bonding, increased self-efficacy, and leadership competencies—have not been tested, despite the promising nature of these youth-involvement activities.

School Climate Change Approaches

This type of prevention program seeks to change the total school environment to be more supportive of nonuse, but also to address many of the mediators for drug use, such as school bonding, self-esteem, association with nonusing friends, a supportive school climate, and positive family relations (Kumpfer & Turner, 1990/1991). School climate change approaches resemble community change coalition approaches but are conducted with an emphasis on the school or school district. Task forces are mobilized to plan, implement, and evaluate locally developed solutions to empirically identified problems derived from a baseline needs assessment. Many different solutions are implemented, including universal interventions for the total school (e.g., school pride days, assemblies, theater performances, school policy changes, curriculum changes, and school structure changes, including cooperative learning), selective interventions for high-risk students (e.g., children of alcoholics groups, theater troupes for high-risk youth, peer leadership classes, new student welcome programs, buddy programs for freshmen, and mentoring programs), and indicated interventions (e.g., peer counseling, teen hotlines for in-crisis youth, and support groups for recovering students).

Project PATHE

This was one of the first comprehensive school climate change programs to be tested and to demonstrate positive results (Gottfredson, 1986). The program involves students, parents, teachers, school officials, and communities in planning teams that follow a specific planning process called the Program Development Evaluation (PDE) method, including a needs assessment, development and implementation of plans to address the substance abuse risk factors, and explicit standards for performance with constant feedback (Gottfredson, 1984; Gottfredson & Gottfredson, 1989). Hence, the school/community partnership teams are free to develop many different strategies and evaluate their effectiveness, making this project the precursor for the popular community partnership approaches. Implemented in junior high schools in Charlotte, South Carolina, this program affected many mediators and actual tobacco, alcohol, and drug use in the participating schools compared to nonparticipating schools.

Coordinated Community Partnership Approaches

In the 1990s, primary prevention specialists and funding sources are stressing a universal community partnership approach involving massive community organizing to create infrastructures to support prevention work. This area, although important as an effective prevention approach, already has been reviewed by the author (see Kumpfer, Whiteside, & Wandersman, NIDA 1997), so less about community partnerships will be included in this overview of prevention.

Community partnership approaches to prevention have become popular in recent years for several reasons:

- Coordinated efforts with non-conflicting messages are thought to be more effective than single-shot programs.

- Drug use or abuse is multicausal and comprehensive; coordinated efforts should address more risk and protective factors.

- Involving many different community organizations, including the media, as shapers of community values, attitudes, and norms, can have an impact on improving a community's norms about alcohol abuse and drug use.

- Local solutions are more effective and more likely to continue operating after the initial funding than programs designed, dictated, or operated by those outside the community.

- Community leaders across the nation believe that wide-scale community involvement of all segments of their communities is required to reduce the drug problem successfully.

This approach seeks to locate "islands of health" in high-risk neighborhoods and communities and to mobilize their combined strength to design locally tailored interventions or environmental change programs to reduce drug use. Community partnerships can mobilize substantial fiscal and voluntary support by recruiting and empowering the civic societies in a community to join them in their "war on drugs." Although schools, law enforcement agencies, alcohol and drug prevention providers, parents, and youth are frequent participants in substance abuse prevention efforts, according to a Join Together study (1993), a number of critically important community organizations have not been very involved, namely labor, business, the media, religious organizations, universities, and transportation. Since this Join Together study was completed, more religious institutions, universities, and the mass media have become involved in partnership activities. Congress recently approved $198 million in matching funds for a special partnership between the White House Office of Drug Control Policy and the Partnership for a Drug-Free America to produce a national drug-free media campaign targeting youth eight to 14 years old.

One of the earliest community partnership approaches for substance abuse prevention was the Midwestern Prevention Project (i.e.,

Project STAR) highlighted in the NIDA (1997) monograph of effective prevention programs. This prevention partnership brought together a number of community leaders in partnership with community foundations (the Kaufman Foundation and the Lilly Foundation). A number of community activities were provided, including a school-based drug prevention curriculum, parent involvement activities, community canvassing and volunteer training, a media campaign involving youth, and health policy changes. The evaluation results were quite positive (Pentz et al., 1989, 1990) and encouraged other foundations and Congress to fund community partnership programs.

Beginning with the Anti-Drug Abuse Act of 1988, Congress tasked CSAP to fund over 250 community partnerships for drug abuse prevention (Davis, 1991). Additional substance abuse prevention community partnerships have been implemented nationwide by the following groups:

- National foundations, such as the Robert Wood Johnson Foundation's Fighting Back and Join Together coalitions, the Annie Casey Family Foundation (which is working with CSAP on the Starting Early/Starting Smart initiative), and the Henry J. Kaiser Family Foundation

- Federal Public Health Service agencies and their special initiatives, such as the National Cancer Institute's COMMIT and ASSIST tobacco and cancer reduction programs (Pierce, Giovino, Hatziandreu, & Shopland, 1989), and the CDC's Planned Approach to Community Health (PATCH) health promotion program (Kreuter, 1992) and the Bureau of Justice Assistance's Weed and Seed and Comprehensive Communities programs

- State and local governments, such as the model programs in Rhode Island and the Communities That Care model (Hawkins, Catalano, & Miller, 1992) implemented originally in Oregon and later in a number of states and local communities through National Performance Review Laboratory or Weed and Seed partnerships

Despite this massive infusion of demand reduction funding into the area of community partnerships, there is still little research demonstrating the effectiveness of these approaches. Although logically appealing, there are few randomized control trials to demonstrate clearly the effectiveness of community partnerships. One of the problems is that it is almost impossible to conduct true randomized control trials with communities. To help with the difficulty in evaluating large communities, geo-mapping methods are now being used to match smaller communities and to evaluate the differential impact of prevention efforts in some communities.

Although a coordinated community approach is more likely to be effective than single-shot school curricula, this massive infusion of funding and effort ignores critical improvements in prevention programming in the Cinderellas of Prevention—family and environmentally based prevention approaches (Kumpfer, 1989).

Family-Focused Universal Prevention Approaches

More risk and protective factors can be addressed when family members are involved in drug prevention approaches. A number of youth social skills training approaches, therefore, have been combined with parent training or family skills training. Examples of school-based, universal family-focused strategies effective in reducing tobacco, alcohol, or drug use include Hawkins and Catalano's Preparing for the Drug-Free Years (Spoth, in press), Parent Drug Education Homework Involvement (Pentz et al., 1989), Iowa Strengthening Families Program (Kumpfer, Molgaard, & Spoth, 1996), and Adolescent Transitions Program (Dishion, Andrews, Kavanagh, & Soberman, 1996; Dishion, Kavanagh, & Kiesner, in press). Each of these is described in more detail in the NIDA publication, *Preventing Drug Use Among Children and Adolescents: A Research-Based Guide* (NIDA, 1997).

To increase the effect size of universal school or community programs, many well-known school-based researchers (e.g., Biglan, Botvin, Dielman/Cherry, Flay, Hawkins, Kumpfer/Spoth, Pentz, and Schinke) currently are testing the efficacy of an added parenting or family component. Family and school-focused programs showcased in the recent NIDA (1997) publication are the Project Family in Iowa, the Seattle Social Development Project (Hawkins et al., 1992), and the Adolescent Transitions Program (Dishion et al., in press) discussed in more detail below.

Effectiveness of Universal Approaches

School-based substance abuse prevention approaches have been reviewed several times (Bangert-Drowns, 1988; Bruvold & Rundall, 1988; Hansen, 1992, 1993; Moskowitz, 1989; Tobler, 1986; Tobler & Stratton, 1997). The most recent published review of effectiveness of

41 school-based substance abuse prevention approaches (Hansen, 1992), including research results from 1980 to 1990, revealed a wide variety of different theoretical bases and intervention approaches. Hansen (1992) classified them into 12 different approaches, including information, decision making, pledges, values clarification, goal setting, stress management, self-esteem building, resistance skills training, life skills training, norm setting, student assistance (peer counseling, peer leadership, professional counseling, hotlines), and alternatives. Social influence programs including resistance skills training, norm setting, and life skills had the largest percentage of positive findings: 51% positive, 38% neutral, and 11% negative. When corrections were made for programs with insufficient power (not enough schools or groups) to detect a significant change, 63% of the programs had positive results, 26% neutral, and 11% negative. After power was corrected, comprehensive school programs were more effective, with 72% positive, 28% neutral, and no negative effects reported. Among the comprehensive programs, two program models B Life Skills Training (Botvin et al., 1990) and STAR (Pentz et al. 1990) B and two other similar programs (SMART and AAPT) contribute to successful outcomes. The information/values clarification programs had mixed results: 30% positive, 40% neutral, and 30% negative outcomes. Affective education also had positive effects (42%) balanced by 25% negative effects and 33% no effect. There were not enough studies with reported results to determine overall effectiveness of the alternatives approach.

Examples of Effective Universal Programs

It appears that the most effective universal prevention programs implemented in schools are those that involve more intensive social or life skills training and often include homework assignments with parents. NIDA has been instrumental in funding research for the development and evaluation of many of these programs. *Preventing Drug Use Among Children and Adolescents: A Research-Based Guide* (NIDA, 1997) includes program descriptions of some of these exemplary school-based prevention programs. The programs listed below are universal research-based programs with positive results in reducing tobacco, alcohol, or drug initiation. Program descriptions appear in the NIDA (1997) "red book" publication:

- Adolescent Alcohol Prevention Trial (AAPT) (Donaldson et al., 1994) is an elementary school classroom program for 5th graders with booster sessions in the seventh grade. It offers normative education and resistance skills training.

- Life Skills Training (LST) Program (Botvin et al., 1990; Botvin, Baker, et al., 1995; Botvin, Schinke, et al., 1995) is a 30-session, three-year, middle school personal and social skills program.

- Project STAR (Pentz, 1995, 1997; Pentz et al., 1989) is a two-year, middle school social influence curriculum, implemented by trained teachers, combined with comprehensive community interventions.

- Seattle Social Development Project (Hawkins, Catalano, & Miller, 1992) is a comprehensive teacher training, social skills training, and parent training program.

Additional examples of effective universal programs funded by other federal agencies (National Institute on Alcohol Abuse and Alcoholism [NIAAA], CSAP, National Cancer Institute [NCI]) include the following:

- Project Northland (Perry et al., 1993; Perry et al., 1996) is a comprehensive program with developmentally appropriate activities for classrooms from elementary school to junior high school. One unique feature is a cartoon series with major characters each year and parent involvement in homework assignments.

- Alcohol Misuse Prevention Project is an alcohol prevention program (Dielman, Shope, Leech, & Butchart, 1989). This middle school classroom program reduced alcohol use significantly, but only in the highest risk youth whose parents allowed them to drink at home (Shope, Kloska, Dielman, & Maharg, 1994). Additionally, these differential results did not show up until the 8th and 9th grades in the annual follow-up study when the control group began escalation of their alcohol use. This "sleeper effect" demonstrates the need for follow-up assessments until the age when youth would normally demonstrate increasing levels of substance use for the population.

- Woodrock Youth Development Project (LoScuito, Freeman, Harrington, Altman, & Lamphear, 1997) is a comprehensive community and school program that includes human relations and skill-building workshops, drug resistance training, and psychosocial family and community supports.

- Say Yes, First (Zavala, 1996) includes training of school staff, comprehensive health education, academic improvement and enhancement programs, parent education and involvement, and drug-free alternative activities.

Crucial Ingredients

All of these prevention programs include teaching social competencies or peer-resistance skills. Some effective programs focus more on broader life skills (Botvin's LST) and some on normative changes (Hansen's All Stars). These theory-based social competency programs differ in a number of ways from other similar school-based programs found to have minimal effects (Tobler, 1986; Tobler & Stratton, 1997), such as DARE (Ennett, 1994; Hansen & McNeal, 1997). They have stronger curricula targeting a larger number of primary risk factors for drug use, improved fidelity to their curricula in implementation, increased dosage or intensity, better training of implementers, more skills-based curricula, and interactive teaching methods.

Tobler and Stratton (1997) conducted a recent meta-analysis of the effectiveness of school-based drug prevention programs. A meta-analysis involves collecting data on all the researched programs, categorizing types, and then comparing effectiveness of different major types of programs by averaging the size of the effects. Some programs have a small effect, some have a moderate effect, and some have a large effect on the precursors of drug use. This statistical analysis revealed that only programs using interactive, skills-training methods as opposed to didactic lecture methods were effective in reducing drug use risk factors and actual alcohol, tobacco, and other drug use. In other words, these universal programs sought to change behaviors by teaching skills and competencies rather than just changing knowledge and attitudes by providing lectures on the consequences of tobacco, alcohol, or drug use.

Donaldson and associates (1996) have conducted an analysis of social influence-based drug abuse prevention programs B the basis for most of the well-researched and successful prevention strategies. They conclude that "this type of programming has produced the most consistently successful preventive effects" (p. 868) with the general population, but may not be as effective with high-risk youth. Unfortunately, most of these programs rely on a mixture of several prevention approaches, so it is difficult to determine the most salient content. Donaldson and associates conclude that the most essential ingredient for success appears to be changing social norms or peer norms rather than training students in refusal skills. They warn against schools or communities implementing only a subset of the lessons of exemplary programs because of the potential of choosing only the less effective lessons.

Parent Involvement Approaches

Parent involvement approaches seek to get parents to learn about substance abuse prevention strategies by having them do homework assignments with their children. School-based prevention programs have had difficulties in attracting parents when they want to involve all parents in a universal intervention. Even when stipends for participation were offered, researchers (Grady, Gersick, & Boratynski, 1985) recruited only about one-third of the eligible parents. If parents are only requested to complete homework assignments at home with their children, parent involvement is higher. Flay and associates (1987) found 94% of students reported that their parents participated in the homework assignments and, more important, that parent involvement may have influenced program success. Perry and associates (1986, 1989) found that 70% of parents reported their adolescents had brought home a parent/adolescent smoking prevention program homework assignment. The results of Project Northland, which focuses on parent involvement in the 6th grade, show that 94% to 98% of the intervention students in 10 school districts reported that they had participated in the parent/child homework assignments (Perry et al., 1993). However, there were no significant effects on smoking or drinking by the end of the 6th grade, possibly because the base rates were very low.

Results from the Midwestern Prevention Program found that about 66% of parents (completing a parent survey about parent involvement) are willing to participate in I-STAR curriculum homework assignments with their children, 23% attended a two-session family skills training program and prevention meetings, 9% served on the parent committee, and 7% participated on the I-STAR Community Advisory Council (Rohrbach et al., in press). The independent contribution of the parent involvement strategy has not been tested in randomized clinical trials and is recommended for further research.

Project Family (Spoth, in press) is a research project that includes evaluating two universal, research-based, family-focused programs: (a) Preparing for the Drug-Free Years (PDFY), a five-session parenting program developed by Hawkins and Catalano (1994) and (b) the Iowa

Strengthening Families Program (ISFP), a seven-session family skills training program developed by Molgaard and Kumpfer (1994), which is a modification for 6th graders of the Strengthening Families Program for 6- to 10-year-olds (Kumpfer, DeMarsh, & Child, 1989). Additionally, this project conducts market research on factors related to family participation and retention as well as a statewide needs assessment for family and community needs.

Results (Spoth, Redmond, & Shin, in press) show positive effects of medium effect sizes of both family programs on child management practices and parent-child affective quality. A 2-year follow-up on ISFP found significant intervention-control differences in positive parent-child affective quality (Spoth, 1997). A one-year follow-up on ISFP showed improvements in critical mediators of substance use, namely increased peer resistance, reduced bonding to antisocial peers, and fewer problem behaviors. Using growth curve analysis, the two-year follow-up data show significant differences between the ISFP and control group in problem behaviors, gateway substance use, minor delinquency, school-related problem behaviors, and affiliation with antisocial peers. Latent transition analysis of dichotomous substance outcomes indicated positive intervention-control differences in probabilities of transitioning to more advanced stages of use. The market research (Spoth & Redmond, 1995; Spoth, Redmond, Haggerty, & Ward, 1995) suggests that parents say they would like flexible scheduling, minimal initial time commitments, contacts with parents' peers, and multiple incentives, such as food, refreshments, and child care.

Seattle Social Development Project (Hawkins et al., 1992) is a universal, comprehensive elementary school program combining teacher training in active classroom management, interactive teaching strategies, and cooperative learning with three developmentally appropriate parent training curricula: "How to Help Your Child Succeed in School," "Catch 'Em Being Good," and "Preparing for the Drug-Free Years." Longitudinal studies found reductions in drug use incidents in school and improvements in other drug use precursors (antisocial behavior, lack of academic skills, alienation and lack of school bonding, and bonding to antisocial others).

Adolescent Transition Program (ATP) (Dishion et al., in press) is a middle school multicomponent program that integrates universal, selective, and indicated approaches to meet the needs of all students and parents. A Family Resource Room is established to disseminate information about risks for substance abuse and effective family management skills through print and video materials. At the selective level, the Family Check-Up provides a family assessment and professional support to help families determine their level of risk. At the indicated level, the Parent Focus curriculum provides direct support through behavioral family therapy, parenting groups, or case management services. Results of a series of intervention trials indicate that the parent interventions are effective in reducing the escalation of drug use in high-risk youth. Also, by testing a youth-only group, with and without the parenting group, and a parenting group only, these researchers discovered that problem behaviors can worsen in child-only groups compared to the parenting-only groups.

General Practice in Universal Prevention Programs

The most popular education programs (DARE, QUEST, Here's Looking At You) are based on combinations of education, affective, social influence, and social skills training approaches. Although they contain some components, such as the social influence content, that have been found to be effective in reducing drug use in adolescents, according to Botvin (1995), their curricula are often poorly implemented and taught by individuals with little or no training or expertise. Hansen (1992) found that even when research-based programs are adopted by schools, they are frequently shortened, which omits crucial elements, and teachers stray from the content by adding their own ideas and material.

DARE Program

DARE, currently the most popular school-based prevention program, is provided to over 6 million students at a cost of over $750 million (Koch, 1994). Most of these students are fifth graders in elementary school; however, DARE has revised its curriculum nine times and now includes seventh and 10th grade boosters. In a recent survey study commissioned by DARE, 97% of the students completing the program made spontaneous positive comments about it. Its popularity with students can be explained partially by the fact that the program gives youth many gifts (e.g., tee shirts, bumper stickers) at graduation, and the police officers drive "hot" DARE cars. Teachers like it because the police officers deliver the program, thus giving the teachers a break in class. Also, it is aggressively marketed, and funding is amply available from local police departments or schools through federal sources such as NIJ and the Department of Education's (DOE) Drug-Free Schools grants.

The curriculum content originally was based on prototype versions of two Project SMART programs (Hansen et al., 1988) and included resistance skills training, self-esteem building, stress management, public commitment, and drug education on consequences. New content includes information on gangs and legal issues and involves seventh and 10th grade booster sessions.

DARE is constantly being revised to include more methods suggested to be effective by other research studies; hence, it is difficult to determine the effectiveness of the current program. Glenn Levant, the founding director of the Los Angeles-based organization, reported at the DARE annual conference attended by 2,300 police officers and educators in Salt Lake City in July 1997 that DARE is now in about 25% of schools nationwide with an annual budget of $210 million. DARE officials recommend that schools adopt the newer 17-week course that is presented in the fifth, seventh, and 10th grades.

DARE officials argue that the recent unfavorable research studies are sales tools for competing antidrug programs. However, a number of the DARE program evaluators are not competitors; they are well-respected researchers in the field. The research conducted on prior versions suggests that DARE has a small but consistently positive impact on student self-reports of reductions in tobacco use (Clayton, Cattarello, & Johnstone, in press; Ennett, Rosenbaum, et al., 1994; Ennett, Tobler, et al., 1994), but not other drugs.

Using hierarchical linear modeling (HLM) to examine how DARE affects 12 hypothesized mediating variables, Hansen and McNeal (Hansen & McNeal, 1997; McNeal & Hansen, 1992) concluded that DARE does not appear to address or affect mediators that offer strong potential paths for intervention effectiveness. Although several mediators were affected mildly by program exposure (e.g., manifest commitment not to use tobacco or alcohol, normative beliefs concerning drug dealing, social skills, and stress management), only manifest commitment was significantly associated with reduced drug use. Conversely, the increase in social skills had a nonsignificant negative impact on drug use. All other mediating variables had no effect (e.g., normative beliefs, lifestyle incongruence, consequence belief, decision skills, resistance skills, self-esteem, stress management, perceived alternatives, goal setting, and assistance skills).

DARE appears to work primarily by enhancing youth's commitment not to use tobacco, alcohol, or other drugs. Unfortunately, as youth move to higher grades, the social and internal pressures to use these substances tend to swamp the early commitment not to use them. Hansen and McNeal (1997) recommend that "the DARE program . . . be replaced by a curriculum that has the potential to target and alter variables that truly mediate substance use and other problem behaviors" (p. 175), such as normative education.

Summary and Research and Practice Recommendations

In general, reviews of the literature or meta-analyses (Hansen, 1992; Moskowitz, 1989; Tobler, 1986) show that "the hoped-for magnitude of effects of school programs are rarely achieved" (Hansen & McNeal, 1997, p. 166). Promising approaches have been identified in reviews of the research (Hansen et al., 1993), but consistently positive effects across different sites appear only for the social influence and life skills approaches (Kumpfer, 1997a, 1997b).

The appropriate response in prevention science now is to examine the reasons for such failures and to design stronger programs. The new Tobler and Stratton (1997) meta-analysis suggests that interactive methods are crucial to effective prevention programming. The social influence or social and life skills curricula involve students more in experiential exercises. Whether involvement, self-discovery, and skill building are critical ingredients in successful universal programs should be tested further in empirical research. Rather than using "black box" evaluation designs of multicomponent programs, research is needed that will allow researchers to dismantle independent variables and determine the relative contribution of the different approaches. Many universal prevention programs are so complex that it is difficult to determine the salient independent variables.

Local etiological research or needs assessments are needed to assure that the selected prevention program is addressing the most salient risk or protective factor mediators in local youth. Hawkins and Catalano (1994) use a similar approach with their Communities That Care community risk factor analysis, except that in addition to existing social indicators, direct baseline assessment of students should be used to determine criteria for matching program content to appropriate mediating processes. This approach was used for Projects PATHE and HI PATHE (Kumpfer, Turner, & Alvarado, 1991); structural equations modeling was used to verify the locally relevant pathways to drug use for males versus females and different ethnic groups (Kumpfer & Turner, 1990/1991).

Schools implementing research-based prevention approaches should seek to implement them with as much fidelity to the original curriculum and process as possible. Efforts should be made to provide sufficient training and to observe facilitators randomly to assure fidelity.

Chapter 64

"Keepin' It REAL" Program Reduces Alcohol, Tobacco, and Marijuana Use

Drug Prevention in Middle Schools

Thirty percent of middle school kids have tried alcohol, tobacco or drugs. But many middle schools often have a mix of children from different ethnic groups. Should these schools have to use drug prevention programs that are targeted to each individual group?

According to a study published in the December issue of *Prevention Science*, middle schools with a mix of Euro-American, Mexican-American and African-American children can use one multicultural curriculum (Keepin' It REAL) to help prevent and delay first-time use of alcohol, tobacco and drugs. Keepin' It REAL, developed by Penn State University and Arizona State University, teaches kids skills to "refuse, explain, avoid and leave," drug use in a way that reflects their traditions, culture and values.

"Schools don't need to use one set of prevention programs for Euro-American children, another set for Mexican-American children and yet another set for African-American children. Our study shows that a program like Keepin' It REAL, which is culturally grounded, can appeal to children of different backgrounds," according to Michael Hecht, PhD, of The Pennsylvania State University. Co-author Flavio Marsiglia, PhD of Arizona State University said the conclusions of their study were based on a survey of more than 6,000 students conducted from 1997–2001 in 10 school districts in Phoenix that used Keepin' It REAL. "Schools from many parts of the country with multi-ethnic kids are already calling to get the program," according to the study authors.

The project was not only successful in reducing alcohol, tobacco and marijuana use between 7th and 8th graders, but it also influenced adolescents' drug use norms and expectations.

Adolescents often think that many of their peers use these substances and that their friends approve when others use them as well. After participating in the Keepin' It REAL program, adolescents did not see as many benefits from substance use, were less approving of substance use, and perceived others, particularly their peers, as less approving.

The researchers said that Keepin' It REAL emphasizes individual values for Euro-American children, family solidarity and family values for Mexican-American children, and communal values for African-American children. The program uses a "from kids, through kids, to kids" approach in the narratives that describe various drug use situations faced by middle school children.

"We started developing Keepin' It REAL by trying to understand not just the different cultures among the kids, but also using some of the protective features of their cultural background. That helped to teach the kids how to say 'no' to drugs in a way that reflected and respected their own culture and the culture of other students," according to Hecht.

Chapter 65

Employee Assistance Programs and Treatment

Many firms have adopted a combination prevention/treatment philosophy. This means that persons detected using prohibited drugs or alcohol are offered a medical regimen to help them give up their drug and/or alcohol abusing lifestyle. An Employee Assistance Program (EAP) can help you properly assess an employee and refer him or her to the appropriate treatment program. Even employers who do not offer treatment to employees who are detected using drugs or alcohol usually encourage those employees to voluntarily seek treatment. EAPs provide a valuable resource for employees to turn to in identifying the proper course of treatment.

Most EAPs also include other employee services, such as financial and legal counseling, exercise and weight reduction programs, stop smoking assistance, and marriage counseling. An EAP is conceived to maximize the health and efficiency of the workforce while conveying a caring attitude on the part of the employer. EAPs often help prevent employees from starting to abuse drugs and/or alcohol by addressing personal problems before they become unmanageable by the employee. EAPs are also excellent tools for supervisors to use when dealing with troubled employees.

EAPs are paid for by the employer and make available to employees specified services. Any company considering an EAP should evaluate for itself the financial factors and success actuaries of such programs

"Employee Assistance Programs and Treatment," Chapter 5 from *Guidelines for a Drug-Free Workforce, 4th Edition*, Summer 2003, Drug Enforcement Administration (DEA), U.S. Department of Justice.

as well as the number of times an employee would be allowed to participate. Some companies set up their EAPs internally, and they are administered by employees of the company. Other companies contract with an outside entity to privately interview troubled employees and, when appropriate, refer them for treatment or counseling.

Companies that choose not to participate directly in an EAP may still offer employees a firm choice of abandoning their drug and/or alcohol abusing lifestyle in return for continued employment. Under this condition, the employer might offer a reasonable time period off the job for the employee to participate in treatment. In the absence of a formal EAP, it is a good idea for employers to maintain a list of treatment facilities that the employee can refer to for help, and to become familiar with the services the facilities offer.

Most health insurance includes some coverage for drug and alcohol treatment, but the uncovered portion of treatment is typically expected to be covered by the employee just as in the case of any other illness. Most employers offer treatment in lieu of termination only once, because offering more than one chance at treatment is not normally cost-effective.

In weighing the costs of rehabilitation, employers should consider the costs of terminating and replacing employees. When an employer has invested a considerable amount in training an employee, sometimes termination can be much more costly than rehabilitation. Consider the value of your employees. If the violating employee is your top sales person, what will happen to the sales of the company if the individual is terminated? Will he or she take along major clients when he or she leaves the company? If the violating employee has specialized skills, what will it cost the company to train a replacement? If the employee is a long-term veteran and has acquired large amounts of knowledge about the overall operation of the company, what is the cost of losing this valuable and versatile person? What about potential legal challenges of terminated employees, such as unemployment claims?

All of these costs must be weighed. And whatever you decide about one employee, you must apply to all of your workforce. Consequences for violations to your policy, and opportunities for rehabilitation treatment, must be applied consistently and in a non-discriminatory manner.

Types of EAPs

Various types of EAPs are available to employers. The most common types include:

- **Internal/In-House Programs:** These are most often found in large companies with substantial resources. The EAP staff is employed by the organization and works on-site with employees.

- **Fixed-Fee Contracts:** Employers contract directly with an EAP provider for a variety of services, e.g., counseling, employee assessment, and educational programs. Fees are usually based on the number of employees and remain the same regardless of how many employees use the EAP.

- **Fee-for-Service Contracts:** Employers contract directly with an EAP provider but pay only when employees use the services. Because this system requires employers to make individual referrals (rather than employees self-referring), care must be taken to protect employee confidentiality.

- **Consortia:** An EAP consortium generally consists of smaller employers who join together to contract with an EAP service provider. The consortium approach lowers the cost per employee.

- **Peer-Based Programs:** Less common than conventional EAPs, peer- or co-worker-based EAPs give education and training, assistance to troubled employees and referrals, all through peers and co-workers. This type of program requires considerable education and training for employees.

Not every EAP will be right for every organization. To determine whether a particular program will meet your specific needs, ask the EAP provider the following questions:

- Do your staff members hold the Certified Employee Assistance Professional (CEAP) credential?

- Do members of your staff belong to a professional EAP association?

- What is the education level of each member of your staff?

- Do you have references we can contact?

- Do you provide on-site employee education and supervisor training services?

- What cost/fee programs do you offer?

- Will you do on-site visits? Are you able to conduct a needs assessment of our organization?

- What types of counseling services are available to employees? How many sessions?

- How easy will it be for employees to use the EAP? Where and how often is the EAP available to employees?

- To which programs and services do you make referrals, and under what circumstances?

- Does the EAP have a system for evaluating the effectiveness of the program?

Professional EAP officials warn employers to shy from unscrupulous EAPs that:

- Own or manage treatment facilities, creating a possible conflict of interest;

- Refer patients to their own facilities or to the same group of facilities, indicating a hidden contract or unethical relationship exists;

- Refuse to allow clients to audit their business transactions or monitor their referrals;

- Lack the Certified Employee Assistance Professional credential.

When weighing employee assistance programs and treatment options, consider the following suggestions:

- Recognize that the identification of a drug or alcohol abuse problem is only the first step and that rehabilitation is the ultimate and most desirable goal. Provide the opportunity, when feasible and appropriate, for employees who test positive to participate in company-sponsored employee assistance and rehabilitation programs. Ensure that the programs include medical monitoring, treatment, re-testing, counseling, and after-care.

- Provide employees with referrals to local counseling and treatment centers as an alternative to, or as a supplement for, company employee assistance programs.

- Insist on a high level of accountability for employees in company-sponsored or company-referred drug rehabilitation programs. Make such programs available only to those employees who acknowledge the existence of a drug and/or alcohol problem. Stress that strict adherence to the requirements of the program and random retesting are the only alternatives to dismissal.

- Address the family and dependent problems of employees who are drug abusers, with emphasis on group, family, personal, and outpatient counseling.

Chapter 66

Drug Testing

Tests to detect drug use can be conducted using various biological specimens. Testing for alcohol is typically conducted by obtaining a breath, blood, or saliva sample. However, when a person is being monitored following treatment for alcoholism, and abstinence is expected, urine may be tested. Testing for drugs other than alcohol is typically conducted using urine samples although some employers use hair samples. Employers regulated by federal testing programs are required to use urine samples only for testing of drugs. Department of Transportation regulations require breath testing for alcohol.

Most employers test applicants and employees in one or more of the following situations:

- During an annual physical;

- Before promotions or transfers;

- Before being placed in—or routinely while in—positions involving money, security, or safety;

- After accidents;

- For past users;

- Following treatment;

"Drug Testing," Chapter 5 from *Guidelines for a Drug-Free Workforce, 4th Edition*, Summer 2003, Drug Enforcement Administration (DEA), U.S. Department of Justice.

- When referred by management through just cause or reasonable suspicion;

- On a random basis.

The only methodology for drug testing approved by the U.S. Department of Health and Human Services is urinalysis.

Urinalysis involves screening urine for the presence of drug metabolites in a relatively simple and inexpensive procedure. Samples with positive results are then subjected to a highly accurate but more expensive confirmation procedure known as gas chromatography/ mass spectrometry (GC/MS). No adverse personnel action should ever be taken before completing the two-step procedure.

Most employers look for a vendor to handle drug testing requirements. In determining how to go about drug testing and what facility to use, consider the following:

- The laboratory should provide guidance in the development of collection procedures to assure that samples are properly obtained and not falsified;

- The vendor should provide all materials for collecting samples as well as specific written instructions for doing so. These may include containers, chain-of-custody and report forms, evidence tape, prepaid tamper-proof mailers and labels. The contract price should include these items as well as courier service. Separate financial arrangements may be needed if a urine collection vendor is required in addition to the laboratory services. If a separate collection vendor is used it should be a facility that specializes in specimen collection for the purpose of workplace drug testing.

- Containers should not contain preservatives that might alter the drugs or metabolites being sought. Containers should also include a built-in temperature strip that is capable of measuring the temperature of the urine sample. This is useful in detecting sample substitutions or other attempts at cheating the test.

- The laboratory and its personnel must comply with state licensing and certification requirements.

- A clear, up-to-date laboratory methods procedure manual must be included. Most reputable laboratories follow the procedural guidelines approved by the U.S. Department of Health and Human Services.

- Tests must be performed only by technicians trained and experienced in the specific drug test procedures.

- The laboratory must furnish an analytical plan to assure that a positive test is followed by a GC/MS confirmatory test and that no results are transmitted to the company based solely on a screening result. In other words, all positives should automatically be submitted for GC/MS confirmation and quantitation.

- The limits of sensitivity and specificity for each test procedure should be defined. Most employers, including non-regulated employers, follow the cutoff levels established by the testing program of the U.S. Department of Transportation. Any change from the laboratory's normal thresholds for detection should be agreed upon in writing.

- The technical and administrative procedures used should differentiate legitimate therapeutic drug use from illicit drug use. In other words, legal medications used by the employee for legitimate medical reasons should be ruled out before a positive is declared. Many employers use the services of a physician known as a Medical Review Officer (MRO) to determine whether legal medications are involved. Employers regulated by the Department of Transportation are required to use an MRO.

- The laboratory should be able to identify any of the normally abused illegal drugs or their metabolites and to offer several "panels" or combination of tests as a cost-effective option to general testing.

- Once the specimen has arrived at the laboratory via approved courier, a confirmed written test result should be delivered within two to three days. Employer actions should never be based upon a verbal test result. Procedures should be established to maintain confidentiality both at the laboratory and in the company, and refrigerated storage of positive samples should be offered by the laboratory.

- Expert testimony in the form of written records and personal appearances concerning results, methodology, and opinions should be available with timely notification.

- Laboratory personnel, technical and managerial, should be subject to a program of drug testing.

497

In conducting drug testing, employers must balance legal liabilities due to lawsuits (brought by unhired applicants and employees who refuse to take the test or who are discharged or disciplined for positive test results) against the well-being of customers, clients, fellow employees, and members of the general public who may be injured or affected by a drug-using employee. Settlements in the former category are usually in the low thousands of dollars, while those in the latter are often in the millions.

Courts are holding more and more companies responsible for mistakes made by poorly trained personnel operating without well-conceived guidelines. As courts have declared, there is enormous liability when a company does nothing or does the wrong thing in the face of the clear evidence of drug and/or alcohol abuse throughout the workplaces of our country.

Many states have drug testing laws that determine what an employer can and cannot do. It is important that employers determine what laws, if any, exist in the states where they conduct business to ensure that the testing rules and procedures established are in compliance with state regulations.

Chapter 67

Ethnic Identification and Cultural Ties May Help Prevent Drug Use

Among Puerto Ricans, African Americans, and Asians, cultural influences and ethnic identification may significantly influence drug use. Studies conducted by National Institute on Drug Abuse (NIDA) researchers in New York City suggest that Puerto Rican and African-American adolescents who strongly identify with their communities and cultures are less vulnerable to risk factors for drug use and benefit more from protective factors than do adolescents without this identification. In San Francisco, NIDA-supported research demonstrated different patterns of drug use among different subgroups of the Asian community. These findings suggest that incorporating ethnic and cultural components into drug abuse prevention programs can make these programs more effective.

In one study, Dr. Judith Brook at the Mount Sinai School of Medicine in New York City examined the extent to which ethnic and cultural factors influenced drug-related behavior in Puerto Rican adolescents. She and her colleagues interviewed 275 males and 280 females aged 16 to 24. The researchers asked the participants to describe the importance in their lives of cultural and ethnic factors such as observation of Hispanic holidays and customs, preference for speaking Spanish or English, feelings of attachment to their ethnic group, ethnic affiliation of their friends, and the value placed on the family. The participants also answered questions designed to assess their

By Patrick Zickler, National Institute on Drug Abuse (NIDA), *NIDA Notes*, Volume 14, Number 3 (September 1999). Reviewed by David A. Cooke, M.D., April 2004.

personal risk for drug use; these risk factors included the use of drugs by parents or siblings, peer use or tolerance of drug use, perception of the riskiness of drug use, and the availability of illegal drugs in their environment. The participants were categorized into stages of drug use: no reported drug use, used alcohol or tobacco only, used marijuana but no other illicit drug, or used illicit drugs other than or in addition to marijuana.

"Other studies have looked at ethnic identification in isolation, not as an interactive part of a young person's cultural and social context," Dr. Brook says. "We wanted to determine the extent to which ethnic and cultural factors might mitigate risk factors or enhance protective factors and lead to lower stages of drug use. We found that strong ethnic identification acts to offset some risks, resulting in less drug use.

"For example, strong identification with Puerto Rican cultural factors offsets drug risks such as a father's drug use, peer tolerance of drugs, and the availability of drugs. Identification with Puerto Rican friends offsets risks associated with family tolerance for drug use and drug availability," Dr. Brook notes.

Ethnic identification also serves to amplify the effect of protective factors, Dr. Brook says. For example, among participants whose siblings were not drug users, those with a strong Puerto Rican affiliation were significantly more likely to be in a lower stage of drug use than those whose affiliation was weaker.

In a related study that focused on late-adolescent African Americans in New York City, Dr. Brook and her colleagues found a similar interaction between ethnic and cultural identification and drug use. The study involved 627 participants—259 male and 368 female—aged 16 to 25 years.

The researchers found that components of ethnic identity—such as awareness of African- American history and tradition, identification with African-American friends, or participation in African-American cultural activities such as Kwanzaa—interacted with other factors to reduce risk or to enhance protection.

"In isolation, few specific components of ethnic identity play a role as main effects on drug use. Instead, they act in combination with family, personality, or peer influences to blunt the negative impact of risk factors and magnify the positive value of protective factors," Dr. Brook says.

"Together, the research with Puerto Rican and African-American populations points out the importance of incorporating ethnic identity into drug programs," Dr. Brook concludes. "It can be a valuable part of drug prevention programs in communities and can also be applied to individual treatment programs."

Cultural Differences Lead to Different Patterns of Drug Use

In another NIDA-supported study, Dr. Tooru Nemoto and his colleagues at the University of California, San Francisco, have identified patterns of drug use among Asian drug users that are unique to ethnicity, gender, age group, and immigrant status.

"Large multiracial studies have not distinguished between Asian ethnic groups," Dr. Nemoto says. "The purpose of our study was to describe the patterns of drug use in Chinese, Filipino, and Vietnamese groups and to assess the relationship between cultural factors and drug use among the groups."

The San Francisco study was based on qualitative interviews with 35 Chinese, 31 Filipino, and 26 Vietnamese drug users who were not enrolled in treatment programs. All participants were 18 years or older, with an average age of 32.5, and had used illicit drugs more than three times per week during the preceding 6 months. Overall, immigrants and women represented 66 percent and 36 percent, respectively. However, all Vietnamese were immigrants.

Overall, participants born in the U.S. began using drugs at an earlier age—15 years—than did immigrant Asians—19 years—and were more likely than immigrants to use more than one drug. In general, women started drug use at about the same age as men—about 17.5 years—but ethnic groups showed a varied pattern. Chinese women began earlier—at 15.2 years—than Chinese men—at 18.5 years. Filipino women began using drugs later—at 15.5 years—than Filipino men—at 13.1 years. Vietnamese women in the study started drug use much later—at 27.8 years—than did Vietnamese men—at 19.9 years.

Dr. Nemoto and his colleagues identified differences in drug use among the ethnic groups. Filipino drug users were most likely to have begun drug use with marijuana, while Vietnamese drug users in the study most often started with crack or powder cocaine. Chinese and Vietnamese were twice as likely as Filipinos to be using crack as their current primary drug. Filipinos were four times more likely to be using heroin than were Chinese or Vietnamese. Filipino study participants were more likely than Chinese or Vietnamese to be injecting and less likely to be smoking drugs. There were also significant differences in the characteristics of drug user networks among the ethnic groups. For example, Filipinos were more than twice as likely as Chinese or Vietnamese participants to use drugs in groups that included members of other races or ethnic groups.

"These differences among ethnic groups have important implications for the way we design programs aimed at Asian drug users," Dr. Nemoto says. "Prevention programs should address the common factors among Asian drug users, such as stigma associated with injection drug use, but we should also be careful to incorporate factors that are unique to each target group."

Part Seven

Additional Help and Information

Chapter 68

Drug Abuse and Addiction Terms

addiction: A chronic, relapsing disease, characterized by compulsive drug seeking and use and by neurochemical and molecular changes in the brain.[1]

anabolic effects: Drug-induced growth or thickening of the body's nonreproductive tract tissues—including skeletal muscle, bones, the larynx, and vocal cords—and decrease in body fat.[1]

analgesics: A group of medications that reduce pain.[1]

androgenic effects: A drug's effects upon the growth of the male reproductive tract and the development of male secondary sexual characteristics.[1]

anorexia: Diminished appetite; aversion to food.[2]

antidepressants: A group of medications used in treating depressive disorders.[1]

ataxia: An inability to coordinate muscle activity during voluntary movement; most often due to disorders of the cerebellum or the posterior columns of the spinal cord; may involve the limbs, head, or trunk.[2]

Terms in this glossary were compiled from various publications of the National Institute on Drug Abuse (NIDA) [1] and reprinted with permission from *Stedman's Medical Dictionary, 27th Edition,* copyright © 2000 Lippincott Williams & Wilkins. All rights reserved.[2]

barbiturate: A type of central nervous system (CNS) depressant often prescribed to promote sleep.[1]

benzodiazepine: A type of CNS depressant prescribed to relieve anxiety; among the most widely prescribed medications, including Valium and Librium.[1]

buprenorphine: A new medication awaiting FDA approval for treatment of opioid addiction. It blocks the effects of opioids on the brain.[1]

central nervous system (CNS): The brain and spinal cord.[2]

CNS depressants: A class of drugs that slow CNS function, some of which are used to treat anxiety and sleeping disorders; includes barbiturates and benzodiazepines.[1]

crack cocaine: A derivative of cocaine, usually smoked, resulting in a brief, intense high. Crack is relatively inexpensive and extremely addictive.[2]

delirium: An altered state of consciousness, consisting of confusion, distractibility, disorientation, disordered thinking and memory, defective perception (illusions and hallucinations), prominent hyperactivity, agitation and autonomic nervous system overactivity; caused by a number of toxic, structural, and metabolic disorders.[2]

depressant: An agent that reduces nervous or functional activity, such as a sedative or anesthetic.[2]

detoxification: A process that allows the body to rid itself of a drug while at the same time managing the individual's symptoms of withdrawal; often the first step in a drug treatment program.[1]

dopamine: A neurotransmitter present in regions of the brain that regulate movement, emotion, motivation, and feelings of pleasure.[1]

drug abuse: Habitual use of drugs not needed for therapeutic purposes, such as solely to alter one's mood, affect, or state of consciousness, or to affect a body function unnecessarily (as in laxative abuse); nontherapeutic use of drugs.[2]

inhalant: A drug (or combination of drugs) with high vapor pressure, carried by an air current into the nasal passage, where it produces its effect.[2]

LAAM (levo-alpha-acetyl-methadol): An approved medication for the treatment of opioid addiction, taken 3 to 4 times a week.[1]

methadone: A long-acting synthetic medication that is effective in treating opioid addiction.[1]

methylphenidate hydrochloride: A central nervous system stimulant used to produce mild cortical stimulation in various types of depressions; commonly used in the treatment of hyperkinetic or hyperactive (attention deficit disorder) children.[2]

narcolepsy: A disorder characterized by uncontrollable episodes of deep sleep.[1]

narcotic hunger: The physiological craving for narcotics.[2]

norepinephrine: A neurotransmitter present in some areas of the brain and the adrenal glands; decreases smooth muscle contraction and increases heart rate; often released in response to low blood pressure or stress.[1]

opioids: Controlled drugs or narcotics most often prescribed for the management of pain; natural or synthetic chemicals based on opium's active component—morphine—that work by mimicking the actions of pain-relieving chemicals produced in the body.[1]

opiophobia: A health care provider's unfounded fear that patients will become physically dependent upon or addicted to opioids even when using them appropriately; can lead to the underprescribing of opioids for pain management.[1]

phencyclidine (PCP): A substance of abuse, used for its hallucinogenic properties, which can produce profound psychologic and behavioral disturbances; the hydrochloride has analgesic and anesthetic properties.[2]

physical dependence: An adaptive physiological state that can occur with regular drug use and results in withdrawal when drug use is discontinued.[1]

placebo: An inactive substance, used in experiments to distinguish between actual drug effects and effects that are expected by the volunteers in the experiments.[1]

polydrug abuse: The abuse of two or more drugs at the same time, such as CNS depressant abuse accompanied by abuse of alcohol.[1]

prescription drug abuse: The intentional misuse of a medication outside of the normally accepted standards of its use.[1]

prescription drug misuse: Taking a medication in a manner other than that prescribed or for a different condition than that for which the medication is prescribed.[1]

psychotherapeutics: Drugs that have an effect on the function of the brain and that often are used to treat psychiatric disorders; can include opioids, CNS depressants, and stimulants.[1]

relapse: Return of the manifestations of a disease after an interval of improvement.[2]

respiratory depression: Depression of respiration (breathing) that results in the reduced availability of oxygen to vital organs.[1]

stimulants: Drugs that enhance the activity of the brain and lead to increased heart rate, blood pressure, and respiration; used to treat only a few disorders, such as narcolepsy and attention-deficit hyperactivity disorder.[1]

tolerance: A condition in which higher doses of a drug are required to produce the same effect as experienced initially.[1]

tranquilizers: Drugs prescribed to promote sleep or reduce anxiety; this National Household Survey on Drug Abuse classification includes benzodiazepines, barbiturates, and other types of CNS depressants.[1]

withdrawal: A variety of symptoms that occur after chronic use of some drugs is reduced or stopped.[1]

Chapter 69

Drug-Related Street Terms

Street Terms for Cocaine

All-American drug
Aspirin (powder cocaine)
Barbs
Basa (crack cocaine)
Base (crack cocaine)
Bernie
Big C
Black rock (crack cocaine)
Candy sugar (powder cocaine)
CDs (crack cocaine)
Coca
Crack
Double bubble
Electric Kool-Aid (crack cocaine)
Flave (powder cocaine)
Florida snow
Foo foo
Gin
Gold dust
Happy dust
Icing
Jelly
Lady
Mama coca
Mojo
Nose stuff
Oyster stew
Paradise
Pariba (powder cocaine)
Pearl
Real tops (crack cocaine)
Rocks (crack cocaine)
Roxanne (crack cocaine)
Scorpion
Sevenup
Snow white
Sugar boogers (powder cocaine)
Twinkie (crack cocaine)
Yam (crack cocaine)
Zip

Terms in this glossary were compiled from various Office of National Drug Control Policy (ONDCP), National Drug Intelligence Center (NDIC), Drug Enforcement Agency (DEA), National Clearinghouse for Alcohol and Drug Information (NCADI), and Drug Policy Information Clearinghouse documents.

Street Terms for Crack

Jelly beans
Rooster
Tornado

Street Terms for Dextromethorphan (DXM)

DXM
Robo
Skittles
Vitamin D
Dex
Tussin

Street Terms for Ecstasy (MDMA)

B-bombs
Bens
Clarity
Conclusion
Cristal
Decadence
Dex
Disco biscuit
E
Essence
Eve
Go
Hug drug
Iboga
Love drug
Morning shot
Pollutants
Scooby snacks
Speed for lovers
Sweeties
Wheels
X

Street Terms for Gamma Hydroxybutyrate (GHB)

Cherry Meth
Fantasy
GBH
Georgia home boy
Great hormones at bedtime
Grievous bodily harm
Liquid E
Liquid Ecstasy
Liquid X
Organic quaalude
Salty water
Scoop
Sleep-500
Soap
Somatomaz
Vita-G

Street Terms for Heroin

Al Capone
Antifreeze
Ballot
Bart Simpson
Big bag
Big H
Brown sugar
Capital H
Cheese
Chip
Crank
Dead on arrival
Dirt
Dr. Feelgood
Ferry dust
George smack
Golden girl
Good horse
Hard candy
Hazel

Hero
Hombre
Horse
HRN
Isda
Jee gee
Joy
Junk
Lemonade
Mexican brown
Nice and easy
Noise
Ogoy
Old Steve
Orange line
P-dope
Pangonadalot
Peg
Perfect high
Poison
Pure
Rawhide
Ready rock
Salt
Sweet dreams
Train
White boy
Zoquete

Street Terms for Inhalants

Air blast
Ames (amyl nitrite)
Amys (amyl nitrite)
Aroma of men (isobutyl nitrite)
Bagging (using inhalants)
Bolt (isobutyl nitrite)
Boppers (amyl nitrite)
Buzz bomb (nitrous oxide)
Climax (isobutyl nitrite)
Discorama
Glading (using inhalant)

Gluey (one who sniffs or inhales glue)
Hardware (isobutyl nitrite)
Hippie crack
Honey oil
Huff
Huffing (sniffing an inhalant)
Kick
Laughing gas (nitrous oxide)
Medusa
Moon gas
Oz
Pearls (amyl nitrite)
Poor man's pot
Poppers (isobutyl nitrite, amyl nitrite)
Quicksilver (isobutyl nitrite)
Rush (isobutyl nitrite)
Shoot the breeze (nitrous oxide)
Snappers (isobutyl nitrite)
Snorting (using inhalant)
Thrust (isobutyl nitrite)
Toncho (octane booster)
Whippets (nitrous oxide)
Whiteout (isobutyl nitrite)

Street Terms for Ketamine

Cat valium
Green K
Honey oil
Jet
K
Ket
Kit kat
Purple
Special K
Special la coke
Super acid
Super C
Vitamin K

511

Street Terms for Khat

Abyssinian tea
African salad
Bushman's tea
Chat
Gat
Kat
Miraa
Oat
Qat
Somali tea
Tohai
Tschat

Street Terms for Lysergic Acid Diethylamide (LSD)

Acid
Acid cube (Sugar cube containing LSD)
Back Breaker
Battery Acid
Candy-flipping (Combining LSD and MDMA)
Come home (End a LSD "trip")
Doses
Dots
Elvis
Flash (LSD with cocaine injection)
Loony Toons
Lucy in the sky with diamonds
Outer Limits (Crack and LSD)
Pane
Superman
Trails (LSD-induced perception of moving objects with trails behind them)
Window pane
Zen

Street Terms for Methadone

Amidone
Chocolate chip cookies (methadone or heroin combined with MDMA)
Fizzies
Street methadone
Wafer

Street Terms for Methamphetamine

Blue meth
Chicken feed
Cinnamon
Crink
Crystal meth
Desocsins
Geep
Granulated orange
Hot ice
Ice
Kaksonjae
L.A. glass
Lemon drop
Meth
OZs
Peanut butter
Sketch
Spoosh
Stove top
Super ice
Tick tick
Trash
Wash
Working man's cocaine
Yellow barn
Yellow powder

Street Terms for OxyContin

40 (a 40-milligram tablet)
80 (an 80-milligram tablet)
Blue
Hillbilly heroin
Kicker
OCs
Ox
Oxy
Oxycotton

Street Terms for Psilocybin

Boomers
Flower flipping (MDMA used
    with psilocybin)
God's flesh
Hippieflip (MDMA used with
    psilocybin)
Hombrecitos
Las mujercitas
Little smoke
Magic mushroom
Mushroom
Mexican mushrooms
Musk
Sacred mushroom
Shrooms

Silly putty
Simple simon

Street Terms for Rohypnol
(from ONDCP)

Circles
Forget me drug
Forget me pill
Getting roached
La Rocha
Lunch money drug
Mexican valium
Pingus
R-2
Reynolds
Rib
Roach-2
Roapies
Robutal
Roofies
Rope
Rophies
Row-shay
Ruffles
Wolfies

Street Terms for Yaba

Crazy medicine
Nazi speed

Chapter 70

Directory of Drug Abuse Information, Prevention, and Treatment Organizations

The resources in this chapter are listed according to the following topics:

- **General Information Resources:** Resources in this section offer information about various substances of abuse, related mental health issues, statistical data, and facts about addiction research. See page 516.

- **Prevention Resources:** Organizations and agencies listed in this section offer information about formal and informal drug prevention efforts in the home, school, community and workplace. See page 525.

- **Treatment Resources:** This section includes resources for information about overcoming addictions and maintaining recovery. See page 539.

- **Drug Policy and Enforcement:** Resources listed in this section provide information about public policy matters and drug enforcement issues. See page 547.

This chapter includes excerpts from "A Topical Listing of Drug-Related Web Sites and Resources," Office of National Drug Control Policy, http://www.whitehousedrugpolicy.gov/links/topical.html along with additional information from the Substance Abuse and Mental Health Services Administration (SAMHSA), the National Institute on Drug Abuse (NIDA), and other sources deemed reliable. Inclusion does not constitute endorsement. All contact information was verified in June 2004.

General Information Resources

Alcohol and Drug Abuse Institute (ADAI)
University of Washington
1107 NE 45th St., Suite 120
Seattle, WA 98105-4631
Phone: 206-543-0937
Fax: 206-543-5473
Website: http://depts.washington.edu/adai
E-mail: adai@u.washington.edu

The ADAI mission is to conduct and support substance abuse research and to disseminate research findings.

American Academy of Child and Adolescent Psychiatry (AACAP)
3615 Wisconsin Ave. NW
Washington, DC 20016-3007
Phone: 202-966-7300
Fax: 202-966-2891
Website: http://www.aacap.org

AACAP provides information about a wide variety of mental health issues, including substance abuse.

American Academy of Pediatrics (AAP)
141 Northwest Point Blvd.
Elk Grove, IL 60007-1098
Phone: 847-434-4000
Fax: 847-434-8000
Website: http://www.aap.org
E-mail: kidsdocs@aap.org

AAP offers information related to all aspects of children's health, including substance abuse prevention and treatment.

American College of Obstetricians and Gynecologists (ACOG)
409 12th St. SW
Washington, DC 20090-6920
Toll-Free: 800-762-2264
Phone: 202-479-0054
Website: http://www.acog.org

ACOG provides information about women's health, including facts about risks related to substance use during pregnancy.

American Medical Association (AMA)
515 N. State St.
Chicago, IL 60610
Toll-Free: 800-621-8335
Website: http://www.ama-assn.org

A professional organization for physicians, the AMA also provides information for patients.

Arrestee Drug Abuse Monitoring Program (ADAM)
National Institute of Justice
810 Seventh St., NW
Washington, DC 20531
Website: http://www.ojp.usdoj.gov/nij/adam

This program tracks trends in the prevalence and type of drug use among booked arrestees in selected urban areas.

Association for Medical Education and Research in Substance Abuse (AMERSA)
125 Whipple St.
3rd Floor, Suite 300
Providence, RI 02908
Phone: 401-349-0000
Fax: 877-418-8769
Website: http://www.amersa.org

AMERSA was founded in 1976 by members of the Career Teachers Program, a multidisciplinary health professional faculty development program supported by the National Institute on Alcohol Abuse and Alcoholism and the National Institute on Drug Abuse.

Center for Alcohol and Addiction Studies (CAAS)
Brown University
Box G-BH
Providence, RI 02912
Phone: 401-444-1800
Fax: 401-444-1850
Website: http://www.caas.brown.edu
E-mail: CAAS@brown.edu

The Center's mission is to promote the identification, prevention, and effective treatment of alcohol and other drug use problems in our society through research, publications, education, and training.

Center for Interventions, Treatment and Addictions Research (CITAR)

Wright State University School of Medicine
216 Medical Sciences Bldg.
3640 Colonel Glenn Highway
Dayton, OH 45435
Phone: 937-775-2850
Website: http://www.med.wright.edu/citar

The Center for Interventions, Treatment and Addictions Research (CITAR) is the focal point for substance abuse-related services, academic research, and services research at the Wright State University School of Medicine. They focus on substance abuse issues in small and mid-sized cities and surrounding suburban and rural communities.

Center for Substance Abuse Research (CESAR)

4321 Hartwick Road, Suite 501
College Park, MD 20740
Phone: 301-405-9770
Fax: 301-403-8342
Website: http://www.cesar.umd.edu
E-mail: cesar@cesar.umd.edu

The mission of this research center is to collect, analyze, and disseminate information on the extent of substance abuse and related problems in Maryland and nationally.

Center for the Neurobiological Investigation of Drug Abuse

Department of Physiology and Pharmacology
Wake Forest University School of Medicine
Medical Center Boulevard
Winston-Salem, NC 27157
Phone 336-716-0083
Fax: 336-716-0237
Website: http://www.bgsm.edu/physpharm/cnida

The purpose of the Center is to provide a research environment that allows investigators with major interests in substance abuse to work together on joint research projects that utilize the broad research expertise of each individual. The internationally recognized faculty with research, training, and service interests related to the actions of drugs of abuse on the brain and the biological basis of drug addiction are the essence of this Center.

Centers for Disease Control and Prevention (CDC)
1600 Clifton Road
MS D-25
Atlanta, GA 30333
Toll-Free: 800-311-3435
Phone: 404-639-3311
Fax: 404-639-7394
Website: http://www.cdc.gov
E-mail: ccdinfo@cdc.gov

The Centers for Disease Control and Prevention (CDC) is recognized as the lead federal agency for protecting the health and safety of people—at home and abroad, providing credible information to enhance health decisions, and promoting health. Information about substance use, its effects on various components of human health, and statistical information is available through the various individual centers that comprise the CDC.

College on Problems of Drug Dependence (CPDD)
3420 N. Broad Street
Philadelphia, PA 19140
Phone: 215-707-3242
Fax: 215-707-1904
Website: http://www.cpdd.vcu.edu

This professional organization of scientists directs its research toward a better understanding of drug abuse and addiction.

DoD Counter-Narcoterrorsim Technology Program Office
17320 Dahlgren Road, Code B07
Dahlgren, VA 22448-5100
Phone: 540-653-2374
Website: http://www.cntpo.com
Website: cntpo@nswc.navy.mil

This Department of Defense program is responsible for developing and demonstrating technology and specific counterdrug system solutions.

Drug Abuse Warning Network (DAWN)
SAMHSA Office of Applied Studies
5600 Fishers Lane, Room 16-105
Rockville, MD 20857
Toll-Free: 800-FYI-DAWN
Phone: 301-443-6239
Website: http://dawninfo.samhsa.gov

519

This site provides information on DAWN, a national public health surveillance system that monitors trends in drug-related emergency department visits and deaths.

DrugAnswer.com
Website: http://www.druganswer.com

This website provides information on inhalants and marijuana in Chinese, Korean, Vietnamese, and Cambodian.

DrugStory.org
Website: http://www.drugstory.org

Sponsored by the Office of National Drug Control Policy, this is an informational resource for entertainment writers and feature journalists.

ePeerVoices.com
Website: http://www.coalitionpathways.com

This website contains information about drugs, alcohol, and tobacco; links to other authoritative websites; and provides young people with the opportunity to talk with peers about related issues.

Freevibe.com
1615 L Street NW, Suite 1000
Washington, DC 20036
Website: http://www.freevibe.com
E-mail: contactus@freevibe.com

This website provides drug-related information and other resources for youth.

HIV.drugabuse.gov
6001 Executive Blvd.
Bethesda, MD 20892-9561
Phone: 301-443-1124
Website: http://hiv.drugabuse.gov
E-mail: information@lists.nida.nih.gov

This National Institute on Drug Abuse (NIDA)-sponsored website explains that an estimated one-third of HIV/AIDS cases are related to injecting drug use and that the use of drugs, injected or not, can endanger one's health and the health of others.

Robert Wood Johnson Foundation
Substance Abuse Resource Center
P.O. Box 2316
Princeton, NJ 08543
Toll-Free: 888-631-9989
Fax: 609-627-6401
Website: http://www.rwjf.org
E-mail: mail@rwjf.org

This center provides information and news about the abuse of alcohol, tobacco, and illegal drugs and efforts to prevent harm from their use.

KidsHealth
Nemours Center for Children's Health Media
1600 Rockland Road
Wilmington, DE 19803
Phone: 302-651-4000
Fax: 302-651-4055
Website: http://kidshealth.org
E-mail: info@kidshealth.org

KidsHealth provides information to parents and children about a wide variety of health-related issues, including substance abuse.

Marijuana-info.org
6001 Executive Blvd.
Bethesda, MD 20892-9561
Phone: 301-443-1124
Website: http://www.marijuana-info.org
E-mail: information@lists.nida.nih.gov

This NIDA-sponsored website addresses common questions regarding the use and effects of marijuana.

Marijuana Policy Project (MPP) Foundation
P.O. Box 77492
Washington, DC 20013
Phone: 202-462-5747
Fax: 202-232-0442
Website: http://www.mpp.org
E-mail: mpp@mpp.org

MPP seeks to have criminal penalties associated with the use of marijuana removed.

Monitoring the Future (MTF)

University of Michigan
412 Maynard
Ann Arbor, MI 48109-1399
Website: http://monitoringthefuture.org
E-mail: MTFinfo@isr.umich.edu

This is an ongoing study of behavior (including drug/alcohol use), attitudes, and values of American secondary students and young adults.

National Association of State Alcohol and Drug Abuse Directors (NASADAD)

808 17th Street NW
Suite 410
Washington, DC 20006
Phone: 202-293-0090
Fax: 202-293-1250
Website: http://www.nasadad.org
E-mail: dcoffice@nasadad.org

This organization strives to foster and support the development of effective alcohol and other drug abuse prevention and treatment programs throughout every state.

National Center for Health Statistics (NCHS)

3311 Toledo Road
Metro IV Building
Hyattsville, MD 20782
Phone: 301-458-4000
Website: http://www.cdc.gov/nchs
E-mail: nchsquery@cdc.gov

NCHS compiles statistics on a wide variety of health related concerns, including substance use, prevention, and treatment.

National Center on Addiction and Substance Abuse at Columbia University (CASA)

633 Third Ave., 19th Floor
New York, NY 10017-6706
Toll-Free: 800-662-HELP (4357)
Phone: 212-841-5200
Website: http://www.casacolumbia.org

This think/action tank engages all disciplines to study every form of substance abuse as it affects society. CASA also offers a library of information related to illegal drugs, tobacco, alcohol, drug policy, and treatment and prevention efficacy.

National Clearinghouse for Alcohol and Drug Information (NCADI)
11420 Rockville Pike
Rockville, MD 20852
Toll-Free: 800-729-6686
Phone: 301-770-5800
Fax: 301-468-7394
TDD: 800-487-4889
Website: http://www.health.org
E-mail: webmaster@health.org

NCADI is the federally funded information service for the Center for Substance Abuse Prevention and other U.S. Department of Health and Human Services agencies.

National Institute of Child Health and Human Development (NICHD)
P.O. Box 3006
Rockville, MD 20847
Toll-Free: 800-370-2943
Phone: 301-496-0536
Fax: 301-496-7101
Website: http://www.nichd.nih.gov
E-mail: NICHDInformationResourceCenter@mail.nih.gov

NICHD is one of the institutes that comprise the National Institutes of Health. The mission of the NICHD is to ensure that every person is born healthy and wanted, that women suffer no harmful effects from reproductive processes, and that all children have the chance to achieve their full potential for healthy and productive lives, free from disease or disability, and to ensure the health, productivity, independence, and well-being of all people through optimal rehabilitation.

National Institute on Alcohol Abuse and Alcoholism (NIAAA)
5635 Fishers Lane, MSC 9304
Bethesda, MD 20892-9304

Phone: 301-496-8176
Website: http://www.niaaa.nih.gov

NIAAA is the lead Institute responsible for research on the causes, consequences, treatment, and prevention of alcohol-related problems.

National Institute on Drug Abuse (NIDA)
6001 Executive Blvd., Room 5213
Bethesda, MD 20892-9561
Phone: 301-443-1124
Website: http://www.nida.nih.gov
E-mail: Information@lists.nida.nih.gov

NIDA supports over 85 percent of the world's research on the health aspects of drug abuse and addiction.

Office of Applied Studies (OAS)
Substance Abuse and Mental Health Services Administration (SAMHSA)
5600 Fishers Lane, Room 16-105
Rockville, MD 20857
Phone: 301-443-6239
Website: http://www.oas.samhsa.gov

OAS collects data on the national prevalence of substance abuse, drug abuse consequences, treatment admissions, and facilities.

Straight Scoop News Bureau
http://www.straightscoop.org

This is an online resource for middle and high school students interested in reporting factual drug-related information.

Substance Abuse and Mental Health Services Administration (SAMHSA)
5600 Fishers Lane
Room 12-105, Parklawn Building
Rockville, MD 20857
Phone: 301-443-4795
Fax: 301-443-0284
Website: http://www.samhsa.gov
E-mail: info@samhsa.gov

SAMHSA offers a broad range of programs focusing on prevention and treatment of the abuse of illicit drugs.

Substance Abuse Librarians and Information Specialists (SALIS)
P.O. Box 9513
Berkeley, CA 94709-0513
Phone: 510-642-5208
Fax: 510-642-7175
Website: http://salis.org
E-mail: salis@arg.org

This is an international association of individuals and organizations with special interests in the exchange and dissemination of alcohol, tobacco, and other drug information.

U.S. Department of Health and Human Services (HHS)
200 Independence Ave. SW
Washington, DC 20201
Toll-Free: 877-696-6775
Phone: 202-619-0257
Website: http://www.hhs.gov

HHS is the United States government's principal agency for protecting the health of all Americans and providing essential human services. More than 300 programs cover a wide spectrum of activities, including substance abuse treatment and prevention.

Web of Addictions
Website: http://www.well.com/user/woa

The Web of Addictions was developed for several reasons: concern about the pro drug use messages in some websites and in some use groups; concern about the extent of misinformation about abused drugs on the internet, particularly on some usenet news groups; and to provide a resource for teachers, students, and others who need information about abused drugs.

Prevention Resources

American Council for Drug Education (ACDE)
164 W. 74th St.
New York, NY 10023
Toll-Free: 800-488-DRUG
Website: http://www.acde.org
E-mail: acde@phoenixhouse.org

This substance abuse prevention organization develops programs and materials based on the most current scientific research on drug use and its impact on society.

Anti-Drug.Com
Website: http://www.theantidrug.com

This website equips parents and other adult caregivers with the tools they need to raise drug-free kids.

Big Brothers Big Sisters of America
230 North 13th St.
Philadelphia, PA 19107
Phone: 215-567-7000
Website: http://www.bbbsa.org
E-mail: enroll@bbbsa.org

This organization provides one-to-one mentoring relationships between adult volunteers and children in over 500 programs throughout the U.S.

Boys and Girls Clubs of America
1230 W. Peachtree Street, NW
Atlanta, GA 30309
Toll-Free: 800-854-CLUB
Phone: 404-487-5700
Website: http://www.bgca.org
E-mail: info@bgca.org

This organization provides a safe place for youth to learn and grow.

Center for Substance Abuse Prevention (CSAP)
5600 Fishers Lane
Room 12-105, Rockwall Building
Rockville, MD 20857
Phone: 301-443-0365
Fax: 301-443-5447
Website: http://prevention.samhsa.gov
E-mail: info@samhsa.gov

CSAP provides national leadership in the development of policies, programs, and services to prevent the onset of illegal drug use, to prevent underage alcohol and tobacco use, and to reduce the negative consequences of using substances. CSAP is one of three centers in the

Substance Abuse and Mental Health Services Administration (SAMHSA) in the U.S. Department of Health and Human Services (HHS).

Check Yourself
Website: http://www.checkyourself.org
E-mail: cyfeedback@drugfree.org

This website, sponsored by Partnership for a Drug-Free America, is designed to lead 15- to 18-year-old recreational drug and alcohol users to reconsider their relationships with their substances of choice and ultimately curtail their use.

Citizens Against Drug Impaired Drivers (CANDID)
P.O. Box 170970
Milwaukee, WI 53217-0705
Toll-Free: 800-929-9077
Phone: 414-352-2043
Fax: 414-352-7080
Website: http://www.candid.org
E-mail: candid@candid.org

CANDID is committed to reducing the number of injuries and fatalities due to drug-impaired drivers by increasing the awareness of the risks involved when driving under the influence of illicit, prescription, or over-the-counter drugs.

Club Drugs
National Institute on Drug Abuse (NIDA)
6001 Executive Blvd.
Bethesda, MD 20892-9561
Phone: 301-443-1124
Website: http://www.clubdrugs.org

This NIDA-sponsored website seeks to alert people to the serious health consequences that can arise from the use of drugs such as MDMA (Ecstasy), GHB, Rohypnol, ketamine, methamphetamine, and LSD.

College Drinking: Changing the Culture
National Institute on Alcohol Abuse and Alcoholism (NIAAA)
6000 Executive Blvd., Wilco Bldg.
Bethesda, MD 20892-7003
Website: http://www.collegedrinkingprevention.gov

This website sponsored by the National Institute on Alcoholism and Alcohol Abuse (NIAAA) provides information on preventing alcohol abuse on college campuses for a variety of audiences including students, parents, and community leaders.

Common Sense
Website: http://www.pta.org/commonsense

Sponsored by the National PTA (Parent Teacher Association), Common Sense provides information about raising children to be alcohol- and drug-free.

Community Anti-Drug Coalitions of America (CADCA)
625 Slaters Lane
Suite 300
Alexandria, VA 22314
Toll-Free: 800-54-CADCA
Fax: 703-706-0565
Website: http://cadca.org

This is a membership organization of over 5,000 anti-drug coalitions working to make their communities safe, healthy, and drug-free.

Drug Abuse Resistance Education (DARE)
9800 La Cienega Blvd.
Suite 401
Inglewood, CA 90301
Toll-Free: 800-223-3273
Phone: 310-215-0575
Fax: 310-215-0180
Website: http://www.dare.com

This police officer-led program of classroom lessons that teaches youth how to resist peer pressure and live drug- and violence-free lives. The website for this anti-drug, anti-violence organization contains a section for kids and a section for parents, teachers, and officers.

Drug Free America Foundation, Inc.
P.O. Box 11298
St. Petersburg, FL 33733-1298
Phone: 727-828-0211
Fax: 727-828-0212
Website: http://www.dfaf.org

The Drug Free America Foundation is a drug prevention organization committed to reducing drug use, addiction, and drug-related injury and death.

Drug-Free Youth in Town (DFYIT)
16201 SW 95 Avenue
Suite 205
Miami, FL 33157
Phone: 305-971-0607
Fax 305-971-4632
Website: http://www.dfyit.org

This organization supports the development of healthy, productive, drug-free youth.

Elks Drug Awareness Resource Center
2750 N. Lakeview Avenue
Chicago, IL 60614-1889
Phone: 773-755-4700
Fax: 773-755-4790
Website: http://www.elks.org/drugs
E-mail: dap@elks.org

This program works to prevent youth drug use through education by reaching parents, teachers, and students in grades four through nine.

Family Guide to Keeping Youth Mentally Healthy and Drug Free
Website: http://family.samhsa.gov

This site was developed to support the efforts of parents and other caregivers to promote mental health and prevent the use of alcohol, tobacco, and illegal drugs among youth.

Fighting Back
Website: http://www.fightingback.org
E-mail: info@fightingback.org

This project was created to test the hypothesis that a broad collaboration of community elements could develop a central strategy to harness and focus their collective resources to significantly reduce their most serious substance abuse problems.

Free to Grow (FTG)
Mailman School of Public Health
Columbia University
722 West 168th Street, 8th Floor
New York, NY 10032
Phone: 212-305-8120
Fax: 212-342-1963
Website: http://www.freetogrow.org
E-mail: info@freetogrow.org

FTG is a national demonstration program testing an innovative approach to two closely related public health problems—substance abuse and child abuse.

General Federation of Women's Clubs (GFWC)
1734 N Street, NW
Washington, DC 20036
Phone: 202-347-3168
Fax: 202-835-0246
Website: http://www.gfwc.org
E-mail: gfwc@gfwc.org

This volunteer service organization promotes education, encourages healthy lifestyles, and stresses civic involvement.

Girls and Boys Town
14100 Crawford St.
Boys Town, NE 68010
Hotline: 800-448-3000
Phone: 402-498-1300 (8 a.m. to 5 p.m. CST Monday through Friday)
Fax: 402-498-1348
Website: http://www.girlsandboystown.org
E-mail: Hotline@girlsandboystown.org

With locations across the U.S., this organization offers help to abused, abandoned, neglected, handicapped, and troubled children.

Girls Incorporated
120 Wall Street
New York, NY 10005-3902
Toll-Free: 800-374-4475
Website: http://www.girlsinc.org

This national nonprofit youth organization provides education programs to millions of American girls, primarily those in high-risk, underserved areas.

Girl Power!
Website: http://www.girlpower.gov
E-mail: gpower@health.org

This site seeks to reinforce and sustain positive values among girls ages 9–14 by targeting health messages to the unique needs, interests, and challenges of girls.

Global Youth Network
P.O. Box 500
A-1400 Vienna
Austria
Phone: +43-1-26060 4244, Fax: +43-1-26060 5928
Website: http://www.unodc.org/youthnet

Run by the United Nations Drug Control Program (UNDCP), the purpose of this project is to increase youth involvement with the international community in developing drug abuse prevention policies and programs.

Help Your Community
Toll-Free: 877-KIDS-313
Website: http://www.helpyourcommunity.org
E-mail: info@helpyourcommunity.org

This online resource educates the public and encourages involvement in community anti-drug coalitions.

Higher Education Center for Alcohol and Other Drug Prevention
Education Development Center, Inc.
55 Chapel Street
Newton, MA 02458-1060
Phone: 800-676-1730, Fax: 617-928-1537
Website: http://www.edc.org/hec
E-mail: HigherEdCtr@edc.org

Established by the U.S. Department of Education, this organization provides support to all institutions of higher education in their efforts to address alcohol and other drug problems.

Hispanic/Latino Portal for Drug Prevention
Website: http://www.latino.prev.info
E-mail: seitzb@indiana.edu

This site provides information on prevention; alcohol, tobacco, and other drugs; HIV/AIDS; general health resources; asset building; and research tools in English, Spanish, and Portuguese.

Indiana Prevention Resource Center (IPRC)
Indiana University
Creative Arts Building
2735 E. 10th St., Room 110
Bloomington, IN 47408-2602
Toll-Free: 800-346-3077 (in Indiana)
Phone: 812-855-1237
Fax: 812-855-4940
Website: http://www.drugs.indiana.edu

IPRC provides resources related to alcohol, tobacco and other drug prevention.

Inhalant Abuse
Alliance for Consumer Education
900 17th Street, NW, Suite 300
Washington, DC 20006
Phone: 202-862-3902
Fax: 202-872-8114
Website: http://www.inhalant.org
E-mail: drugprc@indiana.edu

This site is designed for use by parents and includes information on what inhalant abuse is, the dangers and warning signs of abuse, tips for talking to kids, downloadable brochures and related links.

Join Together Online (JTO)
1 Appleton St., 4th Floor
Boston, MA 02116-5223
Phone: 617-437-1500
Fax: 617-437-9394
Website: http://www.jointogether.org
E-mail: info@jointogether.org

This organization supports community-based efforts to reduce, prevent, and treat substance abuse across the nation.

Leadership to Keep Children Alcohol Free
c/o The CDM Group, Inc.
5530 Wisconsin Avenue, Suite 1600
Chevy Chase, MD 20815-4305
Phone: 301-654-6740
Fax: 301-656-4012
Website: http://www.alcoholfreechildren.org
E-mail: leadership@alcoholfreechildren.org

This coalition strives to prevent the use of alcohol by children ages 9–15.

Misuse of Prescription Pain Relievers Can Kill You
Website: http://www.rx.samhsa.gov

This SAMHSA website provides posters, public service announcements, brochures, news, and other resources on the dangers of prescription pain relievers.

Mothers Against Drunk Driving (MADD)
511 E. John Carpenter Frwy., Suite 700
Irving, TX 75062
Toll-Free: 800-GET-MADD (438-6233)
Phone: 214-744-6233
Fax: 972-869-2206
Website: http://www.madd.org

MADD focuses on looking for effective solutions to the drunk driving and underage drinking problems.

National Association on Alcohol, Drugs and Disability (NAADD)
2165 Bunker Hill Drive
San Mateo, CA 94402-3801
Phone/TTY: 650-578-8047
Fax: 650-286-9205
Website: http://www.naadd.org

NAADD seeks to educate people with disabilities about drug dependency and related issues.

National Crime Prevention Council (NCPC)
1000 Connecticut Ave. NW, 13th Floor
Washington, DC 20036

Phone: 202-466-6272
Fax: 202-296-1356
Website: http://www.ncpc.org
E-mail: webmaster@ncpc.org

NCPC works to ensure safe communities by addressing common sources of crime and violence, including the development of strategies to reduce substance abuse.

National Families in Action (NFIA)

2957 Clairmont Road, NE, Suite 150
Atlanta, GA 30329
Phone: 404-248-9676
Fax: 404-248-1312
Website: http://www.nationalfamilies.org
E-mail: nfia@nationalfamilies.org

NFIA's mission is to help families and communities prevent drug use among children by promoting policies based on science.

National Family Partnership (NFP)

2490 Coral Way, Suite 501
Miami, FL 33145
Toll-Free: 800-705-8997
Phone: 305-856-4886
Fax: 305-856-4815
Website: http://www.nfp.org

The goal of National Family Partnership is to help children grow up drug-free.

National Inhalant Prevention Coalition (NIPC)

2904 Kerbey Lane
Austin, TX 78703
Toll-Free: 800-269-4237
Phone: 512-480-8953
Fax: 512-477-3932
Website: http://www.inhalants.org
E-mail: nipc@io.com

NIPC acts as an inhalant referral and information clearinghouse and strives to promote awareness and recognition of the inhalant abuse problem.

National Youth Anti-Drug Media Campaign
Website: http://www.mediacampaign.org

National Youth Anti-Drug Media Campaign is an initiative launched by the White House Office of National Drug Control Policy (ONDCP) in 1998 to use different media to help promote the avoidance of illicit drugs.

Navy Alcohol and Drug Abuse Prevention Program (NADAP)
Department of the Navy
Navy Personnel Command
PERS-671
5720 Integrity Dr.
Millington, TN 38055-6000
Website: http://navdweb.spawar.navy.mil

The NADAP site provides information and assistance to support drug abuse prevention efforts.

NIDA for Teens: The Science Behind Drug Abuse
6001 Executive Blvd.
Bethesda, MD 20892-9561
Phone: 301-443-1124
Website: http://teens.drugabuse.gov

This site educates adolescents (as well as parents and teachers) on the science behind drug abuse.

NIDA Goes Back to School
6001 Executive Blvd.
Bethesda, MD 20892-9561
Phone: 301-443-1124
Website: http://backtoschool.drugabuse.gov

NIDA Goes Back to School provides information, including the latest science-based drug abuse publications and teaching materials.

Parenting IS Prevention
Website: http://www.parentingisprevention.org
E-mail: pipp@nationalfamilies.org

The mission of this website is to provide accurate information, support, and resources to assist parents and others in raising children to be healthy and drug-free. A list of resources by state is also included.

Parents' Resource Institute for Drug Education (PRIDE)
PRIDE Surveys
166 St. Charles Street
Bowling Green, KY 42101
Phone: 800-279-6361
Fax: 270-746-9598
Website: http://www.pridesurveys.com

This organization is the largest and oldest in the nation devoted to drug- and violence-free youth.

Partnership for a Drug-Free America
405 Lexington Ave., Suite 1601
New York, NY 10174
Phone: 212-922-1560
Fax: 212-922-1570
Website: http://www.drugfreeamerica.org
E-mail: webmail@drugfree.org

The mission of this nonprofit coalition of professionals from the communications industry is to help teens reject substance abuse.

Partnership for Prevention
1015 18th Street NW, Suite 200
Washington, DC 20036
Phone: 202-833-0009
Fax: 202-833-0113
Website: http://www.prevent.org
E-mail: info@prevent.org

Partnership for Prevention seeks to prevent injury and illness by promoting healthy living.

Prevention Pathways
Website: http://preventionpathways.samhsa.gov

This Center for Substance Abuse Prevention website is a gateway to information on prevention programs, program implementation, evaluation technical assistance, online courses, and other prevention resources.

RADAR Network
P.O. Box 2345
Rockville, MD 20847-2345

Toll-Free: 800-729-6686
TDD: 800-487-4889
Website: http://ncadi.samhsa.gov/radar

The mission of the RADAR Network is to strengthen communication, prevention, and treatment activities so that a broad range of organizations can communicate and help each other prevent substance abuse problems.

Reclaiming Futures
National Program Office
Portland State University
527 SW Hall, Suite 400
Portland, OR 97201
Phone: 503-725-8911
Fax: 503-725-8915
Website: http://www.reclaimingfutures.org

This program provides leadership in building community solutions to substance abuse and juvenile delinquency.

Rotary International
One Rotary Center
1560 Sherman Ave.
Evanston, IL 60201
Phone: 847-866-3000
Fax: 847-328-8554 or 847-328-8281
Website: http://www.rotary.org/programs/abuse/index.html

This organization encourages Rotary clubs across the nation to investigate drug and alcohol abuse problems in their communities and identify resources to combat these problems.

School Zone
Website: http://www.whitehousedrugpolicy.gov/schoolzone

This ONDCP-sponsored website contains resources and materials for teachers, coaches, parents, students, and guidance counselors.

Society for Prevention Research
7531 Leesburg Pike, Suite 300
Falls Church, VA 22043
Phone: 703-288-0801
Fax: 703-288-0802
Website: http://www.preventionresearch.org

The focus of this society is broadly defined and concerned with the problems pertaining to the prevention of drug and alcohol abuse, and associated social maladjustment, crime, and behavior disorders.

Students Against Destructive Decisions (SADD)
P.O. Box 800
Marlborough, MA 01752
Toll-Free: 877-SADD-INC
Fax: 508-481-5759
Website: http://www.saddonline.com

SADD is a peer leadership organization dedicated to preventing underage drinking and drug use by focusing attention on the consequences of destructive decisions.

UK Center for Prevention Research
University of Kentucky
School of Public Health, College of Medicine
2365 Harrodsburg Road, Suite B100
Lexington, KY 40504-3381
Phone: 859-257-5588
Fax: 859-257-5592
Website: http://www.uky.edu/RGS/PreventionResearch

This research center, founded in 1987, focuses on understanding and preventing harmful social behaviors.

Wisconsin Clearinghouse for Prevention Resources
1552 University Avenue
Madison, WI 53726-4085
Phone: 608-262-9157
Fax: 608-262-6346
Website: http://wch.uhs.wisc.edu

Wisconsin Clearinghouse for Prevention Resources is part of the University Health Services at the University of Wisconsin-Madison and provides educational materials and training information.

Working Partners for an Alcohol- and Drug-Free Workplace
U.S. Department of Labor
Frances Perkins Building
200 Constitution Avenue, NW
Washington, DC 20210

Toll-Free: 866-4-USA-DOL
TTY: 877-889-5627
Website: http://www.dol.gov/workingpartners

This Department of Labor program provides employers with resources and tools to address the problematic use by employees of alcohol and drugs.

Workplace Resource Center
Toll-Free: 800-WORKPLACE
Website: http://workplace.samhsa.gov

This site provides centralized access to information about drug-free workplaces and related topics.

Treatment Resources

Alcoholics Anonymous (AA)
475 Riverside Drive, 11th Floor
New York, NY 10015
Phone: 212-870-3400
Website: http://www.aa.org

AA is a non-professional, mutual help organization for people seeking to overcome a problem with alcohol.

American Academy of Addiction Psychiatry (AAAP)
1010 Vermont Ave. NW, Suite 710
Washington, DC 20005
Phone: 202-393-4484
Fax: 202-393-4419
Website: http://www.aaap.org
E-mail: info@aaap.org

AAAP was established to help promote excellent quality in the treatment of addictive illnesses.

American Association for the Treatment of Opioid Dependence (AATOD)
217 Broadway, Suite 304
New York, NY 10007
Phone: 212-566-5555
Fax: 212-349-2944
Website: http://www.aatod.org

This organization is dedicated to enhancing the quality of opioid replacement pharmacotherapy for patients and their families.

American Psychiatric Association (APA)
1000 Wilson Blvd.
Suite 1825
Arlington, VA 22209-3901
Phone: 703-907-7300
Website: http://www.psych.org
E-mail: apa@psych.org

A medical society with more than 35,000 members, APA works to ensure appropriate treatment for people with mental health disorders, including disorders related to substance use.

American Society for Addiction Medicine (ASAM)
4601 N. Park Ave.
Upper Arcade #101
Chevy Chase, MD 20815
Phone: 301-656-3920
Fax: 301-656-3815
Website: http://www.asam.org
E-mail: email@asam.org

This organization is the nation's medical specialty society dedicated to educating physicians and improving the treatment of individuals suffering from alcoholism or other addictions.

Center for Substance Abuse Treatment (CSAT)
5600 Fishers Lane
Room 12-105, Rockwall Building
Rockville, MD 20857
Toll-Free: 800-662-HELP
TDD: 800-487-4889
Spanish: 877-767-8432
Phone: 301-443-5700
Fax: 301-443-8751
Website: http://csat.samhsa.gov
E-mail: info@samhsa.gov

CSAT's mission is to expand the availability of effective treatment and recovery services for people with alcohol and drug problems.

Center for Treatment Research on Adolescent Drug Abuse (CTRADA)
University of Miami
P.O. Box 019132
Miami, FL 33101
Phone: 305-243-6434
Website: http://www.miami.edu/ctrada
E-mail: adolescent-drug@miami.edu

CTRADA was established to conduct psychosocial treatment research on adolescent drug abuse, from treatment development to mechanisms, evaluation, and dissemination.

Cocaine Anonymous
3740 Overland Ave., Suite C
Los Angeles, CA 90049
Phone: 310-559-5833
Website: http://www.ca.org
E-mail: cawso@ca.org

Cocaine Anonymous is a non-professional, mutual help organization for people seeking to overcome a problem with cocaine.

Drug Abuse Treatment Outcome Study (DATOS)
Website: http://www.datos.org

The Drug Abuse Treatment Outcome Study (DATOS) is NIDA's third national evaluation of treatment effectiveness. It is based on over 10,000 admissions during 1991–1993 to 96 community-based treatment programs in 11 large U.S. cities.

Dual Recovery Anonymous
World Services Central Office
P.O. Box 8107
Prairie Village, KA 66208
Toll-Free: 877-883-2332
Website: http://draonline.org

Dual Recovery Anonymous is a 12-step organization for people with both chemical dependency and a mental health concern.

Hazelden Foundation
15245 Pleasant Valley Road
Center City, MN 55012-0011

Toll-Free: 800-257-7810
Phone: 651-213-4000
Fax: 651-213-4411
Website: http://www.hazelden.com
E-mail: info@hazelden.org

Hazelden works to help people overcome drug dependency and other related disorders.

Jewish Alcoholics, Chemically Dependent Persons and Significant Others (JACS)
850 Seventh Avenue
New York, NY 10019
Phone: 212-397-4197
Fax: 212-399-3525
Website: http://www.jacsweb.org
E-mail: jacs@jacsweb.org

JACS provides the Jewish community with assistance and information regarding chemical dependency.

Knowledge Application Program (KAP)
Center for Substance Abuse Treatment
Practice Improvement Branch
5600 Fishers Lane, Room 7-214
Rockville, MD 20857
Phone: 301-443-3491
Fax: 301-443-3543
Website: http://www.kap.samhsa.gov

KAP distributes materials about best treatment practices to providers who help individuals seeking substance abuse treatment.

Methamphetamine Treatment Project
UCLA - Integrated Substance Abuse Programs (ISAP)
11050 Santa Monica Blvd., Suite 100
Los Angeles, CA 90025
Phone: 310-312-0500
Fax: 310-312-0538
Website: http://www.methamphetamine.org

The Methamphetamine Treatment Project is a multi-site initiative to study the treatment of methamphetamine dependence.

NAMI, The Nation's Voice on Mental Illness
Colonial Place Three
2107 Wilson Blvd.
Suite 300
Arlington, VA 22201-3042
Toll-Free: 800-950-NAMI
Phone: 703-524-7600
Fax: 703-524-9094
TDD: 703-516-7227
Website: http://www.nami.org

NAMI seeks to ensure that all people with mental health disorders, including addictive disorders, receive appropriate treatment.

Narcotics Anonymous (NA)
P.O. Box 9999
Van Nuys, CA 91409
Phone: 818-773-9999
Fax: 818-700-0700
Website: http://www.na.org
E-mail: customer_service@na.org

NA is a non-professional, mutual help organization for recovering addicts.

National Alliance of Methadone Advocates (NAMA)
435 Second Avenue
New York, NY 10010
Phone: 212-595-NAMA
Website: http://www.methadone.org

The primary objective of NAMA is to advocate for the patient in treatment by destigmatizing and empowering methadone patients. First and foremost, NAMA confronts the negative stereotypes that impact on the self-esteem and worth of many methadone patients with a powerful affirmation of pride and unity.

National Association of Addiction Treatment Providers (NAATP)
313 W. Liberty Street
Suite 129
Lancaster, PA 17603-2748

Phone: 717-392-8480
Fax: 717-392-8481
Website: http://www.naatp.org

NAATP is a professional association that provides leadership in topics related to the treatment of chemical dependency.

National Council on Alcoholism and Drug Dependence (NCADD)
20 Exchange Place, Suite 2902
New York, NY 10005
Toll-Free: 800-NCA-CALL
Phone: 212-269-7797
Fax: 212-269-7510
Website: http://www.ncadd.org
E-mail: national@ncadd.org

NCADD is an advocacy organization for people with addictions and their family members.

National Association of Alcoholism and Drug Abuse Counselors (NAADAC)
901 N. Washington St., Suite 600
Alexandria, VA 22314
Toll-Free: 800-548-0497
Toll-Free Fax: 800-377-1136
Phone: 703-741-7686
Fax: 703-741-7698
Website: http://www.naadac.org

NAADAC is a professional membership organization serving counselors who specialize in the treatment of addiction.

National Association of Lesbian and Gay Addiction Professionals (NALGAP)
901 North Washington St., Suite 600
Alexandria, VA 22314
Phone: 703-465-0539
Website: http://www.nalgap.org
E-mail: clinical@nalgap.org

NALGAP is a professional membership organization seeking to prevent and treat lesbian, gay, bisexual, and transgender chemical dependency.

Parents and Adolescents Recovering Together (PARTS)
P.O. Box 927754
San Diego, CA 92192
Phone: 858-455-0725
Fax: 858-455-0721
Website: http://www.teendrughelp.org
E-mail: parts@teendrughelp.org

PARTS is a nonprofit organization established to help families of adolescents with substance abuse problems.

Paths to Recovery
610 Walnut St., Room 1109
Madison, WI 53726
Phone: 608-265-0063
Fax: 608-263-4523
Website: http://www.pathstorecovery.org
E-mail: info@pathstorecovery.org

Paths to Recovery is an initiative designed to improve the sequence of steps within an organization that lead to patient access to and early engagement in its substance abuse treatment programs.

Secular Organizations for Sobriety (SOS)
SOS National Clearinghouse
The Center for Inquiry-West
4773 Hollywood Blvd.
Hollywood, CA 90026
Phone: 323-666-4295
Fax: 323-666-4271
Website: http://www.secularhumanism.org/sos
E-mail: sos@cfiwest.org

SOS is a non-professional, mutual help organization for people seeking a 12-step style program without spiritual overtones.

SMART Recovery®
7537 Mentor Ave., Suite 306
Mentor, OH 44060
Phone: 440-951-5357
Fax: 440-951-5358
Website: http://www.smartrecovery.org
E-mail: SRMail1@aol.com

SMART Recovery® is an abstinence-based, not-for-profit organization with a sensible self-help program for people having problems with drinking and using drugs. It includes many ideas and techniques to help people change their lives from ones that are self-destructive and unhappy to ones that are constructive and satisfying.

Therapeutic Communities of America (TCA)
1601 Connecticut Ave, NW
Suite 803
Washington, DC 20009
Phone: 202-296-3503
Fax: 202-518-5475
Website: http://www.therapeuticcommunitiesofamerica.org

TCA is a national nonprofit membership association representing substance abuse treatment programs that provide services to substance abuse clients with a diversity of special needs, including those with HIV/AIDS, mothers with children, criminal justice clients, adults with co-occurring mental illnesses, the homeless, and adolescents.

Treatment Facility Locator
Website: http://findtreatment.samhsa.gov

This resource, sponsored by SAMHSA, can help to locate the drug and alcohol abuse treatment programs nearest you.

U.S. Food and Drug Administration (FDA)
5600 Fishers Lane
Rockville, MD 20857-0001
Toll-Free: 888-463-6332
Website: http://www.fda.gov

The Food and Drug Administration is one of the nation's oldest and most respected consumer protection agencies. FDA's mission is to promote and protect the public health by helping safe and effective products reach the market in a timely way and monitoring products for continued safety after they are in use. Medications, including those used in the treatment of addictive disorders, are regulated by the FDA.

Women for Sobriety, Inc.
P.O. Box 618
Quakertown, PA 18951-0618

Phone: 215-536-8026
Fax: 215-538-9026
Website: http://www.womenforsobriety.org

Women for Sobriety is an organization that seeks to assist women in overcoming addiction to alcohol and other substances and to maintain their recovery.

Drug Policy and Enforcement

Bureau of Alcohol, Tobacco, Firearms and Explosives (ATF)
Office of Public and Governmental Affairs
650 Massachusetts Avenue, NW.
Room 8290
Washington, DC 20226
Phone: 202-927-8500
Website: http://www.atf.gov
E-mail: ATFMail@atf.gov

This agency enforces the federal laws and regulations relating to alcohol, tobacco products, firearms, explosives, and arson.

Bureau for International Narcotics and Law Enforcement Affairs (INL)
U.S. Department of State
2201 C Street NW
Washington, DC 20520
Phone: 202-647-4000
Website: http://www.state.gov/g/inl

INL advises departments and agencies within the U.S. government on the development of policies and programs to combat international narcotics and crime.

Civil Air Patrol Counterdrug Operations (CAP)
Website: http://level2.cap.gov/index.cfm?nodeID=5266
E-mail: doc@capnhq.gov

CAP is a civilian nonprofit volunteer organization, that provides aviation-oriented support to U.S. law enforcement agencies.

Customs and Border Protection (CBP)
1300 Pennsylvania Avenue, NW
Washington, DC 20229

Phone: 202-354-1000
Website: http://www.customs.treas.gov

CBP is responsible for apprehending individuals attempting to enter the United States illegally and stemming the flow of illegal drugs and other contraband.

Department of Homeland Security (DHS)
Washington, DC 20528
Website: http://www.dhs.gov

DHS will analyze threats and intelligence, guard U.S. borders and airports, protect the infrastructure, and coordinate emergency response. DHS is also dedicated to protecting the rights of American citizens and enhancing public services, such as natural disaster assistance and citizenship services.

Drug Court Clearinghouse and Technical Assistance Project
Justice Programs Office
School of Public Affairs
American University
Brandywine Building, Suite 100
4400 Massachusetts Avenue, NW
Washington, DC 20016-8159
Phone: 202-885-2875
Fax: 202-885-2885
Website: http://www.american.edu/justice
E-mail: justice@american.edu

This online resource contains listings of drug court materials, activities, information, publications, and technical assistance.

Drug Enforcement Administration (DEA)
U.S. Department of Justice
2401 Jefferson Davis Highway
Alexandria, VA 22301
Toll-Free: 800-DEA-4288
Phone: 202-307-1000
Website: http://www.dea.gov
E-mail: AskDOJ@usdoj.gov

DEA is the lead federal agency for the enforcement of narcotics and controlled substance laws and regulations.

Drug Policy Information Clearinghouse
P.O. Box 6000
Rockville, MD 20849-6000
Toll-Free: 800-666-3332
Fax: 301-519-5212
Website: http://www.whitehousedrugpolicy.gov
E-mail: ondcp@ncjrs.org

Drug Strategies
1150 Connecticut Ave., NW
Suite 800
Washington, DC 20036
Phone: 202-289-9070
Website: http://www.drugstrategies.org
E-mail: dspolicy@aol.com

This website promotes effective approaches to the nation's drug problems and supports efforts to reduce the demand for drugs through prevention, treatment, enforcement, and community initiatives.

Executive Office for Asset Forfeiture (EOAF)
U.S. Department of Treasury
1500 Pennsylvania Ave., NW
Washington, DC 20220
Phone: 202-622-2000
Fax: 202-622-6415
Website: http://www.treas.gov/offices/eotffc/teoaf

This office administers the Treasury Forfeiture Fund, which is the repository for proceeds of assets forfeited under Treasury laws.

Federal Judiciary
Office of Public Affairs
Administrative Office of the U.S. Courts
Washington, DC 20544
Phone: 202-502-2600
Website: http://www.uscourts.gov

The Federal Judiciary deals with drug-related cases and provides court-ordered drug testing, treatment, and supervision of defendants, probationers, and parolees.

Institute for Behavior and Health (IBH)
6191 Executive Boulevard
Rockville, MD 20852
Phone: 301-231-9010
Fax 301-770-6876
Website: http://www.ibhinc.org
E-mail: contactus@ibhinc.org

IBH develops and promotes an array of new, effective, and synergistic anti-drug strategies.

INTERPOL–U.S. National Central Bureau (USNCB)
Washington, DC 20530
Website: http://www.usdoj.gov/usncb
E-mail: USNCB.Web@usdoj.gov

The USNCB exchanges drug-related law enforcement information with the member countries of INTERPOL.

Join Together Online
One Appleton Street, 4th floor
Boston, MA 02116-5223
Phone: 617-437-1500
Fax: 617-437-9394
Website: http://www.jointogether.org/home
E-mail: info@jointogether.org

Join Together Online is a resource to access local elected officials, media guides, and current legislation and issues related to substance abuse.

National Alliance for Model State Drug Laws
700 North Fairfax Street
Suite 550
Alexandria, VA 22314
Phone: 703-836-6100
Fax: 703-836-7495
Website: http://www.natlalliance.org

The Alliance is a resource for governors, state legislators, attorneys general, drug and alcohol professionals, community leaders, the recovering community, and others striving for comprehensive and effective state drug and alcohol laws, policies, and programs.

National Association of Drug Court Professionals (NADCP)
4900 Seminary Rd., Suite 320
Alexandria, VA 22311
Phone: 703-575-9400
Fax: 703-575-9402
Website: http://www.nadcp.org

NADCP advocates the establishment and funding of drug courts and provides for the collection and dissemination of information.

National Association of State Alcohol and Drug Abuse Directors (NASADAD)
808 17th Street NW
Suite 410
Washington, DC 20006
Phone: 202-293-0090
Fax: 202-293-1250
Website: http://www.nasadad.org
E-mail: dcoffice@nasadad.org

NASADAD fosters and supports the development of effective alcohol and other drug abuse prevention and treatment programs throughout every state.

National Conference of State Legislatures
444 North Capitol Street, NW, Suite 515
Washington, DC 20001
Phone: 202-624-5400
Fax: 202-737-1069
Website: http://www.ncsl.org

This is a source for research, informative publications, provocative meetings and seminars on critical state issues.

National Criminal Justice Reference Service (NCJRS)
P.O. Box 6000
Rockville, MD 20849-6000
Toll-Free: 800-851-3420
Phone: 301-519-5500
Fax: 301-519-5212
TTY: 877-712-9279
Website: http://www.ncjrs.org

NCJRS is a federally sponsored information clearinghouse for people involved with research, policy, and practice related to criminal and juvenile justice and drug control.

National Drug Intelligence Center (NDIC)
319 Washington St., 5th Floor
Johnstown, PA 15901
Phone: 814-532-4601
Fax: 814-532-4690
Website: http://www.usdoj.gov/ndic/index.htm
E-mail: NDIC.Contacts@usdoj.gov

NDIC is the nation's principal center for strategic domestic counterdrug intelligence.

National Drug Strategy Network (NDSN)
Criminal Justice Policy Foundation (CJPF)
8730 Georgia Ave., Suite 400
Silver Spring, MD 20910
Phone: 301-589-6020
Fax: 301-589-5056
Website: http://www.ndsn.org
E-mail: NDSN@ndsn.org

NDSN works to identify innovative solutions to a wide spectrum of drug-related issues through the sharing of information.

National Organization for the Reform of Marijuana Laws (NORML)
1600 K St. NW, Suite 501
Washington, DC 20006-2832
Phone: 202-483-5500
Fax: 202-483-0057
Website: http://www.natlnorml.org
E-mail: norml@norml.org

Founded in 1970, NORML works to influence public opinion so that marijuana prohibition will be repealed.

Office of National Drug Control Policy (ONDCP)
P.O. Box 6000
Rockville, MD 20849-6000

Toll-Free: 800-666-3332
Fax: 301-519-5212
Website: http://whitehousedrugpolicy.gov
E-mail: ondcp@ncjrs.org

The White House Office of National Drug Control Policy (ONDCP), a component of the Executive Office of the President, was established by the Anti-Drug Abuse Act of 1988. The principal purpose of ONDCP is to establish policies, priorities, and objectives for the nation's drug control program.

Office of Safe and Drug-Free Schools (OSDFS)
U.S. Department of Education
400 Maryland Ave. SW
Washington, DC 20202
Toll-Free: 800-USA-LEARN
Phone: 202-401-2000
Fax: 202-401-0689
TTY: 800-437-0689
Website: http://www.ed.gov/about/offices/list/osdfs/index.html
E-mail: customerservice@inet.ed.gov

OSDFS administers, coordinates, and recommends policies for improving the quality and excellence of programs and activities that are designed for drug and violence prevention.

Project Safe Neighborhoods (PSN)
Office of Justice Programs
810 Seventh Street, NW
Washington, DC 20531
Website: http://www.psn.gov
E-mail: AskPSN@usdoj.gov

PSN has a nationwide commitment to reduce gun crime in America by networking existing local programs that target gun crime and providing those programs with additional tools necessary to be successful.

Rand Drug Policy Resource Center (DPRC)
1700 Main Street
P.O. Box 2138
Santa Monica, CA 90407-2138
Phone: 310-393-0411
Website: http://www.rand.org/multi/dprc
E-mail: DPRC@rand.org

DPRC conducts research to help community leaders and public officials develop effective drug policies.

U.S. Coast Guard
2100 Second Street, SW
Washington, DC 20593
Phone: 202-267-1587
Website: http://www.uscg.mil

This agency enforces federal laws, including maritime drug interdiction, in the transit and arrival zones with jurisdiction on, under, and over the high seas and U.S. territorial waters.

U.S. Sentencing Commission (USSC)
Office of Public Affairs
One Columbus Circle, NE
Washington, DC 20002-8002
Phone: 202-502-4500
Website: http://www.ussc.gov
E-mail: pubaffairs@ussc.gov

USSC establishes sentencing policies for federal courts, assists in the development of effective policy, and collects, analyzes, and distributes information on sentencing issues.

Index

Index

Page numbers followed by 'n' indicate a footnote. Page numbers in *italics* indicate a table or illustration.

marijuana, continued
  female arrestees *43*
  high school students *43*
  other drug abuse 133–35
  overview 253–62
  prisoners *60*, 61, *62*
  probationers 57–58, *58*, *59*
  prohibition information 107–13
  Schedule I drug 71, 117
  tobacco use 137–41
  usage trends 6
  women *42*, *45*, *46*
  see also medical marijuana
Marijuana-info.org, contact information 521
Marijuana Policy Project (MPP)
  contact information 521
  marijuana prohibition publication 107n
"Marijuana Prohibition Facts" (MPP) 107n
Marinol (dronabinol) 87–88, 120
maternal drug use, fetal brain development 401–7
matrix model, described 348
MDFT *see* multidimensional family therapy
"MDMA (Ecstasy)" (ONDCP) 209n
MDMA (methylenedioxymethamphetamine) *see* ecstasy
Mebaral (mephobarbital) 293
medical detoxification, described 338–39
medical marijuana
  described 87–88
  overview 115–20
  restrictions 108–9
Medusa (slang) 511
mental illness
  prisoners 61, 64
  probationers 59
  social costs 89–90
  substance abuse treatment 351–56
Mepergan (meperidine) 289–90
meperidine 289–90, 291
"Meperidine" (DEA) 289n
mephobarbital 293
meth (slang) 267, 512

methadone
  defined 507
  described 301
  drug addiction treatment 336, 349–50
  effectiveness 329
  overview 263–65
  Schedule II drug 71
  street terms 512
"Methadone Fast Facts: Questions and Answers" (NDIC) 263n
methadone maintenance treatment, described 346–47
methamphetamine
  adolescent drug abuse trends 11, *19*, *26*, *30*
  arrestee drug abuse 57
  brain damage 413–16
  female arrestees *43*
  high school students *43*
  overview 267–78
  Schedule II drug 71
  street terms 512
  usage trends 6–7
  women *42*, *45*, *46*
"Methamphetamine" (ONDCP) 267n
"Methamphetamine and Amphetamines" (DEA) 267n
Methamphetamine Treatment Project, contact information 542
methandrostenolone *313*
methaqualone
  adolescent drug abuse trends *27*, *30*
  Schedule I drug 70
meth labs, described 277–78
methylenedioxymethamphetamine (MDMA) *see* ecstasy
methylphenidate
  described 295
  overview 279–81
methylphenidate hydrochloride, defined 507
methylsulfonylmethane (MSM) 274
Mexican brown (slang) *232*, 511
Mexican mushrooms (slang) 513
Mexican valium (slang) 513
Miller, Shannon 201, 206
miniature spoons 326

Health Reference Series
COMPLETE CATALOG

Adolescent Health Sourcebook

Basic Consumer Health Information about Common Medical, Mental, and Emotional Concerns in Adolescents, Including Facts about Acne, Body Piercing, Mononucleosis, Nutrition, Eating Disorders, Stress, Depression, Behavior Problems, Peer Pressure, Violence, Gangs, Drug Use, Puberty, Sexuality, Pregnancy, Learning Disabilities, and More

Along with a Glossary of Terms and Other Resources for Further Help and Information

Edited by Chad T. Kimball. 658 pages. 2002. 0-7808-0248-9. $78.

"It is written in clear, nontechnical language aimed at general readers. . . . Recommended for public libraries, community colleges, and other agencies serving health care consumers."
— *American Reference Books Annual, 2003*

"Recommended for school and public libraries. Parents and professionals dealing with teens will appreciate the easy-to-follow format and the clearly written text. This could become a 'must have' for every high school teacher." — *E-Streams, Jan '03*

"A good starting point for information related to common medical, mental, and emotional concerns of adolescents." — *School Library Journal, Nov '02*

"This book provides accurate information in an easy to access format. It addresses topics that parents and caregivers might not be aware of and provides practical, useable information." — *Doody's Health Sciences Book Review Journal, Sep-Oct '02*

"Recommended reference source."
— *Booklist, American Library Association, Sep '02*

AIDS Sourcebook, 3rd Edition

Basic Consumer Health Information about Acquired Immune Deficiency Syndrome (AIDS) and Human Immunodeficiency Virus (HIV) Infection, Including Facts about Transmission, Prevention, Diagnosis, Treatment, Opportunistic Infections, and Other Complications, with a Section for Women and Children, Including Details about Associated Gynecological Concerns, Pregnancy, and Pediatric Care

Along with Updated Statistical Information, Reports on Current Research Initiatives, a Glossary, and Directories of Internet, Hotline, and Other Resources

Edited by Dawn D. Matthews. 664 pages. 2003. 0-7808-0631-X. $78.

ALSO AVAILABLE: *AIDS Sourcebook, 1st Edition.* Edited by Karen Bellenir and Peter D. Dresser. 831 pages. 1995. 0-7808-0031-1. $78.

AIDS Sourcebook, 2nd Edition. Edited by Karen Bellenir. 751 pages. 1999. 0-7808-0225-X. $78.

"The 3rd edition of the *AIDS Sourcebook*, part of Omnigraphics' *Health Reference Series*, is a welcome update. . . . This resource is highly recommended for academic and public libraries."
— *American Reference Books Annual, 2004*

"Excellent sourcebook. This continues to be a highly recommended book. There is no other book that provides as much information as this book provides."
— *AIDS Book Review Journal, Dec-Jan 2000*

"Recommended reference source."
— *Booklist, American Library Association, Dec '99*

"A solid text for college-level health libraries."
— *The Bookwatch, Aug '99*

Cited in *Reference Sources for Small and Medium-Sized Libraries, American Library Association, 1999*

Alcoholism Sourcebook

Basic Consumer Health Information about the Physical and Mental Consequences of Alcohol Abuse, Including Liver Disease, Pancreatitis, Wernicke-Korsakoff Syndrome (Alcoholic Dementia), Fetal Alcohol Syndrome, Heart Disease, Kidney Disorders, Gastrointestinal Problems, and Immune System Compromise and Featuring Facts about Addiction, Detoxification, Alcohol Withdrawal, Recovery, and the Maintenance of Sobriety

Along with a Glossary and Directories of Resources for Further Help and Information

Edited by Karen Bellenir. 613 pages. 2000. 0-7808-0325-6. $78.

"This title is one of the few reference works on alcoholism for general readers. For some readers this will be a welcome complement to the many self-help books on the market. Recommended for collections serving general readers and consumer health collections."
— *E-Streams, Mar '01*

"This book is an excellent choice for public and academic libraries."
— *American Reference Books Annual, 2001*

"Recommended reference source."
— *Booklist, American Library Association, Dec '00*

"Presents a wealth of information on alcohol use and abuse and its effects on the body and mind, treatment, and prevention." — *SciTech Book News, Dec '00*

"Important new health guide which packs in the latest consumer information about the problems of alcoholism." — *Reviewer's Bookwatch, Nov '00*

SEE ALSO *Drug Abuse Sourcebook, Substance Abuse Sourcebook*

Allergies Sourcebook, 2nd Edition

Basic Consumer Health Information about Allergic Disorders, Triggers, Reactions, and Related Symptoms, Including Anaphylaxis, Rhinitis, Sinusitis, Asthma, Dermatitis, Conjunctivitis, and Multiple Chemical Sensitivity

Along with Tips on Diagnosis, Prevention, and Treatment, Statistical Data, a Glossary, and a Directory of Sources for Further Help and Information

Edited by Annemarie S. Muth. 598 pages. 2002. 0-7808-0376-0. $78.

ALSO AVAILABLE: *Allergies Sourcebook, 1st Edition.* Edited by Allan R. Cook. 611 pages. 1997. 0-7808-0036-2. $78.

"This book brings a great deal of useful material together. . . . This is an excellent addition to public and consumer health library collections."
— *American Reference Books Annual, 2003*

"This second edition would be useful to laypersons with little or advanced knowledge of the subject matter. This book would also serve as a resource for nursing and other health care professions students. It would be useful in public, academic, and hospital libraries with consumer health collections." — *E-Streams, Jul '02*

■

Alternative Medicine Sourcebook, 2nd Edition

Basic Consumer Health Information about Alternative and Complementary Medical Practices, Including Acupuncture, Chiropractic, Herbal Medicine, Homeopathy, Naturopathic Medicine, Mind-Body Interventions, Ayurveda, and Other Non-Western Medical Traditions

Along with Facts about such Specific Therapies as Massage Therapy, Aromatherapy, Qigong, Hypnosis, Prayer, Dance, and Art Therapies, a Glossary, and Resources for Further Information

Edited by Dawn D. Matthews. 618 pages. 2002. 0-7808-0605-0. $78.

ALSO AVAILABLE: *Alternative Medicine Sourcebook, 1st Edition.* Edited by Allan R. Cook. 737 pages. 1999. 0-7808-0200-4. $78.

"Recommended for public, high school, and academic libraries that have consumer health collections. Hospital libraries that also serve the public will find this to be a useful resource." — *E-Streams, Feb '03*

"Recommended reference source."
—*Booklist, American Library Association, Jan '03*

"An important alternate health reference."
— *MBR Bookwatch, Oct '02*

"A great addition to the reference collection of every type of library." — *American Reference Books Annual, 2000*

Alzheimer's Disease Sourcebook, 3rd Edition

Basic Consumer Health Information about Alzheimer's Disease, Other Dementias, and Related Disorders, Including Multi-Infarct Dementia, AIDS Dementia Complex, Dementia with Lewy Bodies, Huntington's Disease, Wernicke-Korsakoff Syndrome (Alcohol-Reated Dementia), Delirium, and Confusional States

Along with Information for People Newly Diagnosed with Alzheimer's Disease and Caregivers, Reports Detailing Current Research Efforts in Prevention, Diagnosis, and Treatment, Facts about Long-Term Care Issues, and Listings of Sources for Additional Information

Edited by Karen Bellenir. 645 pages. 2003. 0-7808-0666-2. $78.

ALSO AVAILABLE: *Alzheimer's, Stroke & 29 Other Neurological Disorders Sourcebook, 1st Edition.* Edited by Frank E. Bair. 579 pages. 1993. 1-55888-748-2. $78.

ALSO AVAILABLE: *Alzheimer's Disease Sourcebook, 2nd Edition.* Edited by Karen Bellenir. 524 pages. 1999. 0-7808-0223-3. $78.

"This very informative and valuable tool will be a great addition to any library serving consumers, students and health care workers."
—*American Reference Books Annual, 2004*

"This is a valuable resource for people affected by dementias such as Alzheimer's. It is easy to navigate and includes important information and resources."
— *Doody's Review Service, Feb. 2004*

"Recommended reference source."
— *Booklist, American Library Association, Oct '99*

SEE ALSO Brain Disorders Sourcebook

■

Arthritis Sourcebook, 2nd Edition

Basic Consumer Health Information about Osteoarthritis, Rheumatoid Arthritis, Other Rheumatic Disorders, Infectious Forms of Arthritis, and Diseases with Symptoms Linked to Arthritis, Featuring Facts about Diagnosis, Pain Management, and Surgical Therapies

Along with Coping Strategies, Research Updates, a Glossary, and Resources for Additional Help and Information

Edited by Amy L. Sutton. 593 pages. 2004. 0-7808-0667-0. $78.

ALSO AVAILABLE: *Arthritis Sourcebook, 1st Edition.* Edited by Allan R. Cook. 550 pages. 1998. 0-7808-0201-2. $78.

". . . accessible to the layperson."
—*Reference and Research Book News, Feb '99*

Asthma Sourcebook

Basic Consumer Health Information about Asthma, Including Symptoms, Traditional and Nontraditional Remedies, Treatment Advances, Quality-of-Life Aids, Medical Research Updates, and the Role of Allergies, Exercise, Age, the Environment, and Genetics in the Development of Asthma

Along with Statistical Data, a Glossary, and Directories of Support Groups, and Other Resources for Further Information

Edited by Annemarie S. Muth. 628 pages. 2000. 0-7808-0381-7. $78.

"A worthwhile reference acquisition for public libraries and academic medical libraries whose readers desire a quick introduction to the wide range of asthma information." *— Choice, Association of College & Research Libraries, Jun '01*

"Recommended reference source."
— Booklist, American Library Association, Feb '01

"Highly recommended." *— The Bookwatch, Jan '01*

"There is much good information for patients and their families who deal with asthma daily."
— American Medical Writers Association Journal, Winter '01

"This informative text is recommended for consumer health collections in public, secondary school, and community college libraries and the libraries of universities with a large undergraduate population."
— American Reference Books Annual, 2001

Attention Deficit Disorder Sourcebook

Basic Consumer Health Information about Attention Deficit/Hyperactivity Disorder in Children and Adults, Including Facts about Causes, Symptoms, Diagnostic Criteria, and Treatment Options Such as Medications, Behavior Therapy, Coaching, and Homeopathy

Along with Reports on Current Research Initiatives, Legal Issues, and Government Regulations, and Featuring a Glossary of Related Terms, Internet Resources, and a List of Additional Reading Material

Edited by Dawn D. Matthews. 470 pages. 2002. 0-7808-0624-7. $78.

"Recommended reference source."
— Booklist, American Library Association, Jan '03

"This book is recommended for all school libraries and the reference or consumer health sections of public libraries." *— American Reference Books Annual, 2003*

Back & Neck Sourcebook, 2nd Edition

Basic Consumer Health Information about Spinal Pain, Spinal Cord Injuries, and Related Disorders, Such as Degenerative Disk Disease, Osteoarthritis, Scoliosis,

Sciatica, Spina Bifida, and Spinal Stenosis, and Featuring Facts about Maintaining Spinal Health, Self-Care, Pain Management, Rehabilitative Care, Chiropractic Care, Spinal Surgeries, and Complementary Therapies

Along with Suggestions for Preventing Back and Neck Pain, a Glossary of Related Terms, and a Directory of Resources

Edited by Amy L. Sutton. 633 pages. 2004. 0-7808-0738-3 $78.

ALSO AVAILABLE: *Back & Neck Disorders Sourcebook, 1st Edition.* Edited by Karen Bellenir. 548 pages. 1997. 0-7808-0202-0. $78.

"The strength of this work is its basic, easy-to-read format. Recommended."
— Reference and User Services Quarterly, American Library Association, Winter '97

Blood & Circulatory Disorders Sourcebook

Basic Information about Blood and Its Components, Anemias, Leukemias, Bleeding Disorders, and Circulatory Disorders, Including Aplastic Anemia, Thalassemia, Sickle-Cell Disease, Hemochromatosis, Hemophilia, Von Willebrand Disease, and Vascular Diseases

Along with a Special Section on Blood Transfusions and Blood Supply Safety, a Glossary, and Source Listings for Further Help and Information

Edited by Karen Bellenir and Linda M. Shin. 554 pages. 1998. 0-7808-0203-9. $78.

"Recommended reference source."
— Booklist, American Library Association, Feb '99

"An important reference sourcebook written in simple language for everyday, non-technical users. "
— Reviewer's Bookwatch, Jan '99

Brain Disorders Sourcebook

Basic Consumer Health Information about Strokes, Epilepsy, Amyotrophic Lateral Sclerosis (ALS/Lou Gehrig's Disease), Parkinson's Disease, Brain Tumors, Cerebral Palsy, Headache, Tourette Syndrome, and More

Along with Statistical Data, Treatment and Rehabilitation Options, Coping Strategies, Reports on Current Research Initiatives, a Glossary, and Resource Listings for Additional Help and Information

Edited by Karen Bellenir. 481 pages. 1999. 0-7808-0229-2. $78.

"Belongs on the shelves of any library with a consumer health collection." *— E-Streams, Mar '00*

"Recommended reference source."
— Booklist, American Library Association, Oct '99

SEE ALSO *Alzheimer's Disease Sourcebook*

Breast Cancer Sourcebook, 2nd Edition

Basic Consumer Health Information about Breast Cancer, Including Facts about Risk Factors, Prevention, Screening and Diagnostic Methods, Treatment Options, Complementary and Alternative Therapies, Post-Treatment Concerns, Clinical Trials, Special Risk Populations, and New Developments in Breast Cancer Research

Along with Breast Cancer Statistics, a Glossary of Related Terms, and a Directory of Resources for Additional Help and Information

Edited by Sandra J. Judd. 595 pages. 2004. 0-7808-0668-9. $78.

ALSO AVAILABLE: *Breast Cancer Sourcebook, 1st Edition.* Edited by Edward J. Prucha and Karen Bellenir. 580 pages. 2001. 0-7808-0244-6. $78.

"It would be a useful reference book in a library or on loan to women in a support group."
— *Cancer Forum, Mar '03*

"Recommended reference source."
— *Booklist, American Library Association, Jan '02*

"This reference source is highly recommended. It is quite informative, comprehensive and detailed in nature, and yet it offers practical advice in easy-to-read language. It could be thought of as the 'bible' of breast cancer for the consumer." — *E-Streams, Jan '02*

"The broad range of topics covered in lay language make the *Breast Cancer Sourcebook* an excellent addition to public and consumer health library collections."
— *American Reference Books Annual 2002*

"From the pros and cons of different screening methods and results to treatment options, *Breast Cancer Sourcebook* provides the latest information on the subject."
— *Library Bookwatch, Dec '01*

"This thoroughgoing, very readable reference covers all aspects of breast health and cancer.... Readers will find much to consider here. Recommended for all public and patient health collections."
— *Library Journal, Sep '01*

SEE ALSO *Cancer Sourcebook for Women, Women's Health Concerns Sourcebook*

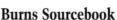

Breastfeeding Sourcebook

Basic Consumer Health Information about the Benefits of Breastmilk, Preparing to Breastfeed, Breastfeeding as a Baby Grows, Nutrition, and More, Including Information on Special Situations and Concerns Such as Mastitis, Illness, Medications, Allergies, Multiple Births, Prematurity, Special Needs, and Adoption

Along with a Glossary and Resources for Additional Help and Information

Edited by Jenni Lynn Colson. 388 pages. 2002. 0-7808-0332-9. $78.

SEE ALSO *Pregnancy & Birth Sourcebook*

"Particularly useful is the information about professional lactation services and chapters on breastfeeding when returning to work.... *Breastfeeding Sourcebook* will be useful for public libraries, consumer health libraries, and technical schools offering nurse assistant training, especially in areas where Internet access is problematic."
— *American Reference Books Annual, 2003*

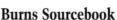

Burns Sourcebook

Basic Consumer Health Information about Various Types of Burns and Scalds, Including Flame, Heat, Cold, Electrical, Chemical, and Sun Burns

Along with Information on Short-Term and Long-Term Treatments, Tissue Reconstruction, Plastic Surgery, Prevention Suggestions, and First Aid

Edited by Allan R. Cook. 604 pages. 1999. 0-7808-0204-7. $78.

"This is an exceptional addition to the series and is highly recommended for all consumer health collections, hospital libraries, and academic medical centers."
— *E-Streams, Mar '00*

"This key reference guide is an invaluable addition to all health care and public libraries in confronting this ongoing health issue."
— *American Reference Books Annual, 2000*

"Recommended reference source."
— *Booklist, American Library Association, Dec '99*

SEE ALSO *Skin Disorders Sourcebook*

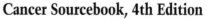

Cancer Sourcebook, 4th Edition

Basic Consumer Health Information about Major Forms and Stages of Cancer, Featuring Facts about Head and Neck Cancers, Lung Cancers, Gastrointestinal Cancers, Genitourinary Cancers, Lymphomas, Blood Cell Cancers, Endocrine Cancers, Skin Cancers, Bone Cancers, Sarcomas, and Others, and Including Information about Cancer Treatments and Therapies, Identifying and Reducing Cancer Risks, and Strategies for Coping with Cancer and the Side Effects of Treatment

Along with a Cancer Glossary, Statistical and Demographic Data, and a Directory of Sources for Additional Help and Information

Edited by Karen Bellenir. 1,119 pages. 2003. 0-7808-0633-6. $78.

ALSO AVAILABLE: *Cancer Sourcebook, 1st Edition.* Edited by Frank E. Bair. 932 pages. 1990. 1-55888-888-8. $78.

New Cancer Sourcebook, 2nd Edition. Edited by Allan R. Cook. 1,313 pages. 1996. 0-7808-0041-9. $78.

Cancer Sourcebook, 3rd Edition. Edited by Edward J. Prucha. 1,069 pages. 2000. 0-7808-0227-6. $78.

"With cancer being the second leading cause of death for Americans, a prodigious work such as this one, which locates centrally so much cancer-related information, is clearly an asset to this nation's citizens and others." — *Journal of the National Medical Association, 2004*

"This title is recommended for health sciences and public libraries with consumer health collections."
— *E-Streams, Feb '01*

". . . can be effectively used by cancer patients and their families who are looking for answers in a language they can understand. Public and hospital libraries should have it on their shelves."
— *American Reference Books Annual, 2001*

"Recommended reference source."
— *Booklist, American Library Association, Dec '00*

Cited in *Reference Sources for Small and Medium-Sized Libraries*, American Library Association, 1999

"The amount of factual and useful information is extensive. The writing is very clear, geared to general readers. Recommended for all levels." — *Choice, Association of College & Research Libraries, Jan '97*

SEE ALSO *Breast Cancer Sourcebook, Cancer Sourcebook for Women, Pediatric Cancer Sourcebook, Prostate Cancer Sourcebook*

Cancer Sourcebook for Women, 2nd Edition

Basic Consumer Health Information about Gynecologic Cancers and Related Concerns, Including Cervical Cancer, Endometrial Cancer, Gestational Trophoblastic Tumor, Ovarian Cancer, Uterine Cancer, Vaginal Cancer, Vulvar Cancer, Breast Cancer, and Common Non-Cancerous Uterine Conditions, with Facts about Cancer Risk Factors, Screening and Prevention, Treatment Options, and Reports on Current Research Initiatives

Along with a Glossary of Cancer Terms and a Directory of Resources for Additional Help and Information

Edited by Karen Bellenir. 604 pages. 2002. 0-7808-0226-8. $78.

ALSO AVAILABLE: *Cancer Sourcebook for Women, 1st Edition.* Edited by Allan R. Cook and Peter D. Dresser. 524 pages. 1996. 0-7808-0076-1. $78.

"An excellent addition to collections in public, consumer health, and women's health libraries."
— *American Reference Books Annual, 2003*

"Overall, the information is excellent, and complex topics are clearly explained. As a reference book for the consumer it is a valuable resource to assist them to make informed decisions about cancer and its treatments." — *Cancer Forum, Nov '02*

"Highly recommended for academic and medical reference collections." — *Library Bookwatch, Sep '02*

"This is a highly recommended book for any public or consumer library, being reader friendly and containing accurate and helpful information."
— *E-Streams, Aug '02*

"Recommended reference source."
— *Booklist, American Library Association, Jul '02*

SEE ALSO *Breast Cancer Sourcebook, Women's Health Concerns Sourcebook*

Cardiovascular Diseases & Disorders Sourcebook, 1st Edition

SEE *Heart Diseases & Disorders Sourcebook, 2nd Edition*

Caregiving Sourcebook

Basic Consumer Health Information for Caregivers, Including a Profile of Caregivers, Caregiving Responsibilities and Concerns, Tips for Specific Conditions, Care Environments, and the Effects of Caregiving

Along with Facts about Legal Issues, Financial Information, and Future Planning, a Glossary, and a Listing of Additional Resources

Edited by Joyce Brennfleck Shannon. 600 pages. 2001. 0-7808-0331-0. $78.

"Essential for most collections."
— *Library Journal, Apr 1, 2002*

"An ideal addition to the reference collection of any public library. Health sciences information professionals may also want to acquire the *Caregiving Sourcebook* for their hospital or academic library for use as a ready reference tool by health care workers interested in aging and caregiving." — *E-Streams, Jan '02*

"Recommended reference source."
— *Booklist, American Library Association, Oct '01*

Child Abuse Sourcebook

Basic Consumer Health Information about the Physical, Sexual, and Emotional Abuse of Children, with Additional Facts about Neglect, Munchausen Syndrome by Proxy (MSBP), Shaken Baby Syndrome, and Controversial Issues Related to Child Abuse, Such as Withholding Medical Care, Corporal Punishment, and Child Maltreatment in Youth Sports, and Featuring Facts about Child Protective Services, Foster Care, Adoption, Parenting Challenges, and Other Abuse Prevention Efforts

Along with a Glossary of Related Terms and Resources for Additional Help and Information

Edited by Dawn D. Matthews. 620 pages. 2004. 0-7808-0705-7. $78.

Childhood Diseases & Disorders Sourcebook

Basic Consumer Health Information about Medical Problems Often Encountered in Pre-Adolescent Children, Including Respiratory Tract Ailments, Ear Infections, Sore Throats, Disorders of the Skin and Scalp, Digestive and Genitourinary Diseases, Infectious Diseases, Inflammatory Disorders, Chronic Physical and Developmental Disorders, Allergies, and More

Along with Information about Diagnostic Tests, Common Childhood Surgeries, and Frequently Used Medications, with a Glossary of Important Terms and Resource Directory

Edited by Chad T. Kimball. 662 pages. 2003. 0-7808-0458-9. $78.

"This is an excellent book for new parents and should be included in all health care and public libraries."
— *American Reference Books Annual, 2004*

Colds, Flu & Other Common Ailments Sourcebook

Basic Consumer Health Information about Common Ailments and Injuries, Including Colds, Coughs, the Flu, Sinus Problems, Headaches, Fever, Nausea and Vomiting, Menstrual Cramps, Diarrhea, Constipation, Hemorrhoids, Back Pain, Dandruff, Dry and Itchy Skin, Cuts, Scrapes, Sprains, Bruises, and More

Along with Information about Prevention, Self-Care, Choosing a Doctor, Over-the-Counter Medications, Folk Remedies, and Alternative Therapies, and Including a Glossary of Important Terms and a Directory of Resources for Further Help and Information

Edited by Chad T. Kimball. 638 pages. 2001. 0-7808-0435-X. $78.

"A good starting point for research on common illnesses. It will be a useful addition to public and consumer health library collections."
— *American Reference Books Annual 2002*

"Will prove valuable to any library seeking to maintain a current, comprehensive reference collection of health resources. . . . Excellent reference."
— *The Bookwatch, Aug '01*

"Recommended reference source."
— *Booklist, American Library Association, July '01*

Communication Disorders Sourcebook

Basic Information about Deafness and Hearing Loss, Speech and Language Disorders, Voice Disorders, Balance and Vestibular Disorders, and Disorders of Smell, Taste, and Touch

Edited by Linda M. Ross. 533 pages. 1996. 0-7808-0077-X. $78.

"This is skillfully edited and is a welcome resource for the layperson. It should be found in every public and medical library." — *Booklist Health Sciences Supplement, American Library Association, Oct '97*

Congenital Disorders Sourcebook

Basic Information about Disorders Acquired during Gestation, Including Spina Bifida, Hydrocephalus, Cerebral Palsy, Heart Defects, Craniofacial Abnormalities, Fetal Alcohol Syndrome, and More

Along with Current Treatment Options and Statistical Data

Edited by Karen Bellenir. 607 pages. 1997. 0-7808-0205-5. $78.

"Recommended reference source."
— *Booklist, American Library Association, Oct '97*

SEE ALSO Pregnancy & Birth Sourcebook

Consumer Issues in Health Care Sourcebook

Basic Information about Health Care Fundamentals and Related Consumer Issues, Including Exams and Screening Tests, Physician Specialties, Choosing a Doctor, Using Prescription and Over-the-Counter Medications Safely, Avoiding Health Scams, Managing Common Health Risks in the Home, Care Options for Chronically or Terminally Ill Patients, and a List of Resources for Obtaining Help and Further Information

Edited by Karen Bellenir. 618 pages. 1998. 0-7808-0221-7. $78.

"Both public and academic libraries will want to have a copy in their collection for readers who are interested in self-education on health issues."
— *American Reference Books Annual, 2000*

"The editor has researched the literature from government agencies and others, saving readers the time and effort of having to do the research themselves. Recommended for public libraries."
— *Reference and User Services Quarterly, American Library Association, Spring '99*

"Recommended reference source."
— *Booklist, American Library Association, Dec '98*

Contagious Diseases Sourcebook

Basic Consumer Health Information about Infectious Diseases Spread by Person-to-Person Contact through Direct Touch, Airborne Transmission, Sexual Contact, or Contact with Blood or Other Body Fluids, Including Hepatitis, Herpes, Influenza, Lice, Measles, Mumps, Pinworm, Ringworm, Severe Acute Respiratory Syndrome (SARS), Streptococcal Infections, Tuberculosis, and Others

Along with Facts about Disease Transmission, Antimicrobial Resistance, and Vaccines, with a Glossary and Directories of Resources for More Information

Edited by Karen Bellenir. 643 pages. 2004. 0-7808-0736-7. $78.

Contagious & Non-Contagious Infectious Diseases Sourcebook

Basic Information about Contagious Diseases like Measles, Polio, Hepatitis B, and Infectious Mononucleosis, and Non-Contagious Infectious Diseases like Tetanus and Toxic Shock Syndrome, and Diseases Occurring as Secondary Infections Such as Shingles and Reye Syndrome

Along with Vaccination, Prevention, and Treatment Information, and a Section Describing Emerging Infectious Disease Threats

Edited by Karen Bellenir and Peter D. Dresser. 566 pages. 1996. 0-7808-0075-3. $78.

Death & Dying Sourcebook

Basic Consumer Health Information for the Layperson about End-of-Life Care and Related Ethical and Legal Issues, Including Chief Causes of Death, Autopsies, Pain Management for the Terminally Ill, Life Support Systems, Insurance, Euthanasia, Assisted Suicide, Hospice Programs, Living Wills, Funeral Planning, Counseling, Mourning, Organ Donation, and Physician Training

Along with Statistical Data, a Glossary, and Listings of Sources for Further Help and Information

Edited by Annemarie S. Muth. 641 pages. 1999. 0-7808-0230-6. $78.

"Public libraries, medical libraries, and academic libraries will all find this sourcebook a useful addition to their collections."

—*American Reference Books Annual, 2001*

"An extremely useful resource for those concerned with death and dying in the United States."

—*Respiratory Care, Nov '00*

"Recommended reference source."

—*Booklist, American Library Association, Aug '00*

"This book is a definite must for all those involved in end-of-life care." —*Doody's Review Service, 2000*

Dental Care & Oral Health Sourcebook, 2nd Edition

Basic Consumer Health Information about Dental Care, Including Oral Hygiene, Dental Visits, Pain Management, Cavities, Crowns, Bridges, Dental Implants, and Fillings, and Other Oral Health Concerns, Such as Gum Disease, Bad Breath, Dry Mouth, Genetic and Developmental Abnormalities, Oral Cancers, Orthodontics, and Temporomandibular Disorders

Along with Updates on Current Research in Oral Health, a Glossary, a Directory of Dental and Oral Health Organizations, and Resources for People with Dental and Oral Health Disorders

Edited by Amy L. Sutton. 609 pages. 2003. 0-7808-0634-4. $78.

ALSO AVAILABLE: *Oral Health Sourcebook, 1st Edition.* Edited by Allan R. Cook. 558 pages. 1997. 0-7808-0082-6. $78.

"This book could serve as a turning point in the battle to educate consumers in issues concerning oral health."

—*American Reference Books Annual, 2004*

"Unique source which will fill a gap in dental sources for patients and the lay public. A valuable reference tool even in a library with thousands of books on dentistry. Comprehensive, clear, inexpensive, and easy to read and use. It fills an enormous gap in the health care literature." —*Reference and User Services Quarterly, American Library Association, Summer '98*

"Recommended reference source."

—*Booklist, American Library Association, Dec '97*

Depression Sourcebook

Basic Consumer Health Information about Unipolar Depression, Bipolar Disorder, Postpartum Depression, Seasonal Affective Disorder, and Other Types of Depression in Children, Adolescents, Women, Men, the Elderly, and Other Selected Populations

Along with Facts about Causes, Risk Factors, Diagnostic Criteria, Treatment Options, Coping Strategies, Suicide Prevention, a Glossary, and a Directory of Sources for Additional Help and Information

Edited by Karen Belleni. 602 pages. 2002. 0-7808-0611-5. $78.

"*Depression Sourcebook* is of a very high standard. Its purpose, which is to serve as a reference source to the lay reader, is very well served."

—*Journal of the National Medical Association, 2004*

"Invaluable reference for public and school library collections alike." —*Library Bookwatch, Apr '03*

"Recommended for purchase."

—*American Reference Books Annual, 2003*

Diabetes Sourcebook, 3rd Edition

Basic Consumer Health Information about Type 1 Diabetes (Insulin-Dependent or Juvenile-Onset Diabetes), Type 2 Diabetes (Noninsulin-Dependent or Adult-Onset Diabetes), Gestational Diabetes, Impaired Glucose Tolerance (IGT), and Related Complications, Such as Amputation, Eye Disease, Gum Disease, Nerve Damage, and End-Stage Renal Disease, Including Facts about Insulin, Oral Diabetes Medications, Blood Sugar Testing, and the Role of Exercise and Nutrition in the Control of Diabetes

Along with a Glossary and Resources for Further Help and Information

Edited by Dawn D. Matthews. 622 pages. 2003. 0-7808-0629-8. $78.

ALSO AVAILABLE: *Diabetes Sourcebook, 1st Edition.* Edited by Karen Bellenir and Peter D. Dresser. 827 pages. 1994. 1-55888-751-2. $78.

Diabetes Sourcebook, 2nd Edition. Edited by Karen Bellenir. 688 pages. 1998. 0-7808-0224-1. $78.

"This edition is even more helpful than earlier versions. . . . It is a truly valuable tool for anyone seeking readable and authoritative information on diabetes."

—*American Reference Books Annual, 2004*

"An invaluable reference." —*Library Journal, May '00*

Selected as one of the 250 "Best Health Sciences Books of 1999." —*Doody's Rating Service, Mar-Apr 2000*

"Provides useful information for the general public."

—*Healthlines, University of Michigan Health Management Research Center, Sep/Oct '99*

". . . provides reliable mainstream medical information . . . belongs on the shelves of any library with a consumer health collection." —*E-Streams, Sep '99*

"Recommended reference source."

—*Booklist, American Library Association, Feb '99*

Diet & Nutrition Sourcebook, 2nd Edition

Basic Consumer Health Information about Dietary Guidelines, Recommended Daily Intake Values, Vitamins, Minerals, Fiber, Fat, Weight Control, Dietary Supplements, and Food Additives

Along with Special Sections on Nutrition Needs throughout Life and Nutrition for People with Such Specific Medical Concerns as Allergies, High Blood Cholesterol, Hypertension, Diabetes, Celiac Disease, Seizure Disorders, Phenylketonuria (PKU), Cancer, and Eating Disorders, and Including Reports on Current Nutrition Research and Source Listings for Additional Help and Information

Edited by Karen Bellenir. 650 pages. 1999. 0-7808-0228-4. $78.

ALSO AVAILABLE: *Diet & Nutrition Sourcebook, 1st Edition.* Edited by Dan R. Harris. 662 pages. 1996. 0-7808-0084-2. $78.

"This book is an excellent source of basic diet and nutrition information." — *Booklist Health Sciences Supplement, American Library Association, Dec '00*

"This reference document should be in any public library, but it would be a very good guide for beginning students in the health sciences. If the other books in this publisher's series are as good as this, they should all be in the health sciences collections."
— *American Reference Books Annual, 2000*

"This book is an excellent general nutrition reference for consumers who desire to take an active role in their health care for prevention. Consumers of all ages who select this book can feel confident they are receiving current and accurate information." — *Journal of Nutrition for the Elderly, Vol. 19, No. 4, '00*

"Recommended reference source."
— *Booklist, American Library Association, Dec '99*

SEE ALSO *Digestive Diseases & Disorders Sourcebook, Eating Disorders Sourcebook, Gastrointestinal Diseases & Disorders Sourcebook, Vegetarian Sourcebook*

Digestive Diseases & Disorders Sourcebook

Basic Consumer Health Information about Diseases and Disorders that Impact the Upper and Lower Digestive System, Including Celiac Disease, Constipation, Crohn's Disease, Cyclic Vomiting Syndrome, Diarrhea, Diverticulosis and Diverticulitis, Gallstones, Heartburn, Hemorrhoids, Hernias, Indigestion (Dyspepsia), Irritable Bowel Syndrome, Lactose Intolerance, Ulcers, and More

Along with Information about Medications and Other Treatments, Tips for Maintaining a Healthy Digestive Tract, a Glossary, and Directory of Digestive Diseases Organizations

Edited by Karen Bellenir. 335 pages. 2000. 0-7808-0327-2. $78.

"This title would be an excellent addition to all public or patient-research libraries."
— *American Reference Books Annual, 2001*

"This title is recommended for public, hospital, and health sciences libraries with consumer health collections." — *E-Streams, Jul-Aug '00*

"Recommended reference source."
— *Booklist, American Library Association, May '00*

SEE ALSO *Diet & Nutrition Sourcebook, Eating Disorders Sourcebook, Gastrointestinal Diseases & Disorders Sourcebook*

Disabilities Sourcebook

Basic Consumer Health Information about Physical and Psychiatric Disabilities, Including Descriptions of Major Causes of Disability, Assistive and Adaptive Aids, Workplace Issues, and Accessibility Concerns

Along with Information about the Americans with Disabilities Act, a Glossary, and Resources for Additional Help and Information

Edited by Dawn D. Matthews. 616 pages. 2000. 0-7808-0389-2. $78.

"It is a must for libraries with a consumer health section." — *American Reference Books Annual 2002*

"A much needed addition to the Omnigraphics *Health Reference Series.* A current reference work to provide people with disabilities, their families, caregivers or those who work with them, a broad range of information in one volume, has not been available until now.... It is recommended for all public and academic library reference collections." — *E-Streams, May '01*

"An excellent source book in easy-to-read format covering many current topics; highly recommended for all libraries." — *Choice, Association of College and Research Libraries, Jan '01*

"Recommended reference source."
— *Booklist, American Library Association, Jul '00*

Domestic Violence Sourcebook, 2nd Edition

Basic Consumer Health Information about the Causes and Consequences of Abusive Relationships, Including Physical Violence, Sexual Assault, Battery, Stalking, and Emotional Abuse, and Facts about the Effects of Violence on Women, Men, Young Adults, and the Elderly, with Reports about Domestic Violence in Selected Populations, and Featuring Facts about Medical Care, Victim Assistance and Protection, Prevention Strategies, Mental Health Services, and Legal Issues

Along with a Glossary of Related Terms and Resources for Additional Help and Information

Edited by Dawn D. Matthews. 628 pages. 2004. 0-7808-0669-7. $78.

ALSO AVAILABLE: *Domestic Violence & Child Abuse Sourcebook, 1st Edition.* Edited by Helene Henderson. 1,064 pages. 2001. 0-7808-0235-7. $78.

"Interested lay persons should find the book extremely beneficial. . . . A copy of *Domestic Violence and Child Abuse Sourcebook* should be in every public library in the United States."
— *Social Science & Medicine, No. 56, 2003*

"This is important information. The Web has many resources but this sourcebook fills an important societal need. I am not aware of any other resources of this type." — *Doody's Review Service, Sep '01*

"Recommended for all libraries, scholars, and practitioners." — *Choice, Association of College & Research Libraries, Jul '01*

"Recommended reference source."
— *Booklist, American Library Association, Apr '01*

"Important pick for college-level health reference libraries." — *The Bookwatch, Mar '01*

"Because this problem is so widespread and because this book includes a lot of issues within one volume, this work is recommended for all public libraries."
— *American Reference Books Annual, 2001*

■

Drug Abuse Sourcebook, 2nd Edition

Basic Consumer Health Information about Illicit Substances of Abuse and the Misuse of Prescription and Over-the-Counter Medications, Including Depressants, Hallucinogens, Inhalants, Marijuana, Stimulants, and Anabolic Steroids

Along with Facts about Related Health Risks, Treatment Programs, Prevention Programs, a Glossary of Abuse and Addiction Terms, a Glossary of Drug-Related Street Terms, and a Directory of Resources for More Information

Edited by Catherine Ginther. 607 pages. 2004. 0-7808-0740-5. $78.

ALSO AVAILABLE: Drug Abuse Sourcebook, 1st Edition. Edited by Karen Bellenir. 629 pages. 2000. 0-7808-0242-X. $78.

"Containing a wealth of information . . . . This resource belongs in libraries that serve a lower-division undergraduate or community college clientele as well as the general public." — *Choice, Association of College and Research Libraries, Jun '01*

"Recommended reference source."
— *Booklist, American Library Association, Feb '01*

"Highly recommended." — *The Bookwatch, Jan '01*

"Even though there is a plethora of books on drug abuse, this volume is recommended for school, public, and college libraries."
— *American Reference Books Annual, 2001*

SEE ALSO Alcoholism Sourcebook, Substance Abuse Sourcebook

Ear, Nose & Throat Disorders Sourcebook

Basic Information about Disorders of the Ears, Nose, Sinus Cavities, Pharynx, and Larynx, Including Ear Infections, Tinnitus, Vestibular Disorders, Allergic and Non-Allergic Rhinitis, Sore Throats, Tonsillitis, and Cancers That Affect the Ears, Nose, Sinuses, and Throat

Along with Reports on Current Research Initiatives, a Glossary of Related Medical Terms, and a Directory of Sources for Further Help and Information

Edited by Karen Bellenir and Linda M. Shin. 576 pages. 1998. 0-7808-0206-3. $78.

"Overall, this sourcebook is helpful for the consumer seeking information on ENT issues. It is recommended for public libraries."
— *American Reference Books Annual, 1999*

"Recommended reference source."
— *Booklist, American Library Association, Dec '98*

■

Eating Disorders Sourcebook

Basic Consumer Health Information about Eating Disorders, Including Information about Anorexia Nervosa, Bulimia Nervosa, Binge Eating, Body Dysmorphic Disorder, Pica, Laxative Abuse, and Night Eating Syndrome

Along with Information about Causes, Adverse Effects, and Treatment and Prevention Issues, and Featuring a Section on Concerns Specific to Children and Adolescents, a Glossary, and Resources for Further Help and Information

Edited by Dawn D. Matthews. 322 pages. 2001. 0-7808-0335-3. $78.

"Recommended for health science libraries that are open to the public, as well as hospital libraries. This book is a good resource for the consumer who is concerned about eating disorders." — *E-Streams, Mar '02*

"This volume is another convenient collection of excerpted articles. Recommended for school and public library patrons; lower-division undergraduates; and two-year technical program students." — *Choice, Association of College & Research Libraries, Jan '02*

"Recommended reference source." — *Booklist, American Library Association, Oct '01*

SEE ALSO Diet & Nutrition Sourcebook, Digestive Diseases & Disorders Sourcebook, Gastrointestinal Diseases & Disorders Sourcebook

■

Emergency Medical Services Sourcebook

Basic Consumer Health Information about Preventing, Preparing for, and Managing Emergency Situations, When and Who to Call for Help, What to Expect in the Emergency Room, the Emergency Medical Team, Patient Issues, and Current Topics in Emergency Medicine

Along with Statistical Data, a Glossary, and Sources of Additional Help and Information

Edited by Jenni Lynn Colson. 494 pages. 2002. 0-7808-0420-1. $78.

"Handy and convenient for home, public, school, and college libraries. Recommended."
— Choice, Association of College and Research Libraries, Apr '03

"This reference can provide the consumer with answers to most questions about emergency care in the United States, or it will direct them to a resource where the answer can be found."
— American Reference Books Annual, 2003

"Recommended reference source."
— Booklist, American Library Association, Feb '03

■

Endocrine & Metabolic Disorders Sourcebook

Basic Information for the Layperson about Pancreatic and Insulin-Related Disorders Such as Pancreatitis, Diabetes, and Hypoglycemia; Adrenal Gland Disorders Such as Cushing's Syndrome, Addison's Disease, and Congenital Adrenal Hyperplasia; Pituitary Gland Disorders Such as Growth Hormone Deficiency, Acromegaly, and Pituitary Tumors; Thyroid Disorders Such as Hypothyroidism, Graves' Disease, Hashimoto's Disease, and Goiter; Hyperparathyroidism; and Other Diseases and Syndromes of Hormone Imbalance or Metabolic Dysfunction

Along with Reports on Current Research Initiatives

Edited by Linda M. Shin. 574 pages. 1998. 0-7808-0207-1. $78.

"Omnigraphics has produced another needed resource for health information consumers."
— American Reference Books Annual, 2000

"Recommended reference source."
— Booklist, American Library Association, Dec '98

■

Environmental Health Sourcebook, 2nd Edition

Basic Consumer Health Information about the Environment and Its Effect on Human Health, Including the Effects of Air Pollution, Water Pollution, Hazardous Chemicals, Food Hazards, Radiation Hazards, Biological Agents, Household Hazards, Such as Radon, Asbestos, Carbon Monoxide, and Mold, and Information about Associated Diseases and Disorders, Including Cancer, Allergies, Respiratory Problems, and Skin Disorders

Along with Information about Environmental Concerns for Specific Populations, a Glossary of Related Terms, and Resources for Further Help and Information

Edited by Dawn D. Matthews. 673 pages. 2003. 0-7808-0632-8. $78.

ALSO AVAILABLE: Environmentally Induced Disorders Sourcebook, 1st Edition. Edited by Allan R. Cook. 620 pages. 1997. 0-7808-0083-4. $78.

"This recently updated edition continues the level of quality and the reputation of the numerous other volumes in Omnigraphics' Health Reference Series."
— American Reference Books Annual, 2004

"Recommended reference source."
— Booklist, American Library Association, Sep '98

"This book will be a useful addition to anyone's library."
— Choice Health Sciences Supplement, Association of College and Research Libraries, May '98

". . . a good survey of numerous environmentally induced physical disorders . . . a useful addition to anyone's library."
— Doody's Health Sciences Book Reviews, Jan '98

". . . provide[s] introductory information from the best authorities around. Since this volume covers topics that potentially affect everyone, it will surely be one of the most frequently consulted volumes in the Health Reference Series."
— Rettig on Reference, Nov '97

■

Environmentally Induced Disorders Sourcebook, 1st Edition

SEE Environmental Health Sourcebook, 2nd Edition

■

Ethnic Diseases Sourcebook

Basic Consumer Health Information for Ethnic and Racial Minority Groups in the United States, Including General Health Indicators and Behaviors, Ethnic Diseases, Genetic Testing, the Impact of Chronic Diseases, Women's Health, Mental Health Issues, and Preventive Health Care Services

Along with a Glossary and a Listing of Additional Resources

Edited by Joyce Brennfleck Shannon. 664 pages. 2001. 0-7808-0336-1. $78.

"Recommended for health sciences libraries where public health programs are a priority."
— E-Streams, Jan '02

"Not many books have been written on this topic to date, and the Ethnic Diseases Sourcebook is a strong addition to the list. It will be an important introductory resource for health consumers, students, health care personnel, and social scientists. It is recommended for public, academic, and large hospital libraries."
— American Reference Books Annual 2002

"Recommended reference source."
— Booklist, American Library Association, Oct '01

"Will prove valuable to any library seeking to maintain a current, comprehensive reference collection of health resources. . . . An excellent source of health information about genetic disorders which affect particular ethnic and racial minorities in the U.S."
— The Bookwatch, Aug '01

Eye Care Sourcebook, 2nd Edition

Basic Consumer Health Information about Eye Care and Eye Disorders, Including Facts about the Diagnosis, Prevention, and Treatment of Common Refractive Problems Such as Myopia, Hyperopia, Astigmatism, and Presbyopia, and Eye Diseases, Including Glaucoma, Cataract, Age-Related Macular Degeneration, and Diabetic Retinopathy

Along with a Section on Vision Correction and Refractive Surgeries, Including LASIK and LASEK, a Glossary, and Directories of Resources for Additional Help and Information

Edited by Amy L. Sutton. 543 pages. 2003. 0-7808-0635-2. $78.

ALSO AVAILABLE: Ophthalmic Disorders Sourcebook, 1st Edition. Edited by Linda M. Ross. 631 pages. 1996. 0-7808-0081-8. $78.

". . . a solid reference tool for eye care and a valuable addition to a collection."
— *American Reference Books Annual, 2004*

■

Family Planning Sourcebook

Basic Consumer Health Information about Planning for Pregnancy and Contraception, Including Traditional Methods, Barrier Methods, Hormonal Methods, Permanent Methods, Future Methods, Emergency Contraception, and Birth Control Choices for Women at Each Stage of Life

Along with Statistics, a Glossary, and Sources of Additional Information

Edited by Amy Marcaccio Keyzer. 520 pages. 2001. 0-7808-0379-5. $78.

"Recommended for public, health, and undergraduate libraries as part of the circulating collection."
— *E-Streams, Mar '02*

"Information is presented in an unbiased, readable manner, and the sourcebook will certainly be a necessary addition to those public and high school libraries where Internet access is restricted or otherwise problematic." — *American Reference Books Annual 2002*

"Recommended reference source."
— *Booklist, American Library Association, Oct '01*

"Will prove valuable to any library seeking to maintain a current, comprehensive reference collection of health resources. . . . Excellent reference."
— *The Bookwatch, Aug '01*

SEE ALSO Pregnancy & Birth Sourcebook

■

Fitness & Exercise Sourcebook, 2nd Edition

Basic Consumer Health Information about the Fundamentals of Fitness and Exercise, Including How to Begin and Maintain a Fitness Program, Fitness as a Lifestyle, the Link between Fitness and Diet, Advice for Specific Groups of People, Exercise as It Relates to

Specific Medical Conditions, and Recent Research in Fitness and Exercise

Along with a Glossary of Important Terms and Resources for Additional Help and Information

Edited by Kristen M. Gledhill. 646 pages. 2001. 0-7808-0334-5. $78.

ALSO AVAILABLE: Fitness & Exercise Sourcebook, 1st Edition. Edited by Dan R. Harris. 663 pages. 1996. 0-7808-0186-5. $78.

"This work is recommended for all general reference collections."
— *American Reference Books Annual 2002*

"Highly recommended for public, consumer, and school grades fourth through college."
— *E-Streams, Nov '01*

"Recommended reference source." — *Booklist, American Library Association, Oct '01*

"The information appears quite comprehensive and is considered reliable. . . . This second edition is a welcomed addition to the series."
— *Doody's Review Service, Sep '01*

"This reference is a valuable choice for those who desire a broad source of information on exercise, fitness, and chronic-disease prevention through a healthy lifestyle." — *American Medical Writers Association Journal, Fall '01*

"Will prove valuable to any library seeking to maintain a current, comprehensive reference collection of health resources. . . . Excellent reference."
— *The Bookwatch, Aug '01*

■

Food & Animal Borne Diseases Sourcebook

Basic Information about Diseases That Can Be Spread to Humans through the Ingestion of Contaminated Food or Water or by Contact with Infected Animals and Insects, Such as Botulism, E. Coli, Hepatitis A, Trichinosis, Lyme Disease, and Rabies

Along with Information Regarding Prevention and Treatment Methods, and Including a Special Section for International Travelers Describing Diseases Such as Cholera, Malaria, Travelers' Diarrhea, and Yellow Fever, and Offering Recommendations for Avoiding Illness

Edited by Karen Bellenir and Peter D. Dresser. 535 pages. 1995. 0-7808-0033-8. $78.

"Targeting general readers and providing them with a single, comprehensive source of information on selected topics, this book continues, with the excellent caliber of its predecessors, to catalog topical information on health matters of general interest. Readable and thorough, this valuable resource is highly recommended for all libraries."
— *Academic Library Book Review, Summer '96*

"A comprehensive collection of authoritative information." — *Emergency Medical Services, Oct '95*

Food Safety Sourcebook

Basic Consumer Health Information about the Safe Handling of Meat, Poultry, Seafood, Eggs, Fruit Juices, and Other Food Items, and Facts about Pesticides, Drinking Water, Food Safety Overseas, and the Onset, Duration, and Symptoms of Foodborne Illnesses, Including Types of Pathogenic Bacteria, Parasitic Protozoa, Worms, Viruses, and Natural Toxins

Along with the Role of the Consumer, the Food Handler, and the Government in Food Safety; a Glossary, and Resources for Additional Help and Information

Edited by Dawn D. Matthews. 339 pages. 1999. 0-7808-0326-4. $78.

"This book is recommended for public libraries and universities with home economic and food science programs." — *E-Streams, Nov '00*

"Recommended reference source."
—*Booklist, American Library Association, May '00*

"This book takes the complex issues of food safety and foodborne pathogens and presents them in an easily understood manner. [It does] an excellent job of covering a large and often confusing topic."
—*American Reference Books Annual, 2000*

Forensic Medicine Sourcebook

Basic Consumer Information for the Layperson about Forensic Medicine, Including Crime Scene Investigation, Evidence Collection and Analysis, Expert Testimony, Computer-Aided Criminal Identification, Digital Imaging in the Courtroom, DNA Profiling, Accident Reconstruction, Autopsies, Ballistics, Drugs and Explosives Detection, Latent Fingerprints, Product Tampering, and Questioned Document Examination

Along with Statistical Data, a Glossary of Forensics Terminology, and Listings of Sources for Further Help and Information

Edited by Annemarie S. Muth. 574 pages. 1999. 0-7808-0232-2. $78.

"Given the expected widespread interest in its content and its easy to read style, this book is recommended for most public and all college and university libraries."
— *E-Streams, Feb '01*

"Recommended for public libraries."
—*Reference & User Services Quarterly, American Library Association, Spring 2000*

"Recommended reference source."
—*Booklist, American Library Association, Feb '00*

"A wealth of information, useful statistics, references are up-to-date and extremely complete. This wonderful collection of data will help students who are interested in a career in any type of forensic field. It is a great resource for attorneys who need information about types of expert witnesses needed in a particular case. It also offers useful information for fiction and nonfiction writers whose work involves a crime. A fascinating compilation. All levels." — *Choice, Association of College and Research Libraries, Jan 2000*

"There are several items that make this book attractive to consumers who are seeking certain forensic data. . . . This is a useful current source for those seeking general forensic medical answers."
—*American Reference Books Annual, 2000*

Gastrointestinal Diseases & Disorders Sourcebook

Basic Information about Gastroesophageal Reflux Disease (Heartburn), Ulcers, Diverticulosis, Irritable Bowel Syndrome, Crohn's Disease, Ulcerative Colitis, Diarrhea, Constipation, Lactose Intolerance, Hemorrhoids, Hepatitis, Cirrhosis, and Other Digestive Problems, Featuring Statistics, Descriptions of Symptoms, and Current Treatment Methods of Interest for Persons Living with Upper and Lower Gastrointestinal Maladies

Edited by Linda M. Ross. 413 pages. 1996. 0-7808-0078-8. $78.

". . . very readable form. The successful editorial work that brought this material together into a useful and understandable reference makes accessible to all readers information that can help them more effectively understand and obtain help for digestive tract problems."
— *Choice, Association of College & Research Libraries, Feb '97*

SEE ALSO *Diet & Nutrition Sourcebook, Digestive Diseases & Disorders, Eating Disorders Sourcebook*

Genetic Disorders Sourcebook, 3rd Edition

Basic Consumer Health Information about Hereditary Diseases and Disorders, Including Facts about the Human Genome, Genetic Inheritance Patterns, Disorders Associated with Specific Genes, such as Sickle Cell Disease, Hemophilia, and Cystic Fibrosis, Chromosome Disorders, such as Down Syndrome, Fragile X Syndrome, and Turner Syndrome, and Complex Diseases and Disorders Resulting from the Interaction of Environmental and Genetic Factors, such as Allergies, Cancer, and Obesity

Along with Facts about Genetic Testing, Suggestions for Parents of Children with Special Needs, Reports on Current Research Initiatives, a Glossary of Genetic Terminology, and Resources for Additional Help and Information

Edited by Karen Bellenir. 777 pages. 2004. 0-7808-0742-1. $78.

ALSO AVAILABLE: Genetic Disorders Sourcebook, 1st Edition. Edited by Karen Bellenir. 642 pages. 1996. 0-7808-0034-6. $78.

Genetic Disorders Sourcebook, 2nd Edition. Edited by Kathy Massimini. 768 pages. 2001. 0-7808-0241-1. $78.

"Recommended for public libraries and medical and hospital libraries with consumer health collections."
— *E-Streams, May '01*

Head Trauma Sourcebook

Basic Information for the Layperson about Open-Head and Closed-Head Injuries, Treatment Advances, Recovery, and Rehabilitation

Along with Reports on Current Research Initiatives

Edited by Karen Bellenir. 414 pages. 1997. 0-7808-0208-X. $78.

Headache Sourcebook

Basic Consumer Health Information about Migraine, Tension, Cluster, Rebound and Other Types of Headaches, with Facts about the Cause and Prevention of Headaches, the Effects of Stress and the Environment, Headaches during Pregnancy and Menopause, and Childhood Headaches

Along with a Glossary and Other Resources for Additional Help and Information

Edited by Dawn D. Matthews. 362 pages. 2002. 0-7808-0337-X. $78.

Health Insurance Sourcebook

Basic Information about Managed Care Organizations, Traditional Fee-for-Service Insurance, Insurance Portability and Pre-Existing Conditions Clauses, Medicare, Medicaid, Social Security, and Military Health Care

Along with Information about Insurance Fraud

Edited by Wendy Wilcox. 530 pages. 1997. 0-7808-0222-5. $78.

Health Reference Series Cumulative Index 1999

A Comprehensive Index to the Individual Volumes of the Health Reference Series, Including a Subject Index, Name Index, Organization Index, and Publication Index

Along with a Master List of Acronyms and Abbreviations

Edited by Edward J. Prucha, Anne Holmes, and Robert Rudnick. 990 pages. 2000. 0-7808-0382-5. $78.

Healthy Aging Sourcebook

Basic Consumer Health Information about Maintaining Health through the Aging Process, Including Advice on Nutrition, Exercise, and Sleep, Help in Making Decisions about Midlife Issues and Retirement, and Guidance Concerning Practical and Informed Choices in Health Consumerism

Along with Data Concerning the Theories of Aging, Different Experiences in Aging by Minority Groups, and Facts about Aging Now and Aging in the Future; and Featuring a Glossary, a Guide to Consumer Help, Additional Suggested Reading, and Practical Resource Directory

Edited by Jenifer Swanson. 536 pages. 1999. 0-7808-0390-6. $78.

SEE ALSO *Physical & Mental Issues in Aging Sourcebook*

Healthy Children Sourcebook

Basic Consumer Health Information about the Physical and Mental Development of Children between the Ages of 3 and 12, Including Routine Health Care, Preventative Health Services, Safety and First Aid, Healthy Sleep, Dental Care, Nutrition, and Fitness, and Featuring Parenting Tips on Such Topics as Bedwetting, Choosing Day Care, Monitoring TV and Other Media, and Establishing a Foundation for Substance Abuse Prevention

Along with a Glossary of Commonly Used Pediatric Terms and Resources for Additional Help and Information.

Edited by Chad T. Kimball. 647 pages. 2003. 0-7808-0247-0. $78.

of timely information on health promotion and disease prevention for children aged 3 to 12."

— American Reference Books Annual, 2004

"The strengths of this book are many. It is clearly written, presented and structured."

— Journal of the National Medical Association, 2004

▪

Healthy Heart Sourcebook for Women

Basic Consumer Health Information about Cardiac Issues Specific to Women, Including Facts about Major Risk Factors and Prevention, Treatment and Control Strategies, and Important Dietary Issues

Along with a Special Section Regarding the Pros and Cons of Hormone Replacement Therapy and Its Impact on Heart Health, and Additional Help, Including Recipes, a Glossary, and a Directory of Resources

Edited by Dawn D. Matthews. 336 pages. 2000. 0-7808-0329-9. $78.

"A good reference source and recommended for all public, academic, medical, and hospital libraries."

— Medical Reference Services Quarterly, Summer '01

"Because of the lack of information specific to women on this topic, this book is recommended for public libraries and consumer libraries."

— American Reference Books Annual, 2001

"Contains very important information about coronary artery disease that all women should know. The information is current and presented in an easy-to-read format. The book will make a good addition to any library."

— American Medical Writers Association Journal, Summer '00

"Important, basic reference."

— Reviewer's Bookwatch, Jul '00

SEE ALSO *Heart Diseases & Disorders Sourcebook, Women's Health Concerns Sourcebook*

▪

Heart Diseases & Disorders Sourcebook, 2nd Edition

Basic Consumer Health Information about Heart Attacks, Angina, Rhythm Disorders, Heart Failure, Valve Disease, Congenital Heart Disorders, and More, Including Descriptions of Surgical Procedures and Other Interventions, Medications, Cardiac Rehabilitation, Risk Identification, and Prevention Tips

Along with Statistical Data, Reports on Current Research Initiatives, a Glossary of Cardiovascular Terms, and Resource Directory

Edited by Karen Bellenir. 612 pages. 2000. 0-7808-0238-1. $78.

ALSO AVAILABLE: *Cardiovascular Diseases & Disorders Sourcebook, 1st Edition.* Edited by Karen Bellenir and Peter D. Dresser. 683 pages. 1995. 0-7808-0032-X. $78.

"This work stands out as an imminently accessible resource for the general public. It is recommended for the reference and circulating shelves of school, public, and academic libraries."

— American Reference Books Annual, 2001

"Recommended reference source."

— Booklist, American Library Association, Dec '00

"Provides comprehensive coverage of matters related to the heart. This title is recommended for health sciences and public libraries with consumer health collections."

— E-Streams, Oct '00

SEE ALSO *Healthy Heart Sourcebook for Women*

▪

Household Safety Sourcebook

Basic Consumer Health Information about Household Safety, Including Information about Poisons, Chemicals, Fire, and Water Hazards in the Home

Along with Advice about the Safe Use of Home Maintenance Equipment, Choosing Toys and Nursery Furniture, Holiday and Recreation Safety, a Glossary, and Resources for Further Help and Information

Edited by Dawn D. Matthews. 606 pages. 2002. 0-7808-0338-8. $78.

"This work will be useful in public libraries with large consumer health and wellness departments."

— American Reference Books Annual, 2003

"As a sourcebook on household safety this book meets its mark. It is encyclopedic in scope and covers a wide range of safety issues that are commonly seen in the home."

— E-Streams, Jul '02

▪

Hypertension Sourcebook

Basic Consumer Health Information about the Causes, Diagnosis, and Treatment of High Blood Pressure, with Facts about Consequences, Complications, and Co-Occurring Disorders, Such as Coronary Heart Disease, Diabetes, Stroke, Kidney Disease, and Hypertensive Retinopathy, and Issues in Blood Pressure Control, Including Dietary Choices, Stress Management, and Medications

Along with Reports on Current Research Initiatives and Clinical Trials, a Glossary, and Resources for Additional Help and Information

Edited by Dawn D. Matthews and Karen Bellenir. 613 pages. 2004. 0-7808-0674-3. $78.

▪

Immune System Disorders Sourcebook

Basic Information about Lupus, Multiple Sclerosis, Guillain-Barré Syndrome, Chronic Granulomatous Disease, and More

Along with Statistical and Demographic Data and Reports on Current Research Initiatives

Edited by Allan R. Cook. 608 pages. 1997. 0-7808-0209-8. $78.

Infant & Toddler Health Sourcebook

Basic Consumer Health Information about the Physical and Mental Development of Newborns, Infants, and Toddlers, Including Neonatal Concerns, Nutrition Recommendations, Immunization Schedules, Common Pediatric Disorders, Assessments and Milestones, Safety Tips, and Advice for Parents and Other Caregivers

Along with a Glossary of Terms and Resource Listings for Additional Help

Edited by Jenifer Swanson. 585 pages. 2000. 0-7808-0246-2. $78.

"As a reference for the general public, this would be useful in any library." — *E-Streams, May '01*

"Recommended reference source."
— *Booklist, American Library Association, Feb '01*

"This is a good source for general use."
— *American Reference Books Annual, 2001*

■

Infectious Diseases Sourcebook

Basic Consumer Health Information about Non-Contagious Bacterial, Viral, Prion, Fungal, and Parasitic Diseases Spread by Food and Water, Insects and Animals, or Environmental Contact, Including Botulism, E. Coli, Encephalitis, Legionnaires' Disease, Lyme Disease, Malaria, Plague, Rabies, Salmonella, Tetanus, and Others, and Facts about Newly Emerging Diseases, Such as Hantavirus, Mad Cow Disease, Monkeypox, and West Nile Virus

Along with Information about Preventing Disease Transmission, the Threat of Bioterrorism, and Current Research Initiatives, with a Glossary and Directory of Resources for More Information

Edited by Karen Bellenir. 634 pages. 2004. 0-7808-0675-1. $78.

■

Injury & Trauma Sourcebook

Basic Consumer Health Information about the Impact of Injury, the Diagnosis and Treatment of Common and Traumatic Injuries, Emergency Care, and Specific Injuries Related to Home, Community, Workplace, Transportation, and Recreation

Along with Guidelines for Injury Prevention, a Glossary, and a Directory of Additional Resources

Edited by Joyce Brennfleck Shannon. 696 pages. 2002. 0-7808-0421-X. $78.

"This publication is the most comprehensive work of its kind about injury and trauma."
— *American Reference Books Annual, 2003*

"This sourcebook provides concise, easily readable, basic health information about injuries. . . . This book is well organized and an easy to use reference resource suitable for hospital, health sciences and public libraries with consumer health collections."
— *E-Streams, Nov '02*

"Practitioners should be aware of guides such as this in order to facilitate their use by patients and their families." — *Doody's Health Sciences Book Review Journal, Sep-Oct '02*

"Recommended reference source."
— *Booklist, American Library Association, Sep '02*

"Highly recommended for academic and medical reference collections." — *Library Bookwatch, Sep '02*

■

Kidney & Urinary Tract Diseases & Disorders Sourcebook

Basic Information about Kidney Stones, Urinary Incontinence, Bladder Disease, End Stage Renal Disease, Dialysis, and More

Along with Statistical and Demographic Data and Reports on Current Research Initiatives

Edited by Linda M. Ross. 602 pages. 1997. 0-7808-0079-6. $78.

■

Learning Disabilities Sourcebook, 2nd Edition

Basic Consumer Health Information about Learning Disabilities, Including Dyslexia, Developmental Speech and Language Disabilities, Non-Verbal Learning Disorders, Developmental Arithmetic Disorder, Developmental Writing Disorder, and Other Conditions That Impede Learning Such as Attention Deficit/ Hyperactivity Disorder, Brain Injury, Hearing Impairment, Klinefelter Syndrome, Dyspraxia, and Tourette Syndrome

Along with Facts about Educational Issues and Assistive Technology, Coping Strategies, a Glossary of Related Terms, and Resources for Further Help and Information

Edited by Dawn D. Matthews. 621 pages. 2003. 0-7808-0626-3. $78.

ALSO AVAILABLE: Learning Disabilities Sourcebook, 1st Edition. Edited by Linda M. Shin. 579 pages. 1998. 0-7808-0210-1. $78.

"The second edition of *Learning Disabilities Sourcebook* far surpasses the earlier edition in that it is more focused on information that will be useful as a consumer health resource."
— *American Reference Books Annual, 2004*

"Teachers as well as consumers will find this an essential guide to understanding various syndromes and their latest treatments. [An] invaluable reference for public and school library collections alike."
— *Library Bookwatch, Apr '03*

Named **"Outstanding Reference Book of 1999."**
— *New York Public Library, Feb 2000*

"An excellent candidate for inclusion in a public library reference section. It's a great source of information. Teachers will also find the book useful. Definitely worth reading."
— *Journal of Adolescent & Adult Literacy, Feb 2000*

"Readable . . . provides a solid base of information regarding successful techniques used with individuals who have learning disabilities, as well as practical suggestions for educators and family members. Clear language, concise descriptions, and pertinent information for contacting multiple resources add to the strength of this book as a useful tool." —*Choice, Association of College and Research Libraries, Feb '99*

"Recommended reference source."
—*Booklist, American Library Association, Sep '98*

"A useful resource for libraries and for those who don't have the time to identify and locate the individual publications." —*Disability Resources Monthly, Sep '98*

■

Leukemia Sourcebook

Basic Consumer Health Information about Adult and Childhood Leukemias, Including Acute Lymphocytic Leukemia (ALL), Chronic Lymphocytic Leukemia (CLL), Acute Myelogenous Leukemia (AML), Chronic Myelogenous Leukemia (CML), and Hairy Cell Leukemia, and Treatments Such as Chemotherapy, Radiation Therapy, Peripheral Blood Stem Cell and Marrow Transplantation, and Immunotherapy

Along with Tips for Life During and After Treatment, a Glossary, and Directories of Additional Resources

Edited by Joyce Brennfleck Shannon. 587 pages. 2003. 0-7808-0627-1. $78.

"Unlike other medical books for the layperson, . . . the language does not talk down to the reader. . . . This volume is highly recommended for all libraries."
—*American Reference Books Annual, 2004*

■

Liver Disorders Sourcebook

Basic Consumer Health Information about the Liver and How It Works; Liver Diseases, Including Cancer, Cirrhosis, Hepatitis, and Toxic and Drug Related Diseases; Tips for Maintaining a Healthy Liver; Laboratory Tests, Radiology Tests, and Facts about Liver Transplantation

Along with a Section on Support Groups, a Glossary, and Resource Listings

Edited by Joyce Brennfleck Shannon. 591 pages. 2000. 0-7808-0383-3. $78.

"A valuable resource."
—*American Reference Books Annual, 2001*

"This title is recommended for health sciences and public libraries with consumer health collections."
—*E-Streams, Oct '00*

"Recommended reference source."
—*Booklist, American Library Association, Jun '00*

■

Lung Disorders Sourcebook

Basic Consumer Health Information about Emphysema, Pneumonia, Tuberculosis, Asthma, Cystic Fibrosis, and Other Lung Disorders, Including Facts about

Diagnostic Procedures, Treatment Strategies, Disease Prevention Efforts, and Such Risk Factors as Smoking, Air Pollution, and Exposure to Asbestos, Radon, and Other Agents

Along with a Glossary and Resources for Additional Help and Information

Edited by Dawn D. Matthews. 678 pages. 2002. 0-7808-0339-6. $78.

"This title is a great addition for public and school libraries because it provides concise health information on the lungs."
—*American Reference Books Annual, 2003*

"Highly recommended for academic and medical reference collections." —*Library Bookwatch, Sep '02*

■

Medical Tests Sourcebook, 2nd Edition

Basic Consumer Health Information about Medical Tests, Including Age-Specific Health Tests, Important Health Screenings and Exams, Home-Use Tests, Blood and Specimen Tests, Electrical Tests, Scope Tests, Genetic Testing, and Imaging Tests, Such as X-Rays, Ultrasound, Computed Tomography, Magnetic Resonance Imaging, Angiography, and Nuclear Medicine

Along with a Glossary and Directory of Additional Resources

Edited by Joyce Brennfleck Shannon. 654 pages. 2004. 0-7808-0670-0. $78.

ALSO AVAILABLE: *Medical Tests, 1st Edition.* Edited by Joyce Brennfleck Shannon. 691 pages. 1999. 0-7808-0243-8. $78.

"Recommended for hospital and health sciences libraries with consumer health collections."
—*E-Streams, Mar '00*

"This is an overall excellent reference with a wealth of general knowledge that may aid those who are reluctant to get vital tests performed."
—*Today's Librarian, Jan 2000*

"A valuable reference guide."
—*American Reference Books Annual, 2000*

■

Men's Health Concerns Sourcebook, 2nd Edition

Basic Consumer Health Information about the Medical and Mental Concerns of Men, Including Theories about the Shorter Male Lifespan, the Leading Causes of Death and Disability, Physical Concerns of Special Significance to Men, Reproductive and Sexual Concerns, Sexually Transmitted Diseases, Men's Mental and Emotional Health, and Lifestyle Choices That Affect Wellness, Such as Nutrition, Fitness, and Substance Use

Along with a Glossary of Related Terms and a Directory of Organizational Resources in Men's Health

Edited by Robert Aquinas McNally. 644 pages. 2004. 0-7808-0671-9. $78.

ALSO AVAILABLE: Men's Health Concerns Sourcebook, 1st Edition. Edited by Allan R. Cook. 738 pages. 1998. 0-7808-0212-8. $78.

"This comprehensive resource and the series are highly recommended."
—*American Reference Books Annual, 2000*

"Recommended reference source."
—*Booklist, American Library Association, Dec '98*

■

Mental Health Disorders Sourcebook, 2nd Edition

Basic Consumer Health Information about Anxiety Disorders, Depression and Other Mood Disorders, Eating Disorders, Personality Disorders, Schizophrenia, and More, Including Disease Descriptions, Treatment Options, and Reports on Current Research Initiatives

Along with Statistical Data, Tips for Maintaining Mental Health, a Glossary, and Directory of Sources for Additional Help and Information

Edited by Karen Bellenir. 605 pages. 2000. 0-7808-0240-3. $78.

ALSO AVAILABLE: Mental Health Disorders Sourcebook, 1st Edition. Edited by Karen Bellenir. 548 pages. 1995. 0-7808-0040-0. $78.

"Well organized and well written."
—*American Reference Books Annual, 2001*

"Recommended reference source."
—*Booklist, American Library Association, Jun '00*

■

Mental Retardation Sourcebook

Basic Consumer Health Information about Mental Retardation and Its Causes, Including Down Syndrome, Fetal Alcohol Syndrome, Fragile X Syndrome, Genetic Conditions, Injury, and Environmental Sources

Along with Preventive Strategies, Parenting Issues, Educational Implications, Health Care Needs, Employment and Economic Matters, Legal Issues, a Glossary, and a Resource Listing for Additional Help and Information

Edited by Joyce Brennfleck Shannon. 642 pages. 2000. 0-7808-0377-9. $78.

"Public libraries will find the book useful for reference and as a beginning research point for students, parents, and caregivers."
—*American Reference Books Annual, 2001*

"The strength of this work is that it compiles many basic fact sheets and addresses for further information in one volume. It is intended and suitable for the general public. This sourcebook is relevant to any collection providing health information to the general public."
—*E-Streams, Nov '00*

"From preventing retardation to parenting and family challenges, this covers health, social and legal issues and will prove an invaluable overview."
—*Reviewer's Bookwatch, Jul '00*

Movement Disorders Sourcebook

Basic Consumer Health Information about Neurological Movement Disorders, Including Essential Tremor, Parkinson's Disease, Dystonia, Cerebral Palsy, Huntington's Disease, Myasthenia Gravis, Multiple Sclerosis, and Other Early-Onset and Adult-Onset Movement Disorders, Their Symptoms and Causes, Diagnostic Tests, and Treatments

Along with Mobility and Assistive Technology Information, a Glossary, and a Directory of Additional Resources

Edited by Joyce Brennfleck Shannon. 655 pages. 2003. 0-7808-0628-X. $78.

". . . a good resource for consumers and recommended for public, community college and undergraduate libraries."
—*American Reference Books Annual, 2004*

■

Muscular Dystrophy Sourcebook

Basic Consumer Health Information about Congenital, Childhood-Onset, and Adult-Onset Forms of Muscular Dystrophy, Such as Duchenne, Becker, Emery-Dreifuss, Distal, Limb-Girdle, Facioscapulohumeral (FSHD), Myotonic, and Ophthalmoplegic Muscular Dystrophies, Including Facts about Diagnostic Tests, Medical and Physical Therapies, Management of Co-Occurring Conditions, and Parenting Guidelines

Along with Practical Tips for Home Care, a Glossary, and Directories of Additional Resources

Edited by Joyce Brennfleck Shannon. 577 pages. 2004. 0-7808-0676-X. $78.

■

Obesity Sourcebook

Basic Consumer Health Information about Diseases and Other Problems Associated with Obesity, and Including Facts about Risk Factors, Prevention Issues, and Management Approaches

Along with Statistical and Demographic Data, Information about Special Populations, Research Updates, a Glossary, and Source Listings for Further Help and Information

Edited by Wilma Caldwell and Chad T. Kimball. 376 pages. 2001. 0-7808-0333-7. $78.

"The book synthesizes the reliable medical literature on obesity into one easy-to-read and useful resource for the general public."
—*American Reference Books Annual 2002*

"This is a very useful resource book for the lay public."
—*Doody's Review Service, Nov '01*

"Well suited for the health reference collection of a public library or an academic health science library that serves the general population." —*E-Streams, Sep '01*

"Recommended reference source."
—*Booklist, American Library Association, Apr '01*

" Recommended pick both for specialty health library collections and any general consumer health reference collection." —*The Bookwatch, Apr '01*

Ophthalmic Disorders Sourcebook, 1st Edition

SEE Eye Care Sourcebook, 2nd Edition

■

Oral Health Sourcebook

SEE Dental Care & Oral Health Sourcebook, 2nd Ed.

■

Osteoporosis Sourcebook

Basic Consumer Health Information about Primary and Secondary Osteoporosis and Juvenile Osteoporosis and Related Conditions, Including Fibrous Dysplasia, Gaucher Disease, Hyperthyroidism, Hypophosphatasia, Myeloma, Osteopetrosis, Osteogenesis Imperfecta, and Paget's Disease

Along with Information about Risk Factors, Treatments, Traditional and Non-Traditional Pain Management, a Glossary of Related Terms, and a Directory of Resources

Edited by Allan R. Cook. 584 pages. 2001. 0-7808-0239-X. $78.

"This would be a book to be kept in a staff or patient library. The targeted audience is the layperson, but the therapist who needs a quick bit of information on a particular topic will also find the book useful."
— *Physical Therapy, Jan '02*

"This resource is recommended as a great reference source for public, health, and academic libraries, and is another triumph for the editors of Omnigraphics."
— *American Reference Books Annual 2002*

"Recommended for all public libraries and general health collections, especially those supporting patient education or consumer health programs."
— *E-Streams, Nov '01*

"Will prove valuable to any library seeking to maintain a current, comprehensive reference collection of health resources. . . . From prevention to treatment and associated conditions, this provides an excellent survey."
— *The Bookwatch, Aug '01*

"Recommended reference source."
— *Booklist, American Library Association, July '01*

SEE ALSO Women's Health Concerns Sourcebook

■

Pain Sourcebook, 2nd Edition

Basic Consumer Health Information about Specific Forms of Acute and Chronic Pain, Including Muscle and Skeletal Pain, Nerve Pain, Cancer Pain, and Disorders Characterized by Pain, Such as Fibromyalgia, Shingles, Angina, Arthritis, and Headaches

Along with Information about Pain Medications and Management Techniques, Complementary and Alternative Pain Relief Options, Tips for People Living with Chronic Pain, a Glossary, and a Directory of Sources for Further Information

Edited by Karen Bellenir. 670 pages. 2002. 0-7808-0612-3. $78.

ALSO AVAILABLE: Pain Sourcebook, 1st Edition. Edited by Allan R. Cook. 667 pages. 1997. 0-7808-0213-6. $78.

"A source of valuable information. . . . This book offers help to nonmedical people who need information about pain and pain management. It is also an excellent reference for those who participate in patient education."
— *Doody's Review Service, Sep '02*

"The text is readable, easily understood, and well indexed. This excellent volume belongs in all patient education libraries, consumer health sections of public libraries, and many personal collections."
— *American Reference Books Annual, 1999*

"A beneficial reference." — *Booklist Health Sciences Supplement, American Library Association, Oct '98*

"The information is basic in terms of scholarship and is appropriate for general readers. Written in journalistic style . . . intended for non-professionals. Quite thorough in its coverage of different pain conditions and summarizes the latest clinical information regarding pain treatment." — *Choice, Association of College and Research Libraries, Jun '98*

"Recommended reference source."
— *Booklist, American Library Association, Mar '98*

■

Pediatric Cancer Sourcebook

Basic Consumer Health Information about Leukemias, Brain Tumors, Sarcomas, Lymphomas, and Other Cancers in Infants, Children, and Adolescents, Including Descriptions of Cancers, Treatments, and Coping Strategies

Along with Suggestions for Parents, Caregivers, and Concerned Relatives, a Glossary of Cancer Terms, and Resource Listings

Edited by Edward J. Prucha. 587 pages. 1999. 0-7808-0245-4. $78.

"An excellent source of information. Recommended for public, hospital, and health science libraries with consumer health collections." — *E-Streams, Jun '00*

"Recommended reference source."
— *Booklist, American Library Association, Feb '00*

"A valuable addition to all libraries specializing in health services and many public libraries."
— *American Reference Books Annual, 2000*

■

Physical & Mental Issues in Aging Sourcebook

Basic Consumer Health Information on Physical and Mental Disorders Associated with the Aging Process, Including Concerns about Cardiovascular Disease, Pulmonary Disease, Oral Health, Digestive Disorders, Musculoskeletal and Skin Disorders, Metabolic Changes, Sexual and Reproductive Issues, and Changes in Vision, Hearing, and Other Senses

Along with Data about Longevity and Causes of Death, Information on Acute and Chronic Pain, Descriptions of Mental Concerns, a Glossary of Terms, and Resource Listings for Additional Help

Edited by Jenifer Swanson. 660 pages. 1999. 0-7808-0233-0. $78.

"This is a treasure of health information for the layperson." — *Choice Health Sciences Supplement, Association of College & Research Libraries, May 2000*

"Recommended for public libraries."
—*American Reference Books Annual, 2000*

"Recommended reference source."
— *Booklist, American Library Association, Oct '99*

SEE ALSO *Healthy Aging Sourcebook*

Podiatry Sourcebook

Basic Consumer Health Information about Foot Conditions, Diseases, and Injuries, Including Bunions, Corns, Calluses, Athlete's Foot, Plantar Warts, Hammertoes and Clawtoes, Clubfoot, Heel Pain, Gout, and More

Along with Facts about Foot Care, Disease Prevention, Foot Safety, Choosing a Foot Care Specialist, a Glossary of Terms, and Resource Listings for Additional Information

Edited by M. Lisa Weatherford. 380 pages. 2001. 0-7808-0215-2. $78.

"Recommended reference source."
— *Booklist, American Library Association, Feb '02*

"There is a lot of information presented here on a topic that is usually only covered sparingly in most larger comprehensive medical encyclopedias."
— *American Reference Books Annual 2002*

Pregnancy & Birth Sourcebook, 2nd Edition

Basic Consumer Health Information about Conception and Pregnancy, Including Facts about Fertility, Infertility, Pregnancy Symptoms and Complications, Fetal Growth and Development, Labor, Delivery, and the Postpartum Period, as Well as Information about Maintaining Health and Wellness during Pregnancy and Caring for a Newborn

Along with Information about Public Health Assistance for Low-Income Pregnant Women, a Glossary, and Directories of Agencies and Organizations Providing Help and Support

Edited by Amy L. Sutton. 626 pages. 2004. 0-7808-0672-7. $78.

ALSO AVAILABLE: *Pregnancy & Birth Sourcebook, 1st Edition.* Edited by Heather E. Aldred. 737 pages. 1997. 0-7808-0216-0. $78.

"A well-organized handbook. Recommended."
— *Choice, Association of College and Research Libraries, Apr '98*

"Recommended reference source."
— *Booklist, American Library Association, Mar '98*

"Recommended for public libraries."
— *American Reference Books Annual, 1998*

SEE ALSO *Congenital Disorders Sourcebook, Family Planning Sourcebook*

Prostate Cancer Sourcebook

Basic Consumer Health Information about Prostate Cancer, Including Information about the Associated Risk Factors, Detection, Diagnosis, and Treatment of Prostate Cancer

Along with Information on Non-Malignant Prostate Conditions, and Featuring a Section Listing Support and Treatment Centers and a Glossary of Related Terms

Edited by Dawn D. Matthews. 358 pages. 2001. 0-7808-0324-8. $78.

"Recommended reference source."
— *Booklist, American Library Association, Jan '02*

"A valuable resource for health care consumers seeking information on the subject. . . .All text is written in a clear, easy-to-understand language that avoids technical jargon. Any library that collects consumer health resources would strengthen their collection with the addition of the *Prostate Cancer Sourcebook*."
— *American Reference Books Annual 2002*

Public Health Sourcebook

Basic Information about Government Health Agencies, Including National Health Statistics and Trends, Healthy People 2000 Program Goals and Objectives, the Centers for Disease Control and Prevention, the Food and Drug Administration, and the National Institutes of Health

Along with Full Contact Information for Each Agency

Edited by Wendy Wilcox. 698 pages. 1998. 0-7808-0220-9. $78.

"Recommended reference source."
— *Booklist, American Library Association, Sep '98*

"This consumer guide provides welcome assistance in navigating the maze of federal health agencies and their data on public health concerns."
— *SciTech Book News, Sep '98*

Reconstructive & Cosmetic Surgery Sourcebook

Basic Consumer Health Information on Cosmetic and Reconstructive Plastic Surgery, Including Statistical Information about Different Surgical Procedures, Things to Consider Prior to Surgery, Plastic Surgery Techniques and Tools, Emotional and Psychological Considerations, and Procedure-Specific Information

Along with a Glossary of Terms and a Listing of Resources for Additional Help and Information

Edited by M. Lisa Weatherford. 374 pages. 2001. 0-7808-0214-4. $78.

"An excellent reference that addresses cosmetic and medically necessary reconstructive surgeries. . . . The

style of the prose is calm and reassuring, discussing the many positive outcomes now available due to advances in surgical techniques."
— *American Reference Books Annual 2002*

"Recommended for health science libraries that are open to the public, as well as hospital libraries that are open to the patients. This book is a good resource for the consumer interested in plastic surgery."
— *E-Streams, Dec '01*

"Recommended reference source."
— *Booklist, American Library Association, July '01*

■

Rehabilitation Sourcebook

Basic Consumer Health Information about Rehabilitation for People Recovering from Heart Surgery, Spinal Cord Injury, Stroke, Orthopedic Impairments, Amputation, Pulmonary Impairments, Traumatic Injury, and More, Including Physical Therapy, Occupational Therapy, Speech/ Language Therapy, Massage Therapy, Dance Therapy, Art Therapy, and Recreational Therapy

Along with Information on Assistive and Adaptive Devices, a Glossary, and Resources for Additional Help and Information

Edited by Dawn D. Matthews. 531 pages. 1999. 0-7808-0236-5. $78.

"This is an excellent resource for public library reference and health collections."
— *American Reference Books Annual, 2001*

"Recommended reference source."
— *Booklist, American Library Association, May '00*

■

Respiratory Diseases & Disorders Sourcebook

Basic Information about Respiratory Diseases and Disorders, Including Asthma, Cystic Fibrosis, Pneumonia, the Common Cold, Influenza, and Others, Featuring Facts about the Respiratory System, Statistical and Demographic Data, Treatments, Self-Help Management Suggestions, and Current Research Initiatives

Edited by Allan R. Cook and Peter D. Dresser. 771 pages. 1995. 0-7808-0037-0. $78.

"Designed for the layperson and for patients and their families coping with respiratory illness. . . . an extensive array of information on diagnosis, treatment, management, and prevention of respiratory illnesses for the general reader."
— *Choice, Association of College and Research Libraries, Jun '96*

"A highly recommended text for all collections. It is a comforting reminder of the power of knowledge that good books carry between their covers."
— *Academic Library Book Review, Spring '96*

"A comprehensive collection of authoritative information presented in a nontechnical, humanitarian style for patients, families, and caregivers."
— *Association of Operating Room Nurses, Sep/Oct '95*

SEE ALSO *Lung Disorders Sourcebook*

Sexually Transmitted Diseases Sourcebook, 2nd Edition

Basic Consumer Health Information about Sexually Transmitted Diseases, Including Information on the Diagnosis and Treatment of Chlamydia, Gonorrhea, Hepatitis, Herpes, HIV, Mononucleosis, Syphilis, and Others

Along with Information on Prevention, Such as Condom Use, Vaccines, and STD Education; And Featuring a Section on Issues Related to Youth and Adolescents, a Glossary, and Resources for Additional Help and Information

Edited by Dawn D. Matthews. 538 pages. 2001. 0-7808-0249-7. $78.

ALSO AVAILABLE: *Sexually Transmitted Diseases Sourcebook, 1st Edition.* Edited by Linda M. Ross. 550 pages. 1997. 0-7808-0217-9. $78.

"Recommended for consumer health collections in public libraries, and secondary school and community college libraries."
— *American Reference Books Annual 2002*

"Every school and public library should have a copy of this comprehensive and user-friendly reference book."
— *Choice, Association of College & Research Libraries, Sep '01*

"This is a highly recommended book. This is an especially important book for all school and public libraries."
— *AIDS Book Review Journal, Jul-Aug '01*

"Recommended reference source."
— *Booklist, American Library Association, Apr '01*

"Recommended pick both for specialty health library collections and any general consumer health reference collection."
— *The Bookwatch, Apr '01*

■

Skin Disorders Sourcebook

Basic Information about Common Skin and Scalp Conditions Caused by Aging, Allergies, Immune Reactions, Sun Exposure, Infectious Organisms, Parasites, Cosmetics, and Skin Traumas, Including Abrasions, Cuts, and Pressure Sores

Along with Information on Prevention and Treatment

Edited by Allan R. Cook. 647 pages. 1997. 0-7808-0080-X. $78.

". . . comprehensive, easily read reference book."
— *Doody's Health Sciences Book Reviews, Oct '97*

SEE ALSO *Burns Sourcebook*

■

Sleep Disorders Sourcebook

Basic Consumer Health Information about Sleep and Its Disorders, Including Insomnia, Sleepwalking, Sleep Apnea, Restless Leg Syndrome, and Narcolepsy

Along with Data about Shiftwork and Its Effects, Information on the Societal Costs of Sleep Deprivation, Descriptions of Treatment Options, a Glossary of Terms, and Resource Listings for Additional Help

Edited by Jenifer Swanson. 439 pages. 1998. 0-7808-0234-9. $78.

"This text will complement any home or medical library. It is user-friendly and ideal for the adult reader."
—*American Reference Books Annual, 2000*

"A useful resource that provides accurate, relevant, and accessible information on sleep to the general public. Health care providers who deal with sleep disorders patients may also find it helpful in being prepared to answer some of the questions patients ask."
—*Respiratory Care, Jul '99*

"Recommended reference source."
—*Booklist, American Library Association, Feb '99*

Smoking Concerns Sourcebook

Basic Consumer Health Information about Nicotine Addiction and Smoking Cessation, Featuring Facts about the Health Effects of Tobacco Use, Including Lung and Other Cancers, Heart Disease, Stroke, and Respiratory Disorders, Such as Emphysema and Chronic Bronchitis

Along with Information about Smoking Prevention Programs, Suggestions for Achieving and Maintaining a Smoke-Free Lifestyle, Statistics about Tobacco Use, Reports on Current Research Initiatives, a Glossary of Related Terms, and Directories of Resources for Additional Help and Information

Edited by Karen Bellenir. 621 pages. 2004. 0-7808-0323-X. $78.

Sports Injuries Sourcebook, 2nd Edition

Basic Consumer Health Information about the Diagnosis, Treatment, and Rehabilitation of Common Sports-Related Injuries in Children and Adults

Along with Suggestions for Conditioning and Training, Information and Prevention Tips for Injuries Frequently Associated with Specific Sports and Special Populations, a Glossary, and a Directory of Additional Resources

Edited by Joyce Brennfleck Shannon. 614 pages. 2002. 0-7808-0604-2. $78.

ALSO AVAILABLE: Sports Injuries Sourcebook, 1st Edition. Edited by Heather E. Aldred. 624 pages. 1999. 0-7808-0218-7. $78.

"This is an excellent reference for consumers and it is recommended for public, community college, and undergraduate libraries."
—*American Reference Books Annual, 2003*

"Recommended reference source."
—*Booklist, American Library Association, Feb '03*

Stress-Related Disorders Sourcebook

Basic Consumer Health Information about Stress and Stress-Related Disorders, Including Stress Origins and Signals, Environmental Stress at Work and Home, Mental and Emotional Stress Associated with Depression, Post-Traumatic Stress Disorder, Panic Disorder, Suicide, and the Physical Effects of Stress on the Cardiovascular, Immune, and Nervous Systems

Along with Stress Management Techniques, a Glossary, and a Listing of Additional Resources

Edited by Joyce Brennfleck Shannon. 610 pages. 2002. 0-7808-0560-7. $78.

"Well written for a general readership, the *Stress-Related Disorders Sourcebook* is a useful addition to the health reference literature."
—*American Reference Books Annual, 2003*

"I am impressed by the amount of information. It offers a thorough overview of the causes and consequences of stress for the layperson. . . . A well-done and thorough reference guide for professionals and nonprofessionals alike."
—*Doody's Review Service, Dec '02*

Stroke Sourcebook

Basic Consumer Health Information about Stroke, Including Ischemic, Hemorrhagic, Transient Ischemic Attack (TIA), and Pediatric Stroke, Stroke Triggers and Risks, Diagnostic Tests, Treatments, and Rehabilitation Information

Along with Stroke Prevention Guidelines, Legal and Financial Information, a Glossary, and a Directory of Additional Resources

Edited by Joyce Brennfleck Shannon. 606 pages. 2003. 0-7808-0630-1. $78.

"This volume is highly recommended and should be in every medical, hospital, and public library."
—*American Reference Books Annual, 2004*

Substance Abuse Sourcebook

Basic Health-Related Information about the Abuse of Legal and Illegal Substances Such as Alcohol, Tobacco, Prescription Drugs, Marijuana, Cocaine, and Heroin; and Including Facts about Substance Abuse Prevention Strategies, Intervention Methods, Treatment and Recovery Programs, and a Section Addressing the Special Problems Related to Substance Abuse during Pregnancy

Edited by Karen Bellenir. 573 pages. 1996. 0-7808-0038-9. $78.

"A valuable addition to any health reference section. Highly recommended."
—*The Book Report, Mar/Apr '97*

". . . a comprehensive collection of substance abuse information that's both highly readable and compact. Families and caregivers of substance abusers will find

the information enlightening and helpful, while teachers, social workers and journalists should benefit from the concise format. Recommended."
—Drug Abuse Update, Winter '96/'97

SEE ALSO *Alcoholism Sourcebook, Drug Abuse Sourcebook*

Surgery Sourcebook

Basic Consumer Health Information about Inpatient and Outpatient Surgeries, Including Cardiac, Vascular, Orthopedic, Ocular, Reconstructive, Cosmetic, Gynecologic, and Ear, Nose, and Throat Procedures and More

Along with Information about Operating Room Policies and Instruments, Laser Surgery Techniques, Hospital Errors, Statistical Data, a Glossary, and Listings of Sources for Further Help and Information

Edited by Annemarie S. Muth and Karen Bellenir. 596 pages. 2002. 0-7808-0380-9. $78.

"Large public libraries and medical libraries would benefit from this material in their reference collections."
— American Reference Books Annual, 2004

"Invaluable reference for public and school library collections alike." *— Library Bookwatch, Apr '03*

Transplantation Sourcebook

Basic Consumer Health Information about Organ and Tissue Transplantation, Including Physical and Financial Preparations, Procedures and Issues Relating to Specific Solid Organ and Tissue Transplants, Rehabilitation, Pediatric Transplant Information, the Future of Transplantation, and Organ and Tissue Donation

Along with a Glossary and Listings of Additional Resources

Edited by Joyce Brennfleck Shannon. 628 pages. 2002. 0-7808-0322-1. $78.

"Along with these advances [in transplantation technology] have come a number of daunting questions for potential transplant patients, their families, and their health care providers. This reference text is the best single tool to address many of these questions. . . . It will be a much-needed addition to the reference collections in health care, academic, and large public libraries."
— American Reference Books Annual, 2003

"Recommended for libraries with an interest in offering consumer health information." *— E-Streams, Jul '02*

"This is a unique and valuable resource for patients facing transplantation and their families."
— Doody's Review Service, Jun '02

Traveler's Health Sourcebook

Basic Consumer Health Information for Travelers, Including Physical and Medical Preparations, Transportation Health and Safety, Essential Information about Food and Water, Sun Exposure, Insect and Snake Bites, Camping and Wilderness Medicine, and Travel with Physical or Medical Disabilities

Along with International Travel Tips, Vaccination Recommendations, Geographical Health Issues, Disease Risks, a Glossary, and a Listing of Additional Resources

Edited by Joyce Brennfleck Shannon. 613 pages. 2000. 0-7808-0384-1. $78.

"Recommended reference source."
— Booklist, American Library Association, Feb '01

"This book is recommended for any public library, any travel collection, and especially any collection for the physically disabled."
— American Reference Books Annual, 2001

Vegetarian Sourcebook

Basic Consumer Health Information about Vegetarian Diets, Lifestyle, and Philosophy, Including Definitions of Vegetarianism and Veganism, Tips about Adopting Vegetarianism, Creating a Vegetarian Pantry, and Meeting Nutritional Needs of Vegetarians, with Facts Regarding Vegetarianism's Effect on Pregnant and Lactating Women, Children, Athletes, and Senior Citizens

Along with a Glossary of Commonly Used Vegetarian Terms and Resources for Additional Help and Information

Edited by Chad T. Kimball. 360 pages. 2002. 0-7808-0439-2. $78.

"Organizes into one concise volume the answers to the most common questions concerning vegetarian diets and lifestyles. This title is recommended for public and secondary school libraries." *— E-Streams, Apr '03*

"Invaluable reference for public and school library collections alike." *— Library Bookwatch, Apr '03*

"The articles in this volume are easy to read and come from authoritative sources. The book does not necessarily support the vegetarian diet but instead provides the pros and cons of this important decision. The *Vegetarian Sourcebook* is recommended for public libraries and consumer health libraries."
— American Reference Books Annual, 2003

Women's Health Concerns Sourcebook, 2nd Edition

Basic Consumer Health Information about the Medical and Mental Concerns of Women, Including Maintaining Health and Wellness, Gynecological Concerns, Breast Health, Sexuality and Reproductive Issues, Menopause, Cancer in Women, the Leading Causes of Death and Disability among Women, Physical Concerns of Special Significance to Women, and Women's Mental and Emotional Health

Along with a Glossary of Related Terms and Directories of Resources for Additional Help and Information

Edited by Amy L. Sutton. 748 pages. 2004. 0-7808-0673-5. $78.

ALSO AVAILABLE: *Women's Health Concerns Sourcebook, 1st Edition.* Edited by Heather E. Aldred. 567 pages. 1997. 0-7808-0219-5. $78.

"Handy compilation. There is an impressive range of diseases, devices, disorders, procedures, and other physical and emotional issues covered . . . well organized, illustrated, and indexed." — *Choice, Association of College and Research Libraries, Jan '98*

SEE ALSO *Breast Cancer Sourcebook, Cancer Sourcebook for Women, Healthy Heart Sourcebook for Women, Osteoporosis Sourcebook*

Workplace Health & Safety Sourcebook

Basic Consumer Health Information about Workplace Health and Safety, Including the Effect of Workplace Hazards on the Lungs, Skin, Heart, Ears, Eyes, Brain, Reproductive Organs, Musculoskeletal System, and Other Organs and Body Parts

Along with Information about Occupational Cancer, Personal Protective Equipment, Toxic and Hazardous Chemicals, Child Labor, Stress, and Workplace Violence

Edited by Chad T. Kimball. 626 pages. 2000. 0-7808-0231-4. $78.

"As a reference for the general public, this would be useful in any library." —*E-Streams, Jun '01*

"Provides helpful information for primary care physicians and other caregivers interested in occupational medicine. . . . General readers; professionals." — *Choice, Association of College & Research Libraries, May '01*

"Recommended reference source." —*Booklist, American Library Association, Feb '01*

"Highly recommended." — *The Bookwatch, Jan '01*

Worldwide Health Sourcebook

Basic Information about Global Health Issues, Including Malnutrition, Reproductive Health, Disease Dispersion and Prevention, Emerging Diseases, Risky Health Behaviors, and the Leading Causes of Death

Along with Global Health Concerns for Children, Women, and the Elderly, Mental Health Issues, Research and Technology Advancements, and Economic, Environmental, and Political Health Implications, a Glossary, and a Resource Listing for Additional Help and Information

Edited by Joyce Brennfleck Shannon. 614 pages. 2001. 0-7808-0330-2. $78.

"Named an Outstanding Academic Title." —*Choice, Association of College & Research Libraries, Jan '02*

"Yet another handy but also unique compilation in the extensive Health Reference Series, this is a useful work because many of the international publications reprinted or excerpted are not readily available. Highly recommended." —*Choice, Association of College & Research Libraries, Nov '01*

"Recommended reference source." —*Booklist, American Library Association, Oct '01*

605

Teen Health Series

*Helping Young Adults Understand, Manage,
and Avoid Serious Illness*

Alcohol Information For Teens

Health Tips About Alcohol And Alcoholism

*Including Facts about Underage Drinking, Preventing
Teen Alcohol Use, Alcohol's Effects on the Brain and
the Body, Alcohol Abuse Treatment, Help for Children
of Alcoholics, and More*

Edited by Joyce Brennfleck Shannon. 400 pages. 2005. 0-7808-0741-3. $58.

Cancer Information for Teens

Health Tips about Cancer Awareness, Prevention, Diagnosis, and Treatment

*Including Facts about Frequently Occurring Cancers,
Cancer Risk Factors, and Coping Strategies for Teens
Fighting Cancer or Dealing with Cancer in Friends or
Family Members*

Edited by Wilma R. Caldwell. 428 pages. 2004. 0-7808-0678-6. $58.

Diet Information for Teens

Health Tips about Diet and Nutrition

*Including Facts about Nutrients, Dietary Guidelines,
Breakfasts, School Lunches, Snacks, Party Food, Weight
Control, Eating Disorders, and More*

Edited by Karen Bellenir. 399 pages. 2001. 0-7808-0441-4. $58.

"Full of helpful insights and facts throughout the book.
. . . An excellent resource to be placed in public libraries
or even in personal collections."
—American Reference Books Annual 2002

"Recommended for middle and high school libraries
and media centers as well as academic libraries that
educate future teachers of teenagers. It is also a suitable
addition to health science libraries that serve patrons
who are interested in teen health promotion and education." *—E-Streams, Oct '01*

"This comprehensive book would be beneficial to collections that need information about nutrition, dietary
guidelines, meal planning, and weight control. . . . This
reference is so easy to use that its purchase is recommended." *—The Book Report, Sep-Oct '01*

"This book is written in an easy to understand format
describing issues that many teens face every day, and
then provides thoughtful explanations so that teens can
make informed decisions. This is an interesting book
that provides important facts and information for
today's teens." *—Doody's Health Sciences
Book Review Journal, Jul-Aug '01*

"A comprehensive compendium of diet and nutrition.
The information is presented in a straightforward,
plain-spoken manner. This title will be useful to those
working on reports on a variety of topics, as well as to
general readers concerned about their dietary health."
— School Library Journal, Jun '01

Drug Information for Teens

Health Tips about the Physical and Mental Effects of Substance Abuse

*Including Facts about Alcohol, Anabolic Steroids, Club
Drugs, Cocaine, Depressants, Hallucinogens, Herbal
Products, Inhalants, Marijuana, Narcotics, Stimulants,
Tobacco, and More*

Edited by Karen Bellenir. 452 pages. 2002. 0-7808-0444-9. $58.

"A clearly written resource for general readers and
researchers alike." *— School Library Journal*

"The chapters are quick to make a connection to their
teenage reading audience. The prose is straightforward
and the book lends itself to spot reading. It should be
useful both for practical information and for research,
and it is suitable for public and school libraries."
— American Reference Books Annual, 2003

"Recommended reference source."
— Booklist, American Library Association, Feb '03

"This is an excellent resource for teens and their parents. Education about drugs and substances is key to
discouraging teen drug abuse and this book provides
this much needed information in a way that is interesting and factual." *—Doody's Review Service, Dec '02*

Fitness Information for Teens

Health Tips about Exercise, Physical Well-Being, and Health Maintenance

*Including Facts about Aerobic and Anaerobic Condi-
tioning, Stretching, Body Shape and Body Image, Sports
Training, Nutrition, and Activities for Non-Athletes*

Edited by Karen Bellenir. 425 pages. 2004. 0-7808-0679-4. $58.

Mental Health Information for Teens

Health Tips about Mental Health and Mental Illness

Including Facts about Anxiety, Depression, Suicide, Eating Disorders, Obsessive-Compulsive Disorders, Panic Attacks, Phobias, Schizophrenia, and More

Edited by Karen Bellenir. 406 pages. 2001. 0-7808-0442-2. $58.

"In both language and approach, this user-friendly entry in the *Teen Health Series* is on target for teens needing information on mental health concerns." — *Booklist, American Library Association, Jan '02*

"Readers will find the material accessible and informative, with the shaded notes, facts, and embedded glossary insets adding appropriately to the already interesting and succinct presentation."
— *School Library Journal, Jan '02*

"This title is highly recommended for any library that serves adolescents and parents/caregivers of adolescents." — *E-Streams, Jan '02*

"Recommended for high school libraries and young adult collections in public libraries. Both health professionals and teenagers will find this book useful."
— *American Reference Books Annual 2002*

"This is a nice book written to enlighten the society, primarily teenagers, about common teen mental health issues. It is highly recommended to teachers and parents as well as adolescents."
— *Doody's Review Service, Dec '01*

Sexual Health Information for Teens

Health Tips about Sexual Development, Human Reproduction, and Sexually Transmitted Diseases

Including Facts about Puberty, Reproductive Health, Chlamydia, Human Papillomavirus, Pelvic Inflammatory Disease, Herpes, AIDS, Contraception, Pregnancy, and More

Edited by Deborah A. Stanley. 391 pages. 2003. 0-7808-0445-7. $58.

"This work should be included in all high school libraries and many larger public libraries. . . . highly recommended."
— *American Reference Books Annual 2004*

"Sexual Health approaches its subject with appropriate seriousness and offers easily accessible advice and information." — *School Library Journal, Feb. 2004*

Skin Health Information For Teens

Health Tips about Dermatological Concerns and Skin Cancer Risks

Including Facts about Acne, Warts, Hives, and Other Conditions and Lifestyle Choices, Such as Tanning, Tattooing, and Piercing, That Affect the Skin, Nails, Scalp, and Hair

Edited by Robert Aquinas McNally. 430 pages. 2003. 0-7808-0446-5. $58.

"This volume, as with others in the series, will be a useful addition to school and public library collections."
— *American Reference Books Annual 2004*

"This volume serves as a one-stop source and should be a necessity for any health collection."
— *Library Media Connection*

Sports Injuries Information For Teens

Health Tips about Sports Injuries and Injury Protection

Including Facts about Specific Injuries, Emergency Treatment, Rehabilitation, Sports Safety, Competition Stress, Fitness, Sports Nutrition, Steroid Risks, and More

Edited by Joyce Brennfleck Shannon. 425 pages. 2003. 0-7808-0447-3. $58.

"This work will be useful in the young adult collections of public libraries as well as high school libraries."
— *American Reference Books Annual 2004*

Suicide Information for Teens

Health Tips about Suicide Causes and Prevention

Including Facts about Depression, Risk Factors, Getting Help, Survivor Support, and More

Edited by Joyce Brennfleck Shannon. 400 pages. 2004. 0-7808-0737-5. $58.

Health Reference Series